Values at the
End of Life

Values at the End of Life

THE LOGIC OF PALLIATIVE CARE

Roi Livne

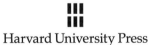

Harvard University Press

Cambridge, Massachusetts

London, England

2019

Library of Congress Cataloging-in-Publication Data

Names: Livne, Roi, 1978– author.
Title: Values at the end of life : the logic of palliative care / Roi Livne.
Description: Cambridge, Massachusetts : Harvard University Press, 2019. |
    Includes bibliographical references and index.
Identifiers: LCCN 2018047863 | ISBN 9780674545175 (alk. paper)
Subjects: LCSH: Terminal care—Economic aspects—United States. | Terminal
    care—Moral and ethical aspects—United States. | Palliative
    treatment—Economic aspects—United States. | Palliative treatment—Moral
    and ethical aspects—United States.
Classification: LCC R726.8 .L58 2019 | DDC 616.02/9—dc23
LC record available at https://lccn.loc.gov/2018047863

To Ashley and Dalia

Value / 'valyo͞o / noun **1** The regard that something is held to deserve; the importance, worth, or usefulness of something; . . . the material or monetary worth of something.
2 A person's principles or standards of behavior; one's judgment of what is important in life.

—Oxford English Dictionary

Contents

Abbreviations

ACA	Patient Protection and Affordable Care Act of 2010
AMA	American Medical Association
CAPC	Center to Advance Palliative Care
CDC	Centers for Disease Control and Prevention
CPR	Cardiopulmonary resuscitation
DNI	Do Not Intubate
DNR	Do Not Resuscitate
DPOA	Durable Power of Attorney
DRG	Diagnosis related group
EMT	Emergency medical technician
ER	Emergency room
ICU	Intensive care unit
IV	Intravenous
LTAC	Long-term acute care facility
MCO	Managed care organization
NHO	National Hospice Organization
NIH	National Institutes of Health
OSI	The Open Society Institute (aka the Open Society Foundation)
PDIA	Project on Death in America

POLST   Physician Order for Life-Sustaining Treatment
RWJF   Robert Wood Johnson Foundation
SUPPORT Study to Understand Prognoses and Preferences for
         Outcomes and Risks of Treatments

Values at the
End of Life

Introduction:

The New Economy of Dying

Individuals in crises do not make life and death decisions on their own. Who shall be saved and who shall die is settled by institutions.

—Mary Douglas, *How Institutions Think*

IN THE SUMMER OF 2011, a nurse at a California hospital sent the Office of Inspector General an impassioned complaint entitled "physician fraud." She wrote about one of the hospital's patients, an 87-year-old woman, describing her as "quadriplegic and in a vegetative state." This woman, I later learned from her medical record, had been uncommunicative and bedbound for many years after a devastating stroke. Like many people in her condition, she developed severe bedsores, which at some point had impelled her family to take her to the hospital. After examining the woman and obtaining her family's consent, one of the hospital's surgeons removed her damaged tissue surgically and provided a course of intravenous antibiotics to control any related infections. The nurse was livid: "I believe that to perform surgeries on an elderly vegetative patient is unethical and costly to Medicare," she wrote in her complaint. "This patient was admitted . . . with no hope to benefit from this hospitalization. . . . [The hospital] and the surgeon, Dr. Wallace, should reimburse Medicare for this futile and unethical behavior." The nurse also notified a hospital ethicist about this complaint. "*Palliative care* [italics mine] should have been asked in from day one," she wrote and added, "I don't actually think anything will happen. There will be no investigation, no penalty, because there is just way too much money made off of the dying bodies of old people. So, my dilemma is, I get paid by this monstrous organization, which I think makes me as much of a whore as Dr. Wallace. It's not a good feeling."

Such misgivings are hardly new. Criticizing U.S. medicine for being aggressive has become a truism, and so has recognizing overdiagnosis, overtreatment, and overspending as chief and stubborn maladies of the U.S. health care system. Explanations for these maladies are plentiful. Back in the 1950s, sociologist Talcott Parsons attributed them to a certain "American culture" that encourages combative medicine. American physicians, Parsons wrote, are "trained and expected to act" in the face of disease, and patients and families want to feel that "something is being done" even when treatment has little to no medical benefit.[1] Some twenty years later, Eliot Freidson concurred that U.S. physicians feel "impelled to do something, if only to satisfy patients who urge [them] to do something when they are in distress."[2] This interventionist "culture" has also drawn attention from journalists: "American medicine is aggressive," wrote Lynn Payer. "American doctors want to *do* something, preferably as much as possible. . . . They often eschew drug treatment in favor of more aggressive surgery, but if they do use drugs they are likely to use higher doses and more aggressive drugs."[3]

Then there is the profit motive—a well-warranted target for much critical scholarship. The U.S. health care system relies on private industry, which operates in several interconnected markets. Many actors in this industry—pharmaceutical companies, medical device producers, and some hospitals and private practitioners—increase their profit margins with the more care they provide. A wholesale economy, unprecedented in its scope, has emerged around diagnosing and treating disease. This economy pours enormous amounts of money into medical research and health care delivery; as a result, extreme interventions have become routine and standard practice.[4]

The problems arising from this economy are particularly pronounced near the end of life. At stake are life and death decisions—whether or not to treat a condition that may be terminal—which are as consequential as medical decisions can be. These decisions are significant financially because they involve very expensive, high-intensity care. But cost aside, providing such care to severely ill patients is morally and medically questionable. It is very hard, for example, to justify putting terminal cancer patients on mechanical ventilators and prolonging their lives, despite great suffering and virtually no chance of long-term survival.[5] In 2009, however, 6.7 percent of Medicare cancer patients whose providers were paid fee-for-service received mechanical ventilation in the month before they died.[6] Such figures make one wonder whether the combination of a capitalist industry, which profits from delivering care, and a culture that glorifies aggressive medicine has led to what the California nurse intimated: dying patients have become victims of medicine's professional hubris and corporations' avarice. Locked in purgatory—incapacitated, seriously ill, not dead and yet not quite alive—they helplessly watch physicians muster cutting-edge technologies that merely prolong their anguish.

This book, however, is not about this economy but about its negation: a counter-economy that aims to put this one in check. It is about clinicians like this nurse; far from being an isolated iconoclast, she expressed sentiments that many people and organizations promote. It is about medical practitioners, ethicists, patient advocates, economists, and corporations who built a social movement, formulated a professional approach, and then gave birth to another multi-billion-dollar health care economy, whose purpose is drawing lines on how far medical care goes near the end of life. The nurse referenced this movement in her complaint: hospice and palliative care.

The ideas and actual practice of hospice and palliative care I will analyze in detail throughout the book. For now, it would suffice to quote the formal definition of the American Board of Medical Specialties, which in 2006 recognized "Hospice and Palliative Care Medicine" as a subspecialty:

> Hospice and Palliative Medicine provides care to prevent and relieve the suffering experienced by patients with life-limiting illnesses. [Specialists work] with an interdisciplinary hospice or palliative care team to optimize quality of life while addressing the physical, psychological, social, and spiritual needs of both patient and family.[7]

A most important part of this definition is what it does *not* include: curing disease and prolonging life. Instead, it emphasizes minimizing suffering and maximizing the quality of life during the time patients have left.

In the United States, *hospice care* takes place outside of hospitals whereas most *palliative care* happens within them.[8] *Hospice* patients are people who physicians have already diagnosed as dying. By Medicare standards, this means they have a predicted life span of six months or less. Hospices cease attempts to prolong these patients' lives and treat them for comfort only. *Palliative care* patients, by contrast, are usually still in the hospital. Many of them are at an earlier stage of their disease and continue to receive care from numerous specialists, which almost certainly involves life-prolonging or life-sustaining measures.[9] The goal of palliative care is to facilitate conversations between patients, families, and clinicians about whether patients' illnesses are terminal, how close to death they are, and how much life-prolonging care they should receive, if any at all. It is a specialty that negotiates and enacts limits on life prolongation.

This specialty has become a remarkable force in U.S. medicine. In 2015, 46 percent of the deaths of Medicare patients took place in hospice, and some 90 percent of the country's large hospitals had an operating palliative care service.[10] A growing number of clinicians from other specialties encounter hospice and palliative care principles in their training, medical journals, conferences, and workplaces; some of them will internalize and apply these principles at the bedside. In media outlets, clinicians and advocates of hospice and palliative care frequently participate in conversations on end-of-life care as authoritative experts. Similarly to the growth in curative medicine and life-prolonging interventions, growth in hospice and palliative medicine has been lubricated with money: by 2017, Medicare paid $16.9 billion to a largely for-profit U.S. hospice industry.[11] The true size and significance of this economy are even greater if we take into account private insurers' payments and the money saved by using hospice and palliative care and avoiding costly life-prolonging treatments.

Two economies therefore face each other: one aims to prolong life and cure disease, and the other focuses on facilitating a "good death" and minimizing suffering. One extracts profit from hospitalizations, medical devices, surgeries, and medications, and the other profits from counteracting life-prolonging care and containing spending on it. One dedicates itself to saving life (or prolonging it), and the other draws on the conviction that life in disability and suffering is not always worth living. People tend to think of the economy as the realm of technical, utilitarian, and somewhat unimaginative quid pro quo monetary exchanges. End-of-life care is one among many examples demonstrating that economic life consists of much more: emotions, conflicting moral values, diverging professional philosophies, and dense social relations.[12]

This book is an account of the counteracting economy, which I will call *the new economy of dying*. It examines the history of this economy's emergence and analyzes its current operations in three California hospitals. At the center of my analysis are hospice and palliative care experts and advocates, who have played a pivotal role in creating this economy through connecting moral views, professional stances, and financial interests. Their endeavors involved a great deal of entrepreneurial work: hospice and palliative care protagonists have spoken to the interests of corporations, garnered endorsements from politicians, and solicited support from funders.[13] They have trained, written to, and spoken with clinicians in nearly all areas in medicine, trying to change how they practice medicine when treating severely ill patients. And they have appealed to the general public and increased popular participation in the new economy of dying by mobilizing current patients, future patients, and their family members to cast doubt on the virtue of life-prolonging treatments in severe illness.

Studying this new economy of dying is important because it has greatly affected how people die in the United States. The topic, however, also has broader significance. For one thing, it teaches us a general lesson about how economies emerge in morally contested areas and what role experts can play in this emergence. Moreover, studying the effort to draw lines on life prolongation sheds light on a major transition into an era where humanity ponders the ultimate reach of progress. Discussions of boundaries and limits—scientific, fiscal, and environmental—are gradually taking the place of the endeavor to advance, grow, and conquer new ground, which has guided modern societies for several centuries.[14] Death is illustrative, in this respect: as Søren Kierkegaard wrote, death "has its own earnestness" because it is the absolute limit on being, the human ability to control life, and the effort to transcend nature.[15] Negotiating when to stop prolonging life means delineating this limit. It means placing a boundary on the reach of human agency—an undertaking of uttermost existential significance.[16]

The enormity of the topic notwithstanding, how U.S. politicians, professionals, and laypeople address it is specific to our time and place. In the spirit of Cicero, who accused Cato of speaking in the Roman Senate "as if he were living in Plato's Republic instead of this cesspit of Romulus," my goal is not to develop ideal and abstract philosophical discussions on human existence, agency, boundaries, and limits.[17] I leave these to ethicists.[18] This book, rather, follows how people and institutions enact limits in the concrete reality of U.S. medicine, polity, and economics: in Congress and in daily newspapers, in the training of medical practitioners and in scholarly journals, in hospital administrators' offices and by patients' deathbeds.[19] These are sites where a project of great proportions takes place, where medical practitioners, policymakers, academics, patients, and family members draw and manage the most categorical limit on human existence: death.

Three Quandaries of Death

When asked about my research, I say that I study death panels. The term is manipulative, to say the least. But it captures the challenges and tensions in setting limits at the end of life in the most poignant and provocative way.

Throughout much of 2009, Americans ferociously debated the Patient Protection and Affordable Care Act (ACA)—a cornerstone piece of health care legislation that became known as "Obamacare." One of the debate's pinnacles was a provision that paid physicians to discuss with patients what life-prolonging and life-sustaining treatments they would and would not want if their medical condition deteriorated. Sarah Palin, the former Republican vice-presidential candidate and an outspoken public figure, vehemently opposed this provision. First on her Facebook page, then in the open editorial section of the *Wall Street Journal*, she bashed the intention to save an estimated $400–500 million through such discussions, saying it would amount to "death panels."[20] This statement echoed a general point the Republican Party was pushing during the period: about a month earlier, House Minority Leader John Boehner and Representative Thaddeus McCotter wrote that the provision "may start us down a treacherous path toward government-encouraged euthanasia."[21] President Obama, on his end, responded that the provision would not "pull the plug on grandma."[22]

Although it was quickly debunked, the death panel allegation persisted—and even won the disreputable "lie of the year" award.[23] It was a very effective lie: a 2011 poll found that 23 percent of U.S. adults thought that the Affordable Care Act gave government the power to make end-of-life decisions on behalf of seniors and 36 percent were unsure.[24] The Obama administration had to remove the provision from the Affordable Care Act, and when it tried to pass a similar regulation a year later, it failed again.[25] In the spring of 2012, as I was shadowing him in a hospital, a palliative care physician told me he could not bill for a conversation he just had with a Medicare patient about end-of-life care. 'This would have been the death panel!' he said sarcastically and wrote in the medical chart that he had managed the patient's pain, which was billable.* At another palliative care service, death panels inspired moments of dark humor: when the service prepared for a staff picnic, one physician suggested printing team shirts that said "I Work for Obama's Death Panel" on the front and "Ask Me about Your Granny" on the back. The death panel became a grotesque trope that painted discussions of policy and care for the dying in macabre colors.

The success of this grotesque trope is revealing. Palin touched upon three major controversial quandaries that the new economy of dying has engendered: how far to go prolonging life, how much money to spend toward this goal, and who should make these decisions. Her allegation was evidently false, but it can serve as a sociological Rorschach test that evinced (and capitalized on) real moral concerns people have about these quandaries. People have feared that emotionally excruciating life-and-death decisions would draw on rigid bureaucratic criteria, that cold monetary calculations would determine who would live and who would die, and that "the state," as a *force majeure,* would violate individuals' autonomy and terminate life-sustaining care unilaterally.[26]

Since the 1960s, social science scholars have produced multiple accounts on death and dying in the United States.[27] Yet the main period that I study—the early 2010s—is different from the periods they examined.

---

* Throughout the book, I use single quotation marks to indicate quotes that I paraphrase from my field notes and double quotation marks to indicate direct quotes, which I audiotaped and transcribed in full. I have adopted this format from Jerolmack (2013).

First, it is a period when these three quandaries congealed into a single political controversy. The first and third quandaries—when life should (not) be prolonged and who should decide on this—have been at the center of public, political, and ethical discussions for several decades. In the 1980s, for example, the U.S. media covered extensively the lengthy campaign to disconnect vegetative Nancy Cruzan from artificial nutrition, and in 1990–2005 right-to-die activists clashed with conservative advocates over the similar case of Terri Schiavo.[28] It was only in the 2000s and 2010s, however, that questions of cost and finance became integral to such discussions, to the extent that a California nurse could argue in a complaint that prolonging the life of an unconscious patient was both "unethical and costly to Medicare."

Second, by the 2010s, the medical profession had assumed an unprecedented role in addressing these quandaries. Although people have been dying under medicine's purview for over a century, medicine did not offer specialized treatment for the dying until the last few decades.[29] Physicians used to treat patients with the goal of avoiding or postponing death; when it became clear to them that death was inevitable, they lost interest in the patient.[30] The development of hospice and palliative care, however, changed this situation by making death and dying major objects of clinical interest. Discussions about the proper ways to manage them medically, ethically, financially, and policy-wise flourished.

This change was palpable and consequential. In the fall of 1965, Elisabeth Kübler-Ross, a young psychiatry professor who would soon become the public face of the U.S. hospice movement, began interviewing dying patients about their feelings, experiences, and needs. The clinicians who treated these patients were hostile to her project, and some of them denied its very legitimacy:

> My phone calls and personal visits to the wards were all in vain. Some physicians said politely that they would think about it, others said they did not wish to expose their patients to such questioning as it might tire them too much. A nurse angrily asked in utter disbelief if I enjoyed telling a twenty-year-old man that he had only a couple of weeks to live! She walked before I could tell her more about our plans.[31]

Despite this resistance, Kübler-Ross's book, *On Death and Dying*, came out in 1969 and became an instant bestseller. Peppered with myriad psychological and sociological observations, it issued a riveting *j'accuse* of modern medicine, condemning it for what the author and many of her contemporaries called "death denial." This denial, Kübler-Ross argued, had devastating consequences: "traditional" medical professionals were untrained and unprepared to talk to terminally ill patients about death and could not help them accept their condition. Instead of acknowledging death and supporting the dying, clinicians treated death as a professional failure, clung onto protocols, tried to treat the untreatable, and caused unnecessary suffering to the terminally ill. The entire medical system, Kübler-Ross argued, was deaf and blind to dying patients' needs and wishes. Many of the patients she interviewed knew they were dying and had no interest in pretending they still had hope for a cure. Pretending, however, was the main thing clinicians had to offer them.[32]

When I launched my own research, however, I encountered a very different reality. For one thing, death was a legitimate—and indeed encouraged—research topic.[33] Without exception, all my interviewees knew what I meant by saying that I studied "end-of-life care," and they all agreed it was an important project.[34] Responding to my interview request, one intensive care unit (ICU) physician complimented me for having found "such an interesting topic to study." She and many of my other interviewees expressed hope that my work would further end-of-life care and increase awareness of the problems posed by care for the dying. Death was also in high demand in my academic community: anonymous reviewers in sociological journals wrote that the topic demanded "close attention by policy-makers and academics alike" and that my project "addresses an important and timely topic." In job interviews, senior faculty who have faced the challenge of caring for aging parents or spouses and confronting end-of-life decisions reflected on how their own experiences compared with my findings. When Harvard University Press offered me my book contract, its social science editor said that the board of editors only wished they could have published the book earlier. Virtually every person that I talked to about my work—interviewees, colleagues, and random people who sat next to me on flights—agreed that studying death and dying was "important," "interesting," and "timely."

The widespread agreement that death and dying pose social and policy problems, which invite research and beg solutions, is the outcome of a process. As with all social problems, death and dying became problematic because certain people constructed them as problematic and promoted particular ways of thinking, speaking, and writing about them.[35] Hospice and palliative care protagonists—Kübler-Ross among them— were the principal actors in promoting this construction. They were not the only ones: bioethicists and right-to-die advocates, for example, had important roles as well, and they will make frequent appearances throughout the book. But hospice and palliative care has been the most consolidated cache of organized clinical knowledge and practices, which framed the problem of death and suggested solutions. The essence of the problem, as advocates defined it, could be summarized in the following way: medicine treats severely ill patients too aggressively, leads to immense suffering and excessive spending, and does so without taking these patients' wishes into account. In the popular media and best-selling books, and among health economists, physicians, journalists, and laypeople, the corollary conclusions have been recited: limits at the end of life should be set, "aggressive" and "extraordinary" measures to prolong life should be moderated, end-of-life spending should be controlled, and patients' wishes should be respected and followed.[36]

I do not seek to criticize this stance but to turn an inquisitive eye toward it. First, I argue that this view has social origins: the argument that prolonged hospital deaths are morally and financially problematic does not explain how people came to see them as problematic, let alone how they problematized them in the particular ways they did. (Similarly, there are countless critical studies on poverty, but very few ask how poverty came to be regarded as problematic.[37]) Second, I show that this view has already impacted health policy, much of the medical profession, and people's attitudes toward death in general. Institutions such as hospices and professional orientations such as palliative care have reshaped professional and public views of death. They transformed Kübler-Ross's *j'accuse* into a new set of expectations from clinicians (and patients) on how to behave when death approaches. They valorized, allowed, and encouraged certain attitudes toward death, while disparaging, disallowing, and marginalizing others.[38] The new economy of dying that they enacted put forth new standards for good, normal, and legitimate care—a new *ars moriendi* that governs how people die and merits renewed examination.[39]

Dying, Economized

I use the term *economization*—and its derivatives *economized* and *economizing*—to unravel two logics that underlie the new economy of dying. This term is multidimensional and carries multiple meanings and connotations.[40] Instead of setting some meanings aside and adopting others, I will deliberately embrace the term's polysemy to illuminate the new economy's compounded nature.

A first meaning of economization originates in ancient Greek philosophy. *Oikonomia*—the art of household management—was of much interest to classical philosophers. Oikonomia's fundamental premise was the abundance of natural resources.[41] Ancient Greeks regarded nature as providing more than what people needed for subsistence: "it is the business of nature to furnish subsistence for each being brought into the world," Aristotle wrote.[42] *Economizing* meant embracing a prudent disposition toward this abundance so that one could use the surplus for non-material ends, such as friendship, politics, and philosophy.[43] In discussing the new economy of dying, I will employ the term *economized dying* to characterize prudency, which people adopt in a similar fashion. Economizing dying would mean embracing a controlled and restrained self-conduct toward the abundant medical interventions that modern medicine makes available.

A second and more widespread meaning of economization originates in neoclassical economics. Economic theorist Lionel Robbins defined economics as "the science which studies human behavior as a relationship between ends and scarce means, which have alternative uses."[44] This definition takes scarcity, not abundance, as the defining feature of economization and sees economic behavior as instrumental and rational: people weigh desired alternatives and choose which ones best serve their goals within the limited resources that they have.[45] Robbins and other neoclassicists applied this logic of economization to virtually all domains of human life. They transformed the rational individual actor into a prototype, arguing that people, households, states, and organizations of various kinds should be modeled, governed, and evaluated as such actors.[46]

Critical theorists have used the term *economization* to characterize these imperial tendencies of economics and the consequent spread of instrumental rational calculations into new domains.[47] Examples range from macroeconomic policies to microsocial interactions. States manage their populations and industries to increase their gross domestic product (GDP).[48] Law schools formulate future plans with the goal of advancing in the ranking of the *U.S. News and World Report*.[49] Individuals make financial decisions while taking into consideration how they affect their credit score.[50] Teenagers try to maximize the "likes" they receive on social media websites. Scholars dedicate their careers to publishing articles in highly ranked journals and maximizing their citation count.[51] All these examples illustrate a pervasive trend, in which people and organizations internalize the neoclassical form of economization and embrace calculated, individuated, and rational self-conduct.[52] In the realm of end-of-life care, economization in its neoclassical sense means formulating the quandaries of dying as a neoclassical problem of optimization. This involves representing patients as individuals, who possess preferences, confront several alternative treatment options, and need to choose how to maximize their utility under a dual state of scarcity—the finitude of resources in the health care economy and the inherent finitude of their life.[53]

Drawing on both forms of economization, the new economy of dying operates as a "regime of valuation," a set of patterned judgments of worth and value that governs the end of life.[54] Most defining of this economy is the judgment that, when it comes to the end of life, less is oftentimes better. This judgment is moral and financial at the same time. On the one hand, it casts doubt on the moral (and medical) value of providing life-prolonging care to severely ill patients; on the other hand, it advocates to economize the spending on this care. Traditionally, modern medicine has targeted disease with maximal technological and scientific capacity, but the new economy of dying presents a rationale to economize dying: restrain, adjust, and appropriate medical interventions, based on evaluations of their morality, cost, and utility.[55] Applying this rationale, however, is full of challenges and contradictions.

Economizing in Practice

Virtually all developed countries have faced rises in medical spending and health care utilization and adopted measures to control them. The U.S. case, however, sheds light on the specific challenge of doing so through a market. Countries with nationalized health care systems could economize through centralized mechanisms, stipulate clear standards for rationing, and require that hospitals and clinicians follow them. An exemplar is the United Kingdom's National Institute for Health and Care Excellence (NICE), which set £30,000 as the maximum recommended spending limit for treatment that prolongs life by one healthy life-year and subjected all exceptions to additional review.[56] By contrast, the U.S. health care system has weak central and direct mechanisms of governance.[57] Decisions on treatment are distributed among numerous organizations— insurers, hospitals, and various physician groups—each with different policies and considerations. When one of them does not approve of a treatment, patients can go to another that does. (Knowing this, pharmaceutical companies have long directed much of their marketing effort to patients.)[58] Ethicists in the United States who attempted to define what would count as nonbeneficial and "medically futile" care have failed to reach a consensus.[59] Their critics specifically targeted the idea of enforcing unilateral definitions of futility on patients.[60] Even Medicare—the federal program that insures patients over the age of 65—does not set clear limits on utilization and spending, in great part due to the country's ruptured political system, where such controversial measures are quickly exploited for political gain.

In the absence of a major centralized governing power, economization in the United States has assumed a diffused form, which draws on changing the intuitions and behaviors of individual patients, clinicians, and organizations.[61] Limits at the end of life are not imposed *extrinsically*, as prohibitions that bind people, but *intrinsically*, through pervading people's professional, financial, and moral outlooks. Analyzing how people and organizations enact limits at the end of life therefore requires examining empirically how this pervasion has occurred—how the new economy of dying has won hearts and minds, making many clinicians, hospitals, administrators, and patients view limits at the end of life as moral, rational, and necessary.

This book does so by analyzing the history of hospice and palliative care and observing the contemporary practice of palliative care. Drawing on both primary and secondary historical sources, I examine how the ideas and practices that underlie the new economy of dying developed over time and how they became influential in U.S. medicine and U.S. society at large. I surveyed books, articles, and reflective essays by hospice and palliative care advocates, hundreds of magazine and newspaper articles and editorials on end-of-life care, all congressional hearings on the topic, publications and activities of advocacy organizations, and academic research that the thriving community of hospice and palliative care has produced since the 1970s.

Between October 2011 and October 2012 I joined three California palliative care services to observe how they limit life prolongation at the bedside. I shadowed members of these services as they discussed diagnoses, prognoses, and care plans with seriously ill patients, their family members, and other hospital clinicians. I sat in on meetings where palliative care practitioners told tearful children, spouses, and at times parents that their "loved one" was terminally ill or dying, and I witnessed the often-slow negotiation over withdrawing treatment that kept this loved one alive. I stood by patients as they were taking their last breaths. I watched and listened to palliative care clinicians interact with other specialists, who disagreed with them on a patient's prospects for recovery. And I interviewed eighty social workers, nurses, chaplains, administrators, and physicians from numerous specialties, who dealt with death in their day-to-day work.

With this mixture of historical, interview, and ethnographic data, I shed light on the different outlooks and practices—professional, financial, and moral—that underlie the economization of dying in public discourse, among clinicians, and at patients' bedsides.

The Professional Outlook

First and foremost, the economization of dying has hinged on changing professional practices and views regarding end-of-life care and fostering a medical intuition that life-prolonging care in severely ill patients should be moderated.

This intuition negated U.S. medicine's long historical trajectory of expansion. Organized medicine obtained a virtual monopoly over U.S. health care services around the turn of the twentieth century. At the height of the modern age, when trust in science peaked, the medical profession drew its authority from a combination of dependence and social legitimacy. Physicians did not have to force people to use their services—people did so voluntarily, out of need and conviction in medicine's powers.[62] The ethos of scientific progress opened the door to boundless professional ambition. Medicine's jurisdiction expanded, and "labels of 'healthy' and 'ill'" became "relevant to an ever-increasing part of human existence."[63] Within its jurisdiction, medicine's interventions multiplied and intensified. By the last decades of the twentieth century, the medical profession seemed to offer patients some treatment or another regardless of a patient's condition. When one line of chemotherapy failed, oncologists could offer a second, third, or even fourth line; when the kidneys decompensated, nephrologists could put the patient on dialysis; when the function of the liver, heart, lungs, kidneys, or pancreas declined, the possibility of transplant surgery was available. When a person's heart and lungs stopped there were emergency care interventions—such as cardiopulmonary resuscitation—that could "bring them back to life."[64] As philosopher Giorgio Agamben suggested, death has become epiphenomenal to medicine: seemingly, death occurs only when physicians withdraw their interventions and allow it to occur.[65]

Reflecting on the development of intensive care—a most emblematic medical frontier—sociologist Robert Zussman observed that "criticisms of intensive care—or, more precisely, of what goes with intensive care—are almost as old as the units themselves."[66] This argument applies to other medical specialties as well. Oncology, surgery, and cardiology introduced innovations that were quickly regarded as mixed blessings because they prolonged human life at the cost of great suffering. Throughout the 1960s and 1970s, numerous critics rebuked medicine for objectifying patients and using them as mere tools of scientific research: "Once a hero, the doctor has now become a villain," observed sociologist Paul Starr.[67] The modern hospital attracted much criticism as well: "clothed with an almost mystical power, yet suffused with a relentless impersonality and a forbidding aura of technical complexity," hospitals and the medicine practiced in them became symbols of dehumanizing professionalism.[68]

The hospice approach very much emerged from this criticism.[69] At times explicitly antiprofessional, hospice pioneers promoted intuition, emotion, and personal attachment between patients and caregivers, and valued singular relationships—as opposed to standardized guidelines—as the most essential features of caregiving.[70] The goals hospices set for themselves—assisting dying people in accepting death and helping them pass away comfortably and with dignity—turned medicine's traditional goals on their heads. They replaced the effort to beat physical decline and postpone mortality with an embrace of death as a natural phenomenon.

Ironically, as hospices developed, their backlash against professionalism transformed into a professional approach itself.[71] It made death and dying an object of great interest for a burgeoning community that involved "doctors and researchers, service providers and grassroots educators, lawyers and writers, politicians and policymakers—a complex of individuals, groups, and formal organizations," similar to what sociologist Steven Epstein observed in the case of AIDS.[72] Just like cancer, heart dysfunction, child medicine, infectious diseases, and intensive care, death and dying became a realm whose management required unique interventions, skills, and expert knowledge.[73] The "correct" way to treat terminal patients became the hospice way: discussing how to phase out life-prolonging treatment, minimize patients' physical and emotional suffering, and help patients reach acceptance.[74]

In the following decades, the professional jurisdiction of hospice practitioners expanded.[75] Palliative care, which developed from hospice in the 1990s, had the goal of starting conversations on death earlier in the disease process, before patients began dying and while they were still in hospital.[76] Its influence gradually extended to general medicine. Primary care physicians are today encouraged to talk to patients about end-of-life care and recommend that they plan for it even if they are healthy.[77]

This professional development of hospice and palliative care is one component of the push to *economize dying*. Hospice and palliative care set forth a medical rationale that puts in check intentions to prolong the lives of seriously ill patients. This rationale stresses that it is morally imperative to question doctors, who pursue treatments that have little chance of succeeding, and to save patients from prolonged and torturous dying processes. Hospice and palliative care clinicians who work inside and outside of hospitals, and hospice organizations which provide designated care for the dying, spread a professionally and morally grounded approach, which pushes to economize dying from within the medical profession.

The Financial Outlook

The second component of economized dying is fiscal: it is the notion that *too much is being spent* on people who approach the end of their life. The solution here has been economizing dying financially: scrutinizing, then reducing expenditure on end-of-life care.

Today's clinicians and hospitals operate in a fundamentally different economy than the economy of the 1960s. The decades after World War II were a period of medical expansion in the United States: following the Hill Burton Act (1946) and against the backdrop of great economic prosperity, the number and size of hospitals increased, new medical schools opened, medical specialization accelerated, and physicians' fees grew rapidly. The growth of the private insurance market and the enactment of Medicare and Medicaid meant that unprecedented amounts of money became available for health care. The commercial, fee-for-service health care market of the period created incentives for physicians and hospitals to increase the reimbursable care that they provided, and by the early 1970s there was evidence of overtreatment.[78] "In a short time," Paul Starr observed, "American medicine seemed to pass from stubborn shortages to irrepressible excess, without ever having passed through happy sufficiency."[79] The physicians and hospitals fighting to prolong life in all circumstances had direct financial incentives to do so.

Evidence that overtreatment still exists in the U.S. health care system is abundant.[80] As the California nurse's complaint letter suggests, some suspect that financial interest drives this overtreatment.[81] Yet since the

1970s, the United States has gradually moved in the opposite direction: policymakers have focused on containing and controlling the increase in spending on health care, eliminating futility, and adopting mechanisms of accountability.[82] On the macro level, they have completely failed: U.S. expenditure on health care has climbed steadily, reaching the unprecedented and internationally incomparable rate of 17.9 percent of the GDP in 2016. Still, the multiple reforms to counteract this rise have had an effect on day-to-day medical practice: managed care organizations pay many providers capitated rates and give incentives to limit utilization.[83] Revisions in the Medicare and Medicaid codes now limit payment for hospitalization days and pressure hospitals to discharge patients early.[84] Health corporations also have adopted cost-effectiveness standards, and they pressure physicians to meet them. Insurance companies send case managers to visit hospitals, review patients' charts, and decline payment for treatments that they deem unnecessary.[85]

In this context, the end of life has become a particularly intriguing site of financial valuation and cost containment. Health economists regularly produce estimates of how much the nation spends on patients in the last months of their lives (see Chapter 2), and newspaper editorials debate the necessity and futility of this spending.[86] Ethicists suggest ways to determine what level of spending near the end of life would be just and appropriate,[87] and people speak of a duty to limit end-of-life spending for future generations' sake.[88]

The end of life has become a realm where moral, professional, and financial values interact with each other in intricate and somewhat unpredictable ways. Financial calculus in this area has become entwined with moral calculus: the further hospice and palliative care advocates went in doubting the moral value of prolonging life in severe illness, the more futile and inefficient it seemed from a financial perspective. By presenting hospice and palliative care as a better and cheaper way of care, advocates connected policymakers' interest in controlling spending and corporations' interest in minimizing their costs with the moral endeavor to limit life prolongation.

The palliative care services that I studied ethnographically consulted on many cases of patients or families who hesitated to sign Do Not Resuscitate (DNR) and Do Not Intubate (DNI) forms, patients who stayed in the hospital for long periods and whose medical condition did not seem to improve, patients who repeatedly came to the hospital for chronic illnesses or infections, and patients with terminal diseases such as cancer, human immunodeficiency virus (HIV), and heart failure in their final stage.[89] All these patients were potentially expensive for hospitals. Their illnesses were likely to result in long hospital stays, whose costs insurance companies were not fully covering. In the 1960s, allowing such patients to die in hospital was common. Glaser and Strauss's classic account from the period, *Time for Dying*, noted that "unless a person dies abruptly . . . the dying trajectory includes a stage of 'last days' and perhaps even 'last weeks'" that are spent waiting and preparing for death in the hospital.[90] The current health care economy has made such waiting periods costly, and many hospital administrations funded palliative care services in hopes that they would encourage seriously ill patients to reflect critically on their desired treatment and help discharge them elsewhere.[91]

The push to economize dying has therefore been financial, moral, and professional. During the decades (1960–1980s) when medicine drew criticism for overtreating patients who had lost realistic hope for cure, people also criticized it for overspending on these patients and driving the health care system and the entire U.S. economy bankrupt. Hospice and palliative care became a moralized financial solution—a way to treat the dying better and more efficiently, which spoke to both policymakers' and corporate administrations' concerns. Yet economizing remained difficult because it required the consent of the patients themselves.

Economized Subjects

Shortly after I began fieldwork, I sat for coffee with Nick, a retired hospice and palliative care physician. 'Things have changed,' he told me. 'It used to be that families and patients were the ones who pushed for less care, and doctors were the ones who wanted to treat as aggressively as possible. Now, it's usually the doctors who want to treat less and the patients who insist on getting more treatment. The culture of the hospital is screaming, "stop," but many patients just don't want to.'

Although I will qualify these observations later in the book, I find them generally accurate.[92] In my fieldwork, I discovered hospital environments that were far more attentive to patients who wanted to eschew life-prolonging care than the environments Kübler-Ross described. The palliative care clinicians that I studied were important in facilitating this change. Walking in Kübler-Ross's footsteps, they actively advocated throughout their hospitals against overly aggressive life-prolonging treatment and for respecting wishes to relinquish acute care. As Nick observed, however, the bulk of their day-to-day work involved conversing with patients and families who were open to aggressive medical interventions that medical teams and hospitals were reluctant to give.

This inversion of clinicians' and patients' stances on end-of-life care—from a situation where many patients pled with doctors to withhold life-prolonging treatment and allow them to die, to a situation where many doctors pled with patients to accept their terminal condition and "let go"—is highly intriguing. It indicates a shift in the center of gravity of economization. Much of the current health care system is oriented toward encouraging patients to accept death and forgo life-prolonging treatment, even when they initially hesitate to do so.[93] At first blush, this seems all too similar to the notorious death panels allegation, but Palin's provocation was far too shallow to capture this economy's true character.[94] What makes the new economy of dying so powerful is that, unlike the death panels imagery, it does not impose external limits on patients, but relies on their consent. It does not base itself on the oppressive power of states or corporations but on grassroots mobilization of clinicians, patients, and families. And it does not force impersonal standards on people, but rather acts through people's own moral conviction that they are doing the right thing.[95]

Individualism, as Bellah and his coauthors put it, is "the first language in which Americans tend to think about their lives."[96] For much of the twentieth century, critics of the medical profession targeted medicine's violations of people's autonomy and individuality. The medical gaze, the argument went, structured medical practice as a spectacle, not a dialogue, and clinicians treated patients as bodies and not people, as objects and not subjects.[97] Critiques of this power dynamic gathered steam during the 1960s and 1970s, when the patient rights movement mobilized people against medical authority.[98] One outcome of this mobilization was a reconfiguration of the medical gaze—a shift that bioethicists, who had a major role in it, described as a transition from *medical pater-nalism* to an orientation that focuses on *patient autonomy*.[99] Medicine adopted a wide array of professional practices that encouraged patients to express themselves, reflect on their condition, voice their fears, and participate in decisions. It enshrined patients as "authors of their own lives," who are capable of "controlling, to some degree, their destiny, fashioning it through successive decisions throughout their life."[100] The main way to pursue and protect the rights of individual patients was facilitating choice.[101] Advance directives, living wills, and other forms and documents recorded patients' wishes and preferences, and declarations such as "A Patient's Bill of Rights" (1973, 1992) and laws such as the Patient Self-Determination Act of 1990 established the right of individual patients to know and influence the treatment they receive.[102] More than just allowing patients a voice in their clinical care, medicine needed, demanded, and incited them to speak.[103]

This focus on the individual patient and the proliferation of clinical practices and legal structures geared toward making people reflect, express themselves, and choose signals the coming of age of a new form of medical power. The question, in this context, is not how this new form of power liberates people from medical authority but how it enables certain patterns of self-expression and self-reflection, disables others, and prompts people to define and voice themselves in new ways.[104]

Palliative care practitioners face the key challenge that Nick highlighted. Although the new economy of dying has grown, making much of the U.S. health care system lean toward economizing dying, many patients and families hesitate to participate in this economization and relinquish life-prolonging care. The push to economize is therefore often at odds with the wish to respect patients' sovereignty and not impose decisions on them. Caroline, a palliative care physician who doubled as the director of her service, described this tension explicitly:

Caroline: If [a family] would feel that "we put [mom] in the grave and we're throwing dirt on her and she's still alive . . .", it's hard to tell me that we should stop. If you look at it from resources—yes, I get that. And can you do this on each person? No, we'll go bankrupt. We already are. . . . You do your best communication, you're hoping that they understand, but if at the end of the day that's how they feel. . . . Yeah,

you can pull out ineffective care policies and probably win, but
I wouldn't sleep well. I don't think palliative care should have that
agenda, to stop all this stuff on everyone because it's not going to
work, ultimately. We have to go where they are . . .

Roi: There's a possibility that patients and families will be feeling that—

Caroline: We might be saving two bucks, instead of really, really facing
something that is inevitable. . . . We have to be careful . . . what do we
say to them?

Roi: What *do* you say to them?

Caroline: Yeah, what's the message? [Sarcastically:] This is the best we can
do, and it's cost-effective, and you know, at least you won't suffer.

Like Caroline, most of the clinicians I interviewed and shadowed
considered economization appropriate and necessary, but were reluctant to
enforce it when patients resisted. Palliative care's way to address this tension
was transforming patients (or their representatives) into agents of economization. Palliative care clinicians did not coerce economization on patients, nor did they employ simple persuasion techniques that convinced
patients of the benefits economizing would have for them. Rather, they
exercised what Nikolas Rose called a *conduct of conduct:* they interacted
with patients as they mulled over their condition, digested it, and formulated their thoughts, in ways that increased the probability that patients
would willingly endorse economization as their own value.[105]

Palliative care practices maintained a delicate balance between force
and consent; to paraphrase Antonio Gramsci, they drew on power that
did "not overwhelm consent" but was backed by it.[106] Empowering
patients—helping them articulate themselves, express their wishes, and
have them followed—was not a mere masking of oppressive clinical (or
corporate) power.[107] Nor did it make patients autonomous individuals,
liberated of all medical power. Facilitating patients' self-expression was
itself a form of medical power because patients and families did not articulate themselves alone—they expressed their values and consolidated
their preferences and stances in family conferences and bedside conversations, where clinicians played a major role.

When successful, the outcome of meetings between palliative care clinicians, patients, and families led to a general agreement not only about
what a patient wanted but also about who the patient *was*.[108] If the patient

herself leaned toward economizing dying, reasoned actively on what she did and did not want to do, and communicated it to the doctors, there was no need to force economization on her. The patient became an economized—and economizing—subject.[109] In Louis Althusser's terms, clinicians *interpellated* patients by recognizing them as reflective and capable beings and inducing them to think and speak of themselves in certain ways.[110] The new economy of dying operated not only through clinicians' moral and professional sense and administrations' financial calculations, but also through the most personal and intimate ways people thought of their own and their family members' wishes, hopes, and personalities.

The three hospitals I studied ethnographically were located in a single metropolitan area in California. "Public Hospital" (or "Public") was the area's safety-net institution. "Private Hospital" (or "Private") was owned by a large, private, not-for-profit corporation. "Academic Hospital" (or "Academic") was a university medical center. I did not find significant differences in how clinicians practiced palliative care in each of these hospitals—a possible testimony to the standardizing power of professional education.[111] However, because the hospitals treated markedly different patient populations (see the methodological appendix), studying them allowed me to see how the new economy of dying operated on different demographics. As I will show in the book's empirical chapters, I found that economization was most likely to be successful, smooth, and effective with populations that we generally recognize as privileged: middle class, highly educated, and white. The people who consented to economize their own dying became part of the new economy of dying; those who resisted it were likely to collide with clinicians who felt they were giving them futile treatment. Both groups, however, experienced the impact of the new economy of dying, which has become sizable and significant enough to influence U.S. deaths in general.

Hospice and palliative care have not achieved complete dominance over managing death and dying in the country.[112] Other patterns of care for the dying still proliferate—from "heroic" medicine, where patients die in ICUs receiving life support until their very last moments, to "death with dignity" (or euthanasia), which several states have made legal.[113] Many deaths, particularly "heroic" ones, occur without palliative care clinicians ever being consulted.[114] At the same time, the possibility of consulting a palliative care specialist or moving a patient to "comfort care" is ever available. Even when physicians do not mention palliative care to patients, federal regulations require, for example, that they inform patients about their right to refuse treatment and fill out an advance directive—two rights that hospice and palliative care advocates have promoted and drawn upon for decades.[115] The new economy of dying has therefore become pervasive and nearly inescapable: structured into formal law and informal institutions, it impacts even those who resist or ignore it.[116]

Structure of the Book

The book has two parts. Chapters 1 to 3 outline the emergence of U.S. end-of-life care and the drive to *economize dying*. This analysis partly draws on historical data. I also included ethnographic and interview data in each chapter to show how the historical trends that the chapters outline manifest in contemporary hospitals. The book's second part, Chapters 4 to 5, is ethnography and interview based. This part documents palliative care practice at the bedside and shows how palliative care works to economize patients' agency.

The first two chapters analyze the professional, institutional, and policy dimensions of the new economy of dying. Chapter 1 examines how the professional outlook of hospice and palliative care informed economization. It follows the development of the hospice and palliative care expertise and the emergence of "end of life" as an object of clinical management. It outlines the history of the U.S. hospice and palliative care movement, its expansion and institutionalization, and its success in spreading and articulating professional doubts over the benefit of invasive treatments in treating seriously ill patients. Chapter 2 focuses on how death and dying became financially significant. It analyzes how the end of life drew the interest of economists, administrators, and policymakers, who viewed end-of-life care as a domain where cost savings could be achieved.

The third chapter analyzes how dying patients' and clinicians' positions on end-of-life care have changed historically, based on data from the archive of a hospital ethics committee. I show how, over the course of its history, the bioethics committee became more preoccupied with patients (or families) who demanded more life-prolonging treatment than their doctors felt comfortable providing. Physicians were the ones who promoted more economized dying processes, and the main challenge in end-of-life care became bringing patients and families to embrace less invasive care and consent to economize dying.

In Chapter 4, I employ the concept of *subjectification*, the interactive process by which palliative care clinicians consolidate a shared sense of who patients *are*. I show that palliative care clinicians did not listen passively to what patients and families wanted but instead worked actively to establish a sense of patients' personhood. I document ethnographically the professional practices that palliative care clinicians employed in this process and show that the clinicians' goal was to elicit patient subjectivities that were reconcilable with the trajectory of economized dying.

Chapter 5 focuses on what I call "taming." Patients and families had various hopes and expectations that did not correspond with what clinicians and hospitals deemed feasible. Based on my ethnography, I outline the practices that palliative care clinicians employed to "tame" patients' and families' wishes. None of these practices *imposed* any agenda on patients. They rather aimed to moderate wishes that did not resonate with the economized dying pattern.

The book's conclusion discusses the concept of economization in some more detail, drawing several parallels between the case of the economization of dying and other economization projects. A description of my methodology, research process, and field sites appears in the appendix. One note, however, is due now. To protect people's privacy, I assigned pseudonyms to all clinicians, hospitals, and patients. In several cases, I also changed some identifiable details while trying to avoid affecting their sociological meaning. I hold the view that anonymizing—or "masking"—should be avoided whenever possible, but the sensitivity of the topic and the possibility that the people involved would be personally affected by this account have merited an exception.[117] Regardless, all the events described in this book happened, and all the people mentioned, quoted, and portrayed in it are as real and imperfect as people are.

CHAPTER 1

The Palliative Care Gaze

At the end of the spectrum is Dr. Pashutin. He has the reputation of a guy who would dialyze a corpse.

—A palliative care physician

I WAS WALKING WITH SCOTT (a palliative care physician) to see a patient, when he spotted in the adjacent room a pale, elderly woman breathing heavily and appearing minimally conscious. Nearly bumping into us, the woman's bedside nurse asked if Scott had come to see her, and Scott responded, 'No, but it looks like I will be called soon.' 'It would make sense,' the nurse agreed, 'but they're discharging her to her nursing facility today.'

About an hour later, sitting at the nurse station, I noticed Scott was splitting his attention between writing a note on his own patient and following two heavy men wearing emergency medical technician (EMT) badges, who had come with an ambulance to drive the woman to the nursing facility. One of them asked the nurse if the patient had a Physician Order for Life-Sustaining Treatment (POLST) form—a bright pink paper that instructs clinicians on whether or not to resuscitate, intubate,* provide artificial nutrition, and rehospitalize a patient if her or his condition declines. Scott interrupted him assertively and said that asking whether the form existed was not enough. 'You should *make* them do a POLST!' he said emphatically. The EMT stepped closer to us and said

---

* Intubation involves inserting a tube into a person's mouth or trachea to open or maintain the airway. The procedure may include connecting the person to a mechanical ventilator.

Scott was completely right, but Scott was still unsatisfied—he insisted that the EMT should demand that everybody be clear about what would happen in any situation that developed. As they continued to talk, the EMT's colleague waved a white piece of paper at him, saying, 'It's okay, this is a legal form.' The EMTs moved the woman to a stretcher and disappeared down the elevator on their way to the ambulance parking.

Some fifteen minutes later, the bedside nurse walked into the station and informed everybody that the ambulance driver called and said they thought the patient was decompensating. 'They're bringing her back to the ER.' 'But they just left!' said another nurse. Scott's loud guffaw could probably be heard in other units, too. 'What did I just tell you?' he asked. 'I always say, don't say what you're *not* going to do if *X* happens; say what you *are* going to do.'

This chapter analyzes how Scott's way of looking at patients—his medical gaze—developed historically and how this gaze affects clinical practice in U.S. hospitals today.[1] Peeking in at an open door of a room he was not called to visit—and without conducting a physical examination, reading the woman's medical chart, or knowing anything about her diagnosis—Scott recognized that she was nearing death. A cardiologist once told me that in 95 percent of the cases, she could recognize cardiac problems just by looking at her patients and listening to their stories; the more elaborate laboratory tests and imaging she used only to formalize her intuitions and fine-tune the diagnosis. Scott exhibited a similar ability within his own expertise when he identified a patient who was at the end of her life just by looking at her. Had he been called to see the patient, he could have also supported what he saw with clinical tests.

But Scott's expertise went beyond clinical diagnosis—it also involved organizational astuteness. Knowing the U.S. health care system, he correctly predicted that without unequivocal instructions stating otherwise, the ambulance staff would turn back to the hospital's emergency room (ER) if the woman's condition declined. What would happen next was harder to predict, and Scott did not want to take the chance. The woman could be assigned to ER physicians who had met her in past hospitalizations and knew her medical problems, but she could also be treated by a team who would see her for the first time. Like Scott, this ER team would not know the woman's medical history, but that team would most likely see a completely different patient than the one Scott saw: a patient in acute medical distress, who required emergency measures to stabilize her condition and save her life.

"If all you have is a hammer," a palliative care nurse who worked with Scott once told me, "everything looks like a nail." Seeing a sick person, nephrologists would tend to think of their medical problems in terms of kidney function, cardiologists would tend to attribute them to the heart, and hepatologists would focus on the liver. From the perspective of emergency medicine specialists working in the ER, a woman whose organs are decompensating needs emergency interventions. They would resuscitate her, intubate her, and connect her to the respirator. They would use vasopressor drugs to sustain her blood pressure. By the time they examined her chart to learn about her preexisting medical problems—which could involve terminal cancer or other incurable and irreversible diseases—the woman would already be connected to life-sustaining machines.

Holding a different "hammer," Scott saw another "nail." Having trained and worked daily as a palliative care specialist, he saw an elderly woman who was at the end of life and needed a specific set of clinical and organizational interventions that would be appropriate to this condition. She needed a POLST, a form that would set clear and legally binding boundaries on the treatments health providers would give her. At the end of her life, medical discussions should focus on when to phase out and how to moderate life-sustaining and life-prolonging interventions. I characterize this medical gaze that takes the *end of life* as its main object of interest as an *economizing gaze* because it represents a regime of valuation, which questions the moral and clinical value of medical interventions. The economizing gaze delimits and checks the abundance of medical interventions that medicine can offer. Palliative care clinicians, the economizing gaze's main carriers in hospitals, have gradually anchored themselves in the U.S. medical profession, in the organizational environments of a record number of hospitals, and in the intuitive moral sense of numerous clinicians, policymakers, and laypeople.

This chapter analyzes how four qualities of this gaze developed. First, the economizing gaze has gradually become formal, professional, and institutional. This means that clinicians today can familiarize themselves with the economizing gaze through formal education and training;

advocates of the gaze can rely on established organizations, rules, and laws; and scholars and practitioners can have careers in the area that the medical profession recognizes and rewards. It also means that a growing number of clinicians accept economized dying as morally virtuous; economization has become the gold standard for treating patients whom physicians identify as approaching the end of life. A second quality of the economizing gaze is its tendency to expand. At first the economizing gaze restricted itself to dying people, like the woman Scott noticed. Later, it reached toward broader populations to include people suffering from diseases that might kill them in the non-immediate future, and healthy people who want to prepare for the inevitable. Third, the economizing gaze has influenced the general public. In an era of commercial health care, in which patients are turned into consumers, advocates of the economizing gaze have tried to create a popular demand for economization. Fourth, for some clinicians, the economized gaze has become an embodied quality. Training as a palliative care physician made Scott capable of *seeing* that a patient was at the end of life. Palliative care is therefore not just a set of professional ideas and moral beliefs, but a concrete capacity to look at patients, notice certain qualities and properties that they have, and treat them accordingly.

In this chapter's first section, I will trace the origins of the economizing gaze in hospices, which were the first comprehensive medical approach to define limiting life-prolonging care as virtuous. I analyze the development of U.S. hospices, which emerged as a grassroots movement from the margins of U.S. medicine and became institutionalized (not without resistance) as a medical specialty during the 1970s and 1980s. The second section examines the expansion of the field's boundaries during the 1990s and the 2000s, when several philanthropic funders invested in developing the palliative care expertise. They extended the economizing gaze's breadth from hospices into hospitals; they trained clinicians like Scott and facilitated hospital environments that would accept them. The third section outlines the efforts of palliative care advocates to popularize their approach and communicate economized dying to the general public. The fourth section draws on ethnographic and interview data to examine how palliative care clinicians internalize the economizing gaze, make it part of their routine practice, and train other clinicians in applying it.

Institutionalizing: The Ascent of U.S. Hospices

Origins of the Field

In 1974, Hospice, Inc., in New Haven, Connecticut, formally admitted the first U.S. hospice patient. Less than forty years later, U.S. hospices were serving an estimated 1.65 million people, and 44.6 percent of all deaths in the country happened under the care of a hospice program.[2] This growth was no less than a revolution: hospice has become the main designated medical institution that manages dying in the United States. The revolution is particularly significant because unlike other medical disciplines that grew during the period (such as intensive care and oncology), hospices did not introduce new technologies or treatments. Hospice is a medical philosophy, not a treatment per se. Although hospice care has not achieved complete dominance in U.S. health care, it has certainly gained much ground remarkably fast.

The origins of hospice can be traced back to "homes for the dying poor," which were mostly founded and run by religious organizations in the nineteenth and twentieth century. Care in these organizations included nursing with "little medical involvement" on the part of physicians.[3] Cicely Saunders—universally recognized as the most prominent early pioneer of modern hospice care—began her career at two of these organizations, Saint Luke's Hospital (opened 1893) and Saint Joseph's Hospital (1905) in London. Saunders trained as a physician in 1951–1958, when, as she wrote, "many of the drugs, whose use we now take for granted, were introduced," making doctors assume an ever-growing agency in treating sick bodies and prolonging people's lives.[4] This was the period that the historians of medicine Harvey McGehee and James Bordley called the "period of explosive growth," in which antibiotics, early chemotherapies, polio vaccines, antipsychotic drugs, and later pacemakers, open-heart surgery, cardiac catheterization, and hemodialysis became part of the medical toolkit.[5] Upon her graduation from medical school, Saunders began a decade's work at Saint Joseph's, a 150-bed hospital that reserved forty to fifty beds for "patients with terminal malignant disease."[6] In this position, she became an active, articulate advocate for dying patients, arguing that their treatment required a distinctive approach to care that was at odds with the direction modern medicine was taking. Medicine's goal was to postpone death as long as possible; when this goal became impossible, doctors saw no reason to continue treatment.[7] "It appears to me," Saunders wrote in 1958, "that many patients feel deserted by their doctors at the end."[8] For one thing, Saunders wanted to guarantee that doctors remained responsible for their patients, even when hope for recovery was lost. For another, she wanted these doctors to provide medical care that suited dying patients' unique needs.

While she was still working at Saint Joseph's, Saunders began preparing her preeminent life project: the foundation of Saint Christopher's Hospice, a free-standing institution located in London that was fully dedicated to the care of the dying. Already a known hospice proponent, Saunders traveled to the United States in 1963, where she divided her time between soliciting donations for Saint Christopher's, lecturing at multiple universities, visiting eighteen medical institutions, and meeting with academic, religious, and medical figures who were interested in the hospice idea. Saunders's charismatic appearances drew hundreds of clinicians and academics to her lectures. Some of them continued to correspond with her, visited Saint Christopher's when it opened, and invited her for subsequent visits in 1965 and 1966.

These lectures outlined the principles of hospice care as Saunders practiced it. First, Saunders defined hospice as focusing on the patient as a *person*, and she criticized medicine's impersonal and technical character, best epitomized in the image of the "specialist without heart" who mechanically treats body parts, not people.[9] Second, Saunders challenged medicine's tendency "to go on pressing for acute, active treatment at a stage when a patient has gone too far and should not be made to return."[10] This, she argued, "is not good medicine. *There is a difference between prolonging living and what can really only be called prolonging dying.*"[11] Instead, Saunders advocated for accepting death as integral to life. Death should be thought of as "life's fulfillment," she said, an event that "helps us find the real meaning" that both the dying and the people mourning them need.[12] Quoting students who worked at Saint Joseph's, she suggested that "death really isn't anything to be frightened of, but a sort of homecoming."[13]

Finally, Saunders envisioned hospices as cohesive communities that would blur boundaries and dismantle hierarchies between professional and nonprofessional work and between clinicians and patients.[14] Although hospice did have a specialized technical component—the use of medications to alleviate patients' physical pain—and although professional physicians were the ones in charge of this component, Saunders insisted that the essence of hospice work lay elsewhere. She promoted hospice as an unorthodox and holistic form of care that addressed physical, emotional, and existential suffering at the same time. Her model was antiprofessional, and it deliberately challenged the compartmentalization of care that medical specialization created.[15] Hospice was interdisciplinary, relied on nursing, combined much general volunteer care work, and had a strong religious component (prayer and religious rituals were daily routines in Saunders's hospice).[16] The drug regimens Saunders used were also unorthodox. Many of her treatments were illegal (she regularly prescribed heroin and was interested in LSD treatments), and others were reminiscent of folk medicine—which Saunders used, quite simply, to make patients happier and more comfortable. Gin was integral to pain treatment at Saint Joseph's, and Saunders encouraged relatives to bring bottles of whiskey to her patients as gifts.[17] Saint Joseph's nurses, Saunders reported, were "young Irish girls who come over and do apprentice nursing with us before they go and get further training elsewhere. Since they have not yet been taught to hurry, as many a trained nurse will, they are well suited to work with dying patients." Saunders described one patient as showing

> her loving response to an *unsophisticated little nurse* who is just enjoying her as she is, demonstrating her pleasure in just meeting her. . . . Now this simplicity is a quality we too often lose, but I notice that the young seem to have it almost by nature, if they choose to come into this kind of work.[18]

Taken together, Saunders's hospice model pushed care for the dying several steps away from mainstream medicine. It doubted the usefulness of specialized clinical care for dying patients, mingled intuition and amateurism in its day-to-day practice, and aspired to replace the clinical settings of the hospital with a mixture of professional and nonprofessional elements. The Victorian tone Saunders adopted when speaking of Saint

Joseph's staff was indicative: young, Irish, "unsophisticated," "little" women, who represented minimal professionalism and maximal ability to care.[19] This was an early, important pillar in the medical economization of death: Saunders questioned the merit of medical interventions for dying patients, and she argued that in certain situations treating less was treating better.

As provocative as they were, these ideas were not completely new to U.S. medicine. In 1940, for example, Harvard physician Alfred Worcester published a poignant essay on the treatment and mistreatment of aging and dying patients.[20] Outlining a comprehensive vision of how to care for the elderly, he called on physicians to accept "ageing as a perfectly natural process" and to refrain from treating the physical decline in old age as a pathology. Care for the elderly, Worcester argued, necessitates "a regressive régime" that gradually moderates medical interventions as the natural decline of patients' bodily functions occurs. He specifically recommended that physicians who found tumors in aged patients should not treat them, given "how common in the aged cancerous tumors are, and also how much less malignant they are than in earlier years."[21] More controversial from a contemporary perspective, Worcester went so far as to define the loss of teeth in old age as a "natural safeguard . . . against overeating," and he argued that dentists and cooks violated this safeguard—"artificial teeth and culinary triumphs are the disguised enemies of a healthy old age."[22] Providing life-prolonging treatment to patients who are naturally dying is a disturbance, Worcester argued, and "all such disturbance of the dying patient is inexcusable."[23]

Not unlike Worcester, many U.S. medical specialists reflected critically on how to properly limit life-prolonging treatments as soon as these treatments became available. In the 1950s, after the invention of chemotherapy, oncology journals printed elaborate discussions on how much chemotherapy was too much. Early chemotherapies were not very effective, and oncologists explicitly referred to their work as "palliative care." In the absence of curative powers, their goal was to control the disease's symptoms, alleviate pain, and at the same time try to prolong life.[24] Saunders actively corresponded with U.S. cancer specialists, and in 1960 she published an article in a six-volume set on cancer treatment.[25] Throughout the 1960s, both physicians and nonphysicians held conferences tackling the question of medicine's limits. "The most difficult problem of medical ethics we are likely to encounter within the next decade," proclaimed René Dubos, is "to what extent can we afford to prolong biological life in individuals who cannot derive either profit or pleasure from existence, and whose survival creates painful burdens for the community?"[26] The resonance of hospice ideas with the intuitions of many non-hospice clinicians continued in the years that followed. In January 1972, North Carolina physician William Poe published in the *New England Journal of Medicine* a sarcastic call to start a new medical specialty—Marantology:

> It should help people endure losing. It should not use silly euphemisms such as rehabilitation and convalescence for its losing patients. It should not send its dear old people to intensive-care units to be treated as winners. It should not embarrass or tempt surgeons to do dramatic things such as operating on dissecting aneurisms. . . . Marantologists are not winners; they have become good losers. . . . There should be an American Journal of Marantology with contributions such as "The Uselessness of Speech Therapy in Mute Octogenarians." . . . What satisfaction could a Marantologist get in his work? . . . He could . . . debunk any number of doctrines propounded by haughty professors who never saw the true end results of their work. He could face honestly the fact of dying and death that our profession as a whole has not yet faced. . . . If I were a dictator, I would dictate that the entire profession have grand rounds in a Marantology ward each fortnight to get a maintenance dose of humility.[27]

These words were printed in one of the most prestigious medical journals in the country. That summer Poe would testify in the first congressional hearing on "Death with Dignity."

In the news magazine of the American Academy of Pediatrics, Dr. Wolf Zuelzer wrote on intensive care unit (ICU) technologies, "When do we turn the machines off? When should we have turned them on in the first place? The beep of the oscillograph is becoming the voice of the new barbarianism."[28] "I have the distinct impression that we are slowly, but perhaps rightly, moving toward choosing death in some instances as a way of avoiding the oppression of misapplied medical technology and of easing the burdens of the sick and their families," declared Yale pediatrician Raymond Duff.[29] Not all these people embraced hospice as a satisfying answer to their questions, yet hospice ideas spoke to issues that concerned them.

Hospice ideas also resonated with general and nonprofessional social and political dynamics in the United States. From the 1950s and to a growing degree during the 1960s and 1970s, public interest in death, dying, and the cultural, political, and moral questions related to them exploded. Historian Peter Filene described this as a "public obsession, [which] had almost a prurient quality to it, as if death had joined the erotic revolution of the sixties."[30] The period's political climate—the iconoclastic, anti-institutional, and antiauthoritative spirit of the civil rights movement—colored this interest in death. Over the course of one decade, public trust in institutions such as the presidency, Congress, the army, universities, and the church plummeted. Modern medicine—an emblem of empathetic and personal care now turned standard, technical, and bureaucratic—was an obvious target. Trust in physicians declined from 72 to 56 percent between 1965 and 1973.[31] Patients' demands to pass away on their own terms, free of professional, institutional, or political coercion, appeared regularly in media outlets, books, and articles. These voices, which came to be known as the Right to Die movement, gained steam during the 1970s as the high profile case of Karen Ann Quinlan unfolded.[32] Many U.S. hospice protagonists were very careful to distinguish themselves from the Right to Die movement, but hospice spoke to the sentiments that fueled its advocacy.[33] The emphasis of hospice on humanizing care, deinstitutionalizing the dying, and personalizing treatment by deprofessionalizing it corresponded to the main criticisms directed at medicine during the period.

In sum, we can attribute the ascent of U.S. hospices to two main factors. First, the U.S. medical profession's preoccupation with both internal and external criticism of medical progress made many clinicians open to alternatives such as hospice. Second, the zeitgeist of ambivalence toward authority and institutions that developed during the period created fertile ground for reformist ideas. In the ensuing years, a "large contingency" of liberal and highly educated professionals and academics began advocating for hospice care, presenting it as a necessary reform.[34]

The Evolution of the Hospice Professional Field

The favorable environment notwithstanding, within U.S. medicine hospice advocates had to fight to make established professionals accept their approach as viable and legitimate.[35] In part, hospices were looked down upon because they were feminized: the public figures promoting them were mostly women, and within the dominant medical patriarchy their emphasis on nursing and amateur volunteer work was dismissed and undervalued.[36] The content of the hospice approach was an additional reason for its marginality: by rejecting many of modern medicine's most basic intuitions, hospice advocates positioned themselves on medicine's margins. The professional institutionalization of hospice care occurred from these margins, where hospice advocates established a professional center whose core uniting principles contradicted conventional medicine.

The first U.S. hospice project began as a pilot program—an "experiment"—at Yale University during the late 1960s. Its most prominent leader, Florence Wald, was appointed Yale's dean of nursing in 1958. An avid supporter of nursing's professional integrity, Wald wanted to establish a distinctive intellectual, research, and clinical nursing approach, which would be independent of medicine and other related disciplines.[37] Saunders's vision of hospice as a comprehensive philosophy of care that placed nursing at its center was very appealing to Wald. She and Saunders met during the latter's 1963 visit to Yale, and they continued to correspond after Saunders returned to London. They met again when Wald reinvited Saunders to Yale as a visiting professor in 1965. In 1967 Wald resigned from her position as dean and traveled to Saint Christopher's Hospice for a sabbatical. When she returned to Yale, she gathered a small group of clinicians and began to work on her own hospice pilot study, which took place in the Yale New Haven Hospital from 1969 to 1971.

Members of Wald's group mostly came from medicine's professional periphery. They belonged to undervalued health professions (nursing and chaplaincy), relatively peripheral medical disciplines (psychiatry and pediatrics), and a social science that health professionals and policymakers all but ignored (anthropology).[38] Most illustrative of the group's character was its members' difficult relationship with the two more "mainstream" physicians who participated in the project, oncologist Ira Goldenberg and internist Robert Scheig.[39] From the pilot project's very beginning, Goldenberg and Scheig criticized Wald's approach for lacking scientific rigor and for focusing too much on bedside care. "I think you have to stop thinking entirely of how it's best to treat the patient and also start thinking about the fact that you're doing a study," Goldenberg told Wald in one particularly heated moment.[40] The group's other members felt Goldenberg and Scheig were reluctant to commit more time to the project because they were avoiding the topic of death and could not accept the centrality of nursing to the hospice model. Within the hospice milieu, these were accusations of blasphemy. "We're really not working through the decisions in a collaborative way," Wald lamented about a year into the project. "I'm thinking that [Goldenberg] thinks . . . that he's the doctor and I'm the nurse."[41]

The Yale pilot study was also regarded with ambivalence within the hospital and the university. One physician criticized Wald's involvement in his patient's care, saying that it was "polarizing" and stifled the creation of a united professional front when the staff met with the patient's family. In 1971, when the pilot was concluded and Wald and her group sought ways to start a permanent hospice service, the hospital administration hesitated. The group decided to pursue a more independent hospice model, similar to Saint Christopher's. As they were looking for funding sources, Wald and Edward Dobihal—a chaplain who had been central to the project from its beginning—found that state agencies were as ambivalent as the professionals. They met with a representative from the Department of Health, Education and Welfare in Washington, D.C., and applied to multiple federal programs for care of the poor, disabled, and the elderly—all showed little support for hospice care. Most contemptuous in his rejection was Arthur Jarvis of the Connecticut State Department of Health, who said the group's application was "fuzzy" and expressed concern over their way of "segregating" terminally ill patients. He recommended that Wald and her colleagues "go to a mountain top somewhere; I might give you a lot of nuns just so I don't have to be involved and see what you're doing."[42]

This blend of rejection from the medical establishment on the one hand, and resonance with the intuitions, feelings, and interests of numerous clinicians and nonclinicians of the period on the other, was a key characteristic of U.S. hospices' development in their first two decades (1970s–1980s). Hospice advocates were torn between quixotic iconoclasm, which took the rejection of institutionalized medicine as its defining feature, and a more pragmatic drive to formalize and professionalize hospice in order to establish it as a medical specialty, spread its message, and expand it. Gradually, they distanced themselves from the former and inched toward the latter.

In 1971, Wald and her group founded the independent Hospice, Inc., which quickly became a national professional hub. The leaders of Hospice, Inc., had a tight relationship with Saunders, who advised them in the months leading up to its opening. Even in a new field, whose promoters rejected authority and formal codes of professional reputation, proximity to a founding mother meant prestige. The year Hospice, Inc., opened Wald and her colleagues organized the first "annual hospice day" in New Haven, Connecticut—a national conference that attracted 150 to 200 attendees.[43] They spoke at events as practitioners representing not only themselves or their institution but the hospice approach in general.[44] Several other groups of clinicians also began organizing hospice programs, but none could match the organizational power of Hospice, Inc.: by 1973 it had more than 200 members, friends, and advisors, including representatives from business, city planning, insurers, and a community health care center. The Rockefeller Foundation, Wald wrote to Saunders, was "strongly interested in picking up the big tab."[45]

In 1975 Hospice, Inc., created the National Advisory Council, whose declared purpose was to promote hospice "by replication of New Haven's Hospice."[46] Hospice, Inc., made itself a prototype, and by the end of the decade New Haven was a Mecca for hospice care: a 1978 congressional report found fifty-nine health care organizations "providing at least one hospice-type service" and seventy-three organizations "were in various stages of planning."[47] That same year, Hospice, Inc., was guiding some 100 local hospice groups from all over the country.[48] Somewhat paradoxically, the antiprofessional ideas of care that challenged institutional hierarchies were now spreading from a professional center.

Through the 1960s, as hospices were acquiring their professional shape, dying people—and hospital patients in particular—were being studied by the hundreds. The U.S. Public Health Service's Division of Nursing funded three major projects on death and dying: the Yale pilot program, sociologists Barney Glaser and Anselm Strauss's studies on hospital deaths, and another study by Ray Duff and August Hollingshead on patients' and families' experiences in hospitals.[49] Across the Atlantic, Cicely Saunders documented the treatment and dying trajectories of 1,100 patients in Saint Joseph's Hospice and built a database of clinical notes and interviews with these patients.[50] The U.S. psychiatrist Elisabeth Kübler-Ross interviewed dozens of dying patients and mapped the psychological phases that they passed through.[51]

There was a growing body of data, analysis, and theoretical concepts related to "death and dying," which inspired a flourishing medical and intellectual discourse on the topic. Universities offered courses, seminars, and workshops in thanatology, and multiple popular and scholarly books explored the cultural, historical, sociological, psychological, and spiritual aspects of death. Academic and professional publications in the area thrived. The *International Journal for the Study of Death and Dying* (OMEGA) published its first issue in 1970. The *Hospice Journal* and the *American Journal of Hospice Care* began publishing in 1984, followed by the *Journal of Pain and Symptom Management* (1986) and later the *Journal of Palliative Medicine* (1998), *Journal of Hospice and Palliative Nursing* (1999), and *Palliative and Supportive Care* (2003). "Death and dying" was topicalized.[52] It became a target of research and clinical practice as well as an existential category. Terminally ill people, living in great proximity to death, were managed as subjects with unique physiological, psychological, and spiritual characteristics and needs (see Figure 1.2).[53]

The further hospices crystalized professionally, the more distinctive they became from other forms of medical care. Early hospice ideas did not reflect such a contrast. In her practice, lectures, and writing, Cicely Saunders often spoke about reforms necessary to patient care in general: being attentive to both physical and nonphysical needs, facilitating better communication between physicians, nurses, and patients, and not abandoning patients when a cure became unachievable. Hospice was meant to affect all medical specialties in all institutions, not to isolate and restrict itself to a bounded professional jurisdiction.[54] But hospice advocacy achieved the opposite outcome. Needing to prove to funders and policy-makers that they had a unique contribution that other medical disciplines were not providing, the advocates found themselves delineating special-ized characteristics of their approach.[55] In grant proposals, the New Haven group defined hospice as "offering specialized, coordinated terminal care, which focused on quality of life for patients who were unable to be cured or rehabilitated."[56] The decision of Hospice, Inc., to part ways with Yale's medical center added an organizational differentiation. Hospice care be-came the opposite of "curative care," which hospitals provided. Physi-cians either treated patients to cure or focused on alleviating their pain and refrained from invasive, life-prolonging treatment.

This binary manifested in the criticisms of conventional physicians. During the first congressional hearing on "Death with Dignity," which featured a host of hospice advocates, Dr. Laurence Foye from the Veterans Administration in Bethesda, Maryland, argued categorically against lim-iting life-prolonging care:

> Every physician can . . . describe a number of patients for whom he predicted a rapidly fatal outcome—saying, "I knew they were going to die"—and was wrong. The patient who was told by his doctor that he had 6 months to live but is alive years later is legendary. . . . If a physician withholds maximum effort from patients he considers hopelessly ill, he will unavoidably withhold maximum effort from an occasional patient who could have been saved. Patients will die because of the physician's decision not to treat actively. This approach and concern cannot be fostered or condoned, legally or otherwise.[57]

Advances in medical research made such positions highly intuitive in fields that were on the cutting edge of medical research. Contrary to their predecessors, oncologists in the 1970s saw curing cancer as merely a matter of time, so they contended that life should be prolonged and death postponed to the longest extent possible.[58] "A recently developed group of specialists in death and dying are teaching physicians how to accept the mortality of man," warned the editorial of a leading clinical cancer journal. "While this new philosophy certainly has merit, . . . it must never become an excuse for lack of aggression in saving lives and lack of knowledge about what can be done to preserve a life."[59] An oncologist echoed, "In the last several years we have seen the development of a 'death and dying' cult that is antitherapy and antitherapist. These 'patient advocates' often fail to recognize that oncologists who are technically skilled also have a genuine humanitarian concern with their patients."[60] These rancorous reflections, directed from one of the most prestigious medical specialties to medicine's margins, show that these margins had developed a coherent and sufficiently significant set of ideas to become a center in their own right, worthy of criticizing.

These margins also knew how to organize themselves and act politically. In 1978, after the founding of the National Hospice Association, hospice proponents began federal and state level advocacy. Over the next four years, they lobbied for creating a special hospice benefit (see Chapter 2) and battled the other advocacy organizations—specifically the National Hospital Organization and to some extent the National Association for Home Health Agencies—that claimed they were providing similar services.[61] When Congress authorized a Medicare benefit in 1982, it formalized a separation between hospice and other forms of care. The benefit defined hospice as care "provided to a terminally ill individual" by an interdisciplinary program and specified what services needed to be included in it.[62] Because the legislation approved payment for two periods of ninety days, it established that hospice patients would be people with a prognosis of six months or less.[63] The distinctiveness of hospice and of dying patients was now inscribed in regulation, and Medicare paid hospice organizations to treat hospice patients with hospice methods.

The emergence of social fields, as sociologist Pierre Bourdieu observed, is a hierarchical process: fields are spaces that have a core and periphery, which hierarchize people along their differential endowment with pertinent cultural, symbolic, social, and economic capital.[64] By the beginning of the 1990s, the professional field of hospice care was established: it had widely recognized clinical principles, professional associations that promoted those principles and clinicians who practiced them, examinations that certified the clinicians, free-standing organizations that hired the clinicians, a public insurer that paid the organizations, and patients whose condition required hospice care. There were people who achieved centrality in the field—clinicians and researchers who published in hospice journals and advocates who assumed leadership positions in the professional association. One could pursue a hospice career and be rewarded with recognition from a thriving professional and clinical community.

Expansion: Projecting Death in America

Hospice was the center of the first phase in the history of economized dying in the United States: a grassroots movement that became more professional, formal, and institutional. The second phase in this history involved a far more coordinated, top-down mobilization that expanded the economizing gaze into hospitals and blurred the distinction between dying and non-dying patients. What drove this mobilization were monetary contributions from some of the largest philanthropic organizations in the country.

Over eleven years (1994–2005), the Robert Wood Johnson Foundation (henceforth RWJF), the Open Society Institute (OSI), and several other funders invested more than $220 million in transforming how U.S. clinicians, hospitals, policymakers, and society at large thought about, approached, and managed death.[65] These initiatives' comprehensiveness was impressive. They supported clinicians advocating to change care for the dying in their institutions, scholars who would study the topic, and professors who would teach about it. The initiatives funded professional associations for hospice and palliative care, organizations that "educated" communities about death and dying, policy organizations that authored reports and promoted policy change, artists and authors whose work engaged death, and organizations that sustained the field after it had exhausted its seed money. This mobilization created a new medical subspecialty called *palliative care*, which economized dying in hospitals and made clinicians, administrators, and policymakers more favorable toward end-of-life care.

Greater Commitment and More Forceful Measures

During the early 1980s, as a retrospective RWJF account tells us, many of the foundation's leaders began reflecting on "personal experiences" they had had with care of the dying.[66] These experiences made them concerned that "elderly, fatally ill persons were likely to be vigorously treated in intensive care units, at great financial cost and suffering, even if their families objected."[67] The leaders convened a meeting on the topic in 1985, and then invited William Knaus and Joanne Lynn, who over the next three years consolidated a design for the "Study to Understand Prognoses and Preferences for Outcomes and Risks of Treatment," also known as the SUPPORT study. SUPPORT quickly became the field's most ambitious flagship project: with a $29 million budget, its research team comprised dozens of clinicians, who studied 9,105 severely ill patients in five hospitals.[68]

In their first two years of research (starting in 1989), the SUPPORT team worked on proving the need to change end-of-life care in hospitals. Examining over 4,000 cases of seriously ill hospital patients, they found that only 47 percent of the physicians whose patients would refuse cardiopulmonary resuscitation (CPR) were aware of this preference, and that about half of those patients did not have formal Do Not Resuscitate (DNR) orders. Nearly half of the DNR orders that did exist were filed two days or less before the patients died; among the patients who died in the hospital, 38 percent had spent 10 days or more in the ICU, and 46 percent received mechanical ventilation in the last three days of their life. No less indicative was that half of all conscious patients who died in hospital "experienced moderate or severe pain at least half the time during their last 3 days."[69] In the SUPPORT principal investigators' eyes, these data added up to a grim picture: conventional U.S. medicine was oblivious to death. It treated patients aggressively and invasively until the very last moments of life, fighting to extend life even after all realistic hope for recovery or improvement was lost. This failure to recognize dying patients' needs and acknowledge their preferences happened even when the patients or their family members had stated them clearly. Now that it had been rigorously demonstrated and was more pertinent than ever, medicine's ineptitude in treating dying patients invited new specialized interventions to economize dying.

SUPPORT's second phase intended to demonstrate the efficacy of two interventions. The first intervention aimed to increase doctors' awareness of their patients' prognosis. The second aimed to improve doctors' communication with their patients. The researchers split 4,804 additional participants into an intervention and a control group. The physicians in the intervention group received data about their patients' six-month survival rate, the expected outcomes from CPR, and their patients' predicted level of disability. In addition, the intervention group included trained nurses who talked to patients and their families about their prognosis, inquired about pain, clarified the likely outcomes of attempted resuscitation, brought up the possibility of writing an advance directive, and reported the conversation back to the physicians.[70]

RWJF had so much faith in these interventions that it prepared a major media campaign to advertise their success before the results had been clarified. But the study did not obtain the expected results. The physicians in the intervention group did *not* file DNR forms earlier than in the control group. The resource usage and number of ICU days were similar in both groups. The patients in the intervention group were slightly *more* likely to report pain. As SUPPORT's principal investigators summarized, "the intervention had no impact on any of [the] designated targets."[71] But perhaps the most perplexing finding was that the patients and families in both groups expressed satisfaction with the treatment they received.[72]

The first article the SUPPORT researchers published began with the declaration that the wish to economize dying originated from the patients themselves. "Many Americans today fear they will lose control over their lives if they become critically ill, and their dying will be prolonged and impersonal. This has led to an increasingly visible right-to-die movement."[73] Much of the data they collected, however, indicated otherwise. Only 30.6 percent of the patients asked to relinquish CPR in the event of a cardiac arrest.[74] Some of the patients still wanted other forms of life-prolonging therapy, such as intensive care.[75] By the first SUPPORT article's conclusion, the researchers' tone changed:

> One could conclude that physicians, patients, and families are fairly comfortable with the current situation. Certainly, most patients and families indicated they were satisfied, no matter what happened to them. . . . Perhaps physicians and patients in this study acknowledged problems with the care of seriously ill patients as a group. However, when involved with their own situation or engaged in the

care of their individual patients, they felt they were doing the best they could, were satisfied they were doing well, and did not wish to directly confront problems or face choices.[76]

In the eyes of the researchers, the patients were a part of the problem as well as its victims. The conclusion was unequivocal: "to improve the experience of seriously ill and dying patients, greater individual and societal commitment and more proactive and forceful measures may be needed."[77] With its media campaign ready to launch and study results that completely contradicted it, RWJF had to change plans.[78] It reoriented the campaign to emphasize "how entrenched problems are in care at the end of life" and stress "the urgency to address this issue."[79] The campaign presented SUPPORT's failure as reflecting negatively not on the attempt to economize dying but on the physicians who refused to embrace it and the patients who did not recognize the benefits it offered them.

The media campaign carried this framing to network television studios and newspaper headlines, and SUPPORT very much marked the direction the entire field took in the next decade. Its unprecedentedly rich and detailed data set yielded over sixty-two research articles by the decade's end, followed by many others in the next years.[80] No less importantly, it was a compass for the extensive projects that followed it, starting in the mid-1990s.

Most prominent among these was the Project on Death in America (PDIA), which the Open Society Institute (OSI) announced several months before SUPPORT's results went public. PDIA's official history used a very familiar narrative to describe what motivated it: the personal experiences of OSI's founding president, George Soros, whose mother passed away two years earlier. Soros found his mother's dying process far more satisfying than what he had experienced with his father decades earlier. He felt that he and his family were more "present" and supportive of his mother and wanted to facilitate similar experiences by promoting institutional change. In the early 1990s, some twenty years after the opening of Hospice, Inc., finding professional figures interested in the care of the dying was fairly easy, and OSI officials quickly gathered a professional board to lead the project. Soros's words at PDIA's unveiling event in New York echoed arguments that hospice advocates since Saunders had made: "We have created a medical culture so intent on curing disease and prolonging life that it fails to provide support during one of life's most empathic phases—death. Advances in high technology interventions have deluded doctors and patients alike into believing that the inevitable can be delayed almost indefinitely."[81] Dying shall be economized.

Against the backdrop of SUPPORT's findings, PDIA's board decided "that it was essential to change the culture of medicine in hospital and nursing homes, where 80 percent of Americans die."[82] Expanding specialized care of the dying beyond the institutional confines of hospice and into the bastions of curative medicine meant redrawing professional jurisdictions: "palliative care" became the name of end-of-life medicine practiced in hospitals. Its professional authority crossed a delicate line: hospices treated patients who were unquestionably dying, but palliative care engaged in decisions on *whether* patients were dying, how far away they were from death, whether a clear line between serious and terminal illness could be drawn, and what type of care would be appropriate given their prognosis. Discussion of death moved toward the gray areas where death's imminence and the likelihood of cure or improvement were less certain.

Building a Professional Field

PDIA's most central initiative was the Faculty Scholars Program, which began in 1995 with the goal to identify professional leaders "who could change medical culture from the inside."[83] The program admitted eighty-seven fellows in eight cohorts over nine years of existence. Its highly selective character reflected its organizers' deliberate strategy to create a professional elite and build the field from the top. Funders were explicit about this strategy:

> For a medical field to gain legitimacy it should be built into prestigious organizations . . . as well as backed by highly respected professionals with top-ranked academic backgrounds. . . . Standards

and certification are important as well. . . . Physicians listen best to other physicians, particularly those within the same specialty. . . . [The] call for action was heard because the experts involved were powerful enough to affect [*sic*] change. . . . In line with this analysis, staff from RWJF and PDIA developed what they called an "elite strategy."[84]

PDIA created a hub of professional leaders, paid their salaries for two years, and supported their research. No less importantly, it promoted "the visibility and prestige of [the fellows] in end-of-life care and enhanced their effectiveness as academic leaders, role models, and mentors."[85] In effect, the Faculty Program crowned its fellows as leaders by providing them the prerogative and resources to delineate the specialty's boundaries and principles.

The program acted on several fronts. First, it fostered scholarly discourse on "end of life." Its fellows authored over 2,000 articles by 2003 and raised more than $113 million for research in the area.[86] The term "end of life" became visible in leading medical journals during these years (Figure 1.1), and it gradually replaced "death and dying" as the field's main object of management (Figure 1.2). This replacement reflected a shift in the field's center of gravity, from hospice to palliative care. Hospices treated death and dying—a clearly demarcated group of terminal patients. Palliative care, by contrast, referred to the end of life—a broader and more open-ended group. Because, as the cliché goes, "today is the first day of the rest of your life," virtually everyone could be considered a target for palliative care.

Second, the faculty program trained fellows to become agents of change in their hospitals once they graduated, and its ultimate goal was to establish "at least three permanent faculty members who promote end-of-life care in all 144 U.S. medical schools."[87] "Medical students learn by watching interns, residents, and faculty who are further along in their career," reflected PDIA board member Peter Selwyn; "the culture will change when these role models embrace palliative care."[88] Empowering a cadre of role models and replanting them in their hospitals was an effort to impact not only research but also clinical practice.

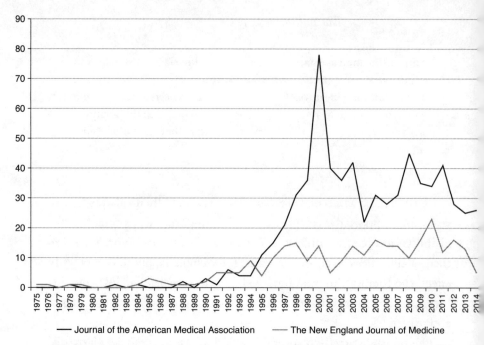

Figure 1.1. Number of articles mentioning "end of life" in top U.S. medical journals.

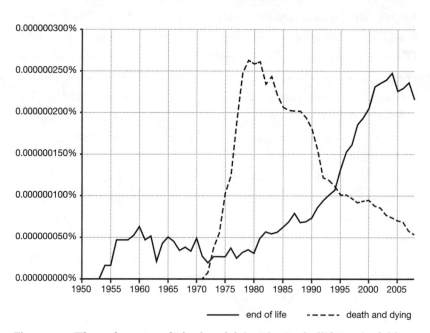

Figure 1.2. The replacement of "death and dying" by "end of life" as the field's main concern (1950–2008). Source: Google Books Ngram Viewer. Corpus: American English, smoothing 3 (http://books.google.com/ngrams).*

* For an explanation of the values on the Y-axis, see https://books.google.com/ngrams/info

Finally, program fellows advanced more general educational projects. A number of studies they authored reviewed medical textbooks in a variety of specialties and pointed to "major deficiencies" in their discussion of "care of the dying."[89] In 1999, PDIA and RWJF cosponsored a conference that gathered doctors, nurses, textbook writers, editors, publishers, and advocates to discuss strategies to change the situation. Several years later, PDIA announced the deficiencies "have largely been identified and addressed, and clear guidelines for end-of-life care context have been instituted."[90]

PDIA helped disseminate its fellows' work. Before the program began, two of its board members—Kathleen Foley and Robert Burt—had already lobbied the Institute of Medicine to write *Approaching Death*, a comprehensive report on end-of-life care.[91] Burt later said that while the Institute of Medicine did not do much independent research, editing *Approaching Death* involved contacting the National Institutes of Health and other organizations and inquiring about the research they had done in the area. This had the impact of "shaming the National Institutes of Health about their funding for research," he said. "So they would come in one after another and they would tell us they're doing nothing."[92] PDIA distributed more than 4,000 copies of *Approaching Death* "to diverse constituencies" and cosponsored other synthesizing reports the Institute of Medicine published on the topic.[93]

The further end-of-life care professionalized, the more hierarchical, physician-oriented, and male-dominated it became: 60 percent of PDIA's faculty fellows were men, and the women were clustered in the less prestigious nursing profession.[94] Only nine of the faculty fellows were nurses, and all but one were women. (The faculty fellows program's chair later attributed the low number of nurse fellows to the physicians' dominance in the review committee.)[95] Many of PDIA's nursing and social work initiatives took place outside the Faculty Fellows Program. The palliative care field was interdisciplinary but not transdisciplinary—it fostered cooperation between different professions, but it did not blur professional boundaries the way the early hospice movement had aspired to do. Beyond everything, leaders of the faculty program evaluated nursing and social work initiatives along physician-centric standards, which were not sensitive to the peculiarities of these professional fields. There were far fewer publication opportunities for nurses and social workers, and given the relative dearth of resources in these fields, it was harder to mobilize people to join the community.

In 1999, PDIA funded the Nursing Leadership Consortium on End-of-Life Care, which convened forty-three participants representing twenty-three nursing specialty organizations, as well as other organizations, to develop a collaborative end-of-life "nursing agenda."[96] The consortium led to the establishment of the National Nursing Leadership Academy at Johns Hopkins University. In line with PDIA's general top-down approach, it envisioned the academy as a center for palliative care nursing "leaders" who would publish in nursing journals, present papers at professional conferences, and design curricula for nursing schools as well as for continued professional education.[97] The nine nurses who participated in the Faculty Scholars Program also contributed toward these goals. Two of them, Marianne Matzo and Deborah Witt Sherman, developed palliative care nursing curricula, and together with other nurses authored two textbooks on palliative care nursing.[98] This group also initiated the End of Life Nursing Education Consortium (ELNEC), a curriculum on end-of-life care that trained thousands of palliative and nonpalliative care nurses over the ensuing years.

PDIA's engagement with social work was even more separate from its flagship Faculty Scholars Program. The faculty program did not include a single social worker, but in 2000 PDIA launched the Social Work Leadership Development Awards, with the now-usual goal of developing "leaders in the field." The awards supported forty-two social workers (82 percent of them women) in 2000–2003, who organized conferences, symposia, training manuals, certification programs, and fellowships[99]—all meant to add content on palliative care, end-of-life care, and bereavement to social work education. Much of this work culminated in 2011 with the publication of the *Oxford Textbook of Palliative Social Work*, which two of the program's graduates edited; many of the book's eighty-four chapters were authored by other program graduates.[100]

These projects received far less funding than the physician-focused and male-dominated projects. PDIA leaders criticized the National Nursing Leadership Academy for what they thought were modest outcomes compared with the Faculty Scholars Program. (In the first three years, the academy published eighteen related articles in nursing journals, organized six national conferences on nursing and palliative care, and advanced two organizations that wrote curricula.) Historian David Clark, whom PDIA commissioned to write its history, mentioned that the nursing consortium "was an initiative where it was hard to trace major tangible outcomes and obvious 'products' were difficult to identify."[101] The social work projects suffered from similar difficulties. In 1999, for example, PDIA launched a "community and bereavement initiative," which funded multiple bereavement programs in schools, prisons, and a variety of community organizations. It was virtually impossible to present quantified outcomes from such projects, which made it very hard for the organizers to secure additional funding. Years later, Robert Burt, who was in charge of the initiative, said that "nothing lasting" came out of it.[102] Given PDIA's constitutive influence on the entire end-of-life care field, its emphasis on educating and empowering physicians—and its consequent marginalization of the professions (nursing and social work) and people (women) who were central to the field in its beginning—resulted in long-lasting hierarchies.

Part of PDIA's effort to sustain this professional center involved supporting palliative care associations and organizations. PDIA's series of "exit grants," which it awarded when the project ended in 2003, gave the highest support to the American Academy of Hospice and Palliative Medicine—the most central palliative care physician organization in the country. Smaller grants were given to the Hospice and Palliative Nurses Association, the National Hospice and Palliative Care Organization, and Harvard Medical School's Program in Palliative Care Education and Practice—all organizations that would promote the field on educational, scholarly, and institutional fronts. The PDIA grant to the American Board of Hospice and Palliative Medicine was particularly suggestive. It supported creating "standards for fellowship programs in palliative care and . . . begin[ing] the lengthy application to establish palliative medicine as a subspecialty."[103] In 2006, the American Board of Medical Specialties formally recognized "Hospice and Palliative Care" as a subspecialty; in the next years, physicians wishing to specialize in hospice and palliative care had to work for a year as fellows and pass a formal board examination.

The field's resourcefulness attracted many young professionals. One PDIA fellow told me that as a young physician he was interested in bio-ethics, but the existence of a developed and well-funded palliative care field changed his trajectory:

> Suddenly there was a lot of interest, not only on the part of Soros, but the Robert Wood Johnson Foundation and a couple of other major private funders, in end-of-life issues and death and dying. And then that spurred a certain amount of interest from public funders, too. So there was a big shift. A lot of people who had initially been inter-ested in medical ethics suddenly found themselves as end-of-life and palliative care specialists, because that's where the money was.

Like hospice before it, palliative care became a career. Physicians could train in it, publish in numerous journals, apply for research funding, and teach on the topic; starting in the late 1990s and to a greater degree the 2000s, they could work as palliative care specialists in hospi-tals. In 2000–2005, the number of palliative care programs in U.S. hos-pitals increased from 632 (15 percent of the hospitals in the country) to 1,240 (30 percent).[104] As I mentioned in the introduction, by 2015, 90 percent of the large hospitals in the country (over 300 beds) had a pal-liative care service.[105] This growth owed much to the organizations that had, in one way or another, originated from PDIA. Particularly notable was the Center to Advance Palliative Care (CAPC), a national organ-ization led by PDIA fellow Diane Meier, which promoted palliative care programs throughout the country. CAPC developed training curricula for palliative care teams and offered seminars to clinicians who were starting palliative care services, which instructed them on how to ad-vance the service within the hospital, present it to administrations, and establish relationships with other hospital clinicians. In its effort to pro-mote palliative care expertise, CAPC began grading U.S. states by their level of palliative care services. In 2015, two-thirds of the states received A and B grades, and the rest got Cs and Ds (none failed).[106] With two exceptions (Florida and New Mexico), the latter group included tradi-tionally red states, a possible testimony to the movement's progressive leanings.[107]

"We've gotten ourselves a real field of palliative care," said Susan Block in 2003 when PDIA concluded its operations.[108] The field was at the same time professional and organizational: palliative care had relatively clear and recognized principles, and clinicians could be counted as its opponents or proponents.[109] The field had a turf that defined it—the *end of life*—and was broader than *death and dying,* which hospices managed. The specialty at the field's center had particular health institutions where it was anchored—hospitals—and palliative care advocates continued work on expanding it to new institutions, such as nursing homes, long-term acute care facilities, and outpatient clinics. Health organizations, policymakers, individual clinicians, and even states could count as open or closed to end-of-life care, and palliative care advocates could praise, shame, and grade them.

Creating Demand: Transforming the Culture of Death

If the Faculty Scholars Program aimed to create a supply for palliative care—professionals who delivered it, and hospitals that employed them—other PDIA engagements sought to create a demand by organizing and mobilizing a public who would want to receive palliative care services. In 1995, when PDIA announced its grant program, it listed among its focus areas "arts and humanities" and "educational programs for the public about death and dying." Focus on these areas reflected PDIA's ambition to "transform the culture of death." They aimed to increase the topic's visibility in public discourse, cultivate public sentiments that would support economized dying, and inspire existential reflections on the use and misuse of medicine, on what counts as a good and bad death, and on patients' wishes and expectations from medical personnel. Consider these efforts as attempts to tackle the great dissonance the SUPPORT study had confronted—the fact that despite experiencing torturous dying trajectories, patients and their families were still happy with the care they received. These projects aimed to engage the wider U.S. public in end-of-life discourse. The goal was to stimulate what an RWJF report called "an impassioned consumer movement" that would pressure the medical profession, health care institutions, and policymakers to economize dying.[110]

As an example, the project of a Montana physician, Ira Byock, which RWJF and PDIA began funding in 1996, engaged an entire town—Missoula, Montana—in an effort to improve end-of-life care. Byock first created "a picture of dying, death, and bereavement in Missoula" by observing 250 families who were experiencing death over the course of one year. He gathered data on how a variety of health care institutions in the town cared for dying people. "Because this area had been so neglected in American life, most dying people and their families expect very little palliative care, and as a result make few demands for better treatment," wrote historian David Clark. One of Byock's main goals was therefore to *create* public expectations and encourage people to demand more palliative care.[111]

Another project was the Vermont Voices on Care of the Dying. Researchers from the Vermont Ethics Network interviewed 388 Vermont residents in forty-two focus groups, asking them about their experiences with "end-of-life care for someone they knew intimately." The report summarized their answers in nine concise statements, which ostensibly expressed public expectations of medical personnel who treat severely ill and dying patients. Among these statements, which were all written in first person plural: "When we are ourselves approaching the condition of being dying persons, we want to hear about it sooner and more clearly than people do now—but we want to be told in a way that is sensitive to our varying abilities to absorb bad news"; "We want to have adequate opportunity to understand the various care options that are available, and then to choose what fits us best"; "We want, while still relatively well, to have the help of doctors and nurses in preparing advance directives that will really work to bring us the kind of care we would want when we can no longer speak for ourselves"; and "Critically—we hope our caregivers never forget that we are all unique individuals; that no generality applies easily to any of us; and that we need a unique partnership with those who are helping us."[112]

Sociologist Stefan Timmermans observed that the hospice and palliative care movement has "catered to [the] cultural model of 'good' death," which involves pain and symptom management, conscious decision making, preparation for death, and the achievement of "closure."[113] Here we see that palliative care protagonists not only catered passively to the model but actively articulated it, spread it, and persuaded people of its virtue. These initiatives incited thousands of people to think about their expectations from end-of-life care, voice them, and demand that they be followed. They mobilized people to be part of an end-of-life discourse. Even healthy people, once they expressed preferences on how they would like to be treated when facing serious illness, became subjects of end-of-life care. Some fifteen years after PDIA launched, while sitting in on a lecture for advocates who promote the use of advance directive forms, I heard this idea presented to hospital clinicians:

> By the way, the last time I checked—let me know if I'm wrong—a hundred percent of us will die [laughter]. Everybody. So there's no way out, and you can remind your patients that accidents happen. How many people say, "Oh, I might be hit by a bus"? You might *be* hit by a bus. Especially when you're in our town, and you ride your bike—that's really true. And there are a lot of young bicyclists who have been hit by buses, or other things, and I care for many of them. None of them had an Advance Directive, and I've seen the pain that their families went through. It's so important: it would have helped them so much if they had known what their loved one would have wanted before they were comatose.

PDIA supported organizations similar to this, such as the Medicare Rights Center, which worked to "educate" consumers, families, caregivers, professional counselors, and clinicians "about Medicare hospice and home health benefits for the terminally ill."[114] They not only encouraged people to think and document their end-of-life preferences but also gave them practical information on how to pursue these preferences.

PDIA allocated another budget to support artwork on death. In 1998, historian, ethicist, and PDIA board member David Rothman began chairing PDIA's Arts and Humanities Initiative, which in the next years supported projects of "video, photography, poetry essays, dance, and artwork to express individual and community experiences of illness, death, and grief and to encourage conversation and thoughtful reflection."[115] Among the fifteen projects it funded were the art exhibit, book, and documentary *Aging in America: The Years Ahead*, and fabric panels by artist

Deidre Scherer.[116] The documentary *Auburn* followed the lives of elderly people aged 80 to 100 in Auburn, Nebraska. Alan Shapiro's spectacular poetry book, *The Dead Alive and Busy* (2000), dwelled on family relations around aging, physical decay, serious illness, and death. And Lisa Schnell's 2004 work "Learning How to Tell" recounted her grieving after her daughter's death.[117] Similarly to other non-medical initiatives, the investments in culture and the arts encountered much criticism within the PDIA board. "We probably wouldn't have funded some of those people . . . as far as our mission to move the field forward and be more visible is concerned, we would have been more discriminating and tougher," said Patricia Prem, social worker and close friend of George Soros, who played a pivotal role as a PDIA board member.[118]

Less doubted were the investments in media campaigns and popular media productions. In 1997, RWJF created the "Last Acts" campaign, which ran through national and local media outlets, as well as through a coalition of professional and community organizations. Last Acts worked with journalists, authors, reporters, documentarians, television and radio producers, and newsletter and industry publication editors "to encourage their participation in addressing the culture and experience of dying in America."[119] One of the campaign's most famous outcomes was Bill Moyers's PBS documentary series *On Our Own Terms: Moyers on Dying*, which aired in 2000 and had an estimated audience of 19 million people.[120] When Moyers applied for PDIA support, the review committee noticed that "about 90 percent of the people he was going to interview . . . were PDIA grantees"—a figure that indicated the program's immense influence on the field. PDIA feared that funding Moyers "would look too self-serving," so he ultimately relied on support from RWJF. The series had a $2.6 million production budget, in addition to $2.5 million that was allocated to "outreach." Seventy national organizations and numerous local television stations facilitated and coordinated public discussion on the series, which also drew a great deal of coverage in national newspapers and magazines. The Barnes and Noble bookstore chain featured the program on its website and offered its customers a selection of books on end-of-life care in 900 stores. Local "coalitions" on end-of-life care held over 300 town hall meetings and public discussion forums about the series, making it the most influential popular cultural product on death and dying since

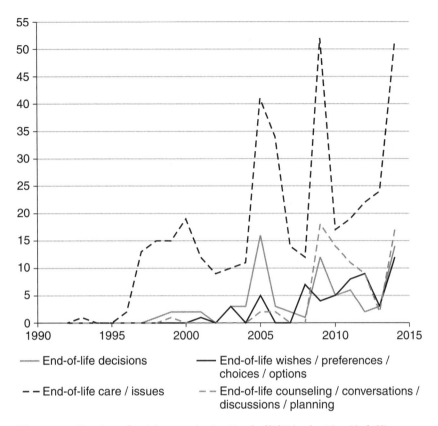

Figure 1.3. Number of articles mentioning "end of life" in the *New York Times* (1990–2014).

Elisabeth Kübler-Ross's bestseller *On Death and Dying*.[121] This orchestrated, generously funded buzz would stimulate the media's interest in "end of life." Starting in the mid-1990s, media discussions of "end of life," which previously had been nonexistent, became very common (Figure 1.3).

To be clear, I am not arguing that public and professional concerns over how people die in the United States derived solely from the monetary investments of OSI, RWJF, and other philanthropic organizations. As shown, critical discourse on death and dying predated these investments and, one could argue, inspired them. (For example, George Soros could not have reflected critically on how his father died without having experienced the opposite dying trajectory of his mother, who had joined the Hemlock Society and died at home, surrounded by family.)[122] I do argue, however, that these investments acted on sentiments that already existed in the United States, particularly among middle-class and highly educated populations, enhanced them, and brought them to larger social groups. Furthermore, the investments have transformed these general sentiments into a hierarchical and institutionalized professional field, which advocated for economizing dying.

Analyzed in context, this movement's raison d'être lay in counteracting the greater historical trajectory that U.S. health care has taken toward a more technologically advanced medicine. The ethos of medical progress, infused with the ever growing power of what Arnold Relman famously called "the medical-industrial complex," set U.S. medicine on a seemingly infinite course of expansion to advance one medical frontier after the other.[123] By the 1990s, big pharmaceutical companies, medical device producers, and biotech industries had grown into an enormous economy that had immense influence on health care delivery. With these industries' sponsorship, the number of clinical trials of various treatments and technologies skyrocketed. In the 1990s, over $50 billion was spent annually on medical research, yielding over 250,000 controlled clinical trials and an estimated 2 million medical articles.[124] (OSI and RWJF's contributions seem modest compared to these amounts, although palliative care is inherently cheaper.) Once this vast research enterprise established the usefulness of various drugs and devices, physicians and patients somewhat automatically embraced them as the new norms of treatment. This is what anthropologist Sharon Kaufman called "ordinary medicine": taken-for-granted sets of life-prolonging and death-postponing medical practices that both physicians and patients use unquestioningly. The "chain of connections among science, politics, industry, and insurance," Kaufman argued, is the foundation of this ordinary medicine, which "offers no inherent facility, no clue or advice for physicians with which to evaluate when *more* is no better and for putting on the brakes."[125]

I argue that "clues" and "advice," which negate this trajectory, have developed elsewhere, in a very organized fashion. The professionalization of hospice and palliative care, its spread into health care institutions, and its influence over policymaking are certainly not complete. But they have conquered sufficient ground to provide a pertinent alternative for a growing number of clinicians. For many clinicians palliative care has itself become ordinary medicine—a taken-for-granted knowledge that they practice unquestioningly. "The good news," said PDIA Associate Director Mary Callaway, "is that nobody is against us—nobody thinks it's a bad idea to improve care for the dying."[126] It has become almost universally clear that treating the dying less aggressively and invasively means improving care.

Embodied Economization

Perhaps the most powerful feature of economization was that, beyond relying on institutions, laws, and formal certifications, it succeeded in pervading many clinicians' intuitive and practical judgment. These clinicians were not only intellectually persuaded that economizing dying was the best form of care they could give. They also internalized the economizing gaze as an embodied quality. It set them to look at patients in certain ways and to see certain properties in them. In Bourdieu's terms, the economizing gaze was a "practical belief": not an "adherence to a set of instituted dogmas and doctrines" (which would count as a "belief") but "a state of the body . . . a durable way of standing, speaking, walking, and thereby feeling and thinking."[127]

I examine this embodiment in two ways. First, I look at how the professional experiences of palliative care clinicians in the hospital predisposed them to look at patients in an economizing way, and I show the differences between the palliative care clinicians' gaze and the more standard medical gaze of other clinicians. Second, I examine how palliative care clinicians educated young physicians and spread their way of looking at patients in the hospital.

Seeing the "End of Life"

There is an interesting intricacy in the palliative care gaze. On the one hand, with some resonance to Cicely Saunders's ideas, palliative care is an integrative perspective, which aims to transcend the sequestration of care that specialization created. Time and again, I heard palliative care clinicians criticize other specialists who they thought were looking at the small technical details in the function of individual organ systems instead of at "the big picture." "The specialty services . . . are really more focused on . . . [say,] this person's heart," one social worker told me, who then emulated a dramatic speech: "'What's going on with this person's heart?' You're reading ICU notes, and I'm like, Are [they] talking about a human being, or are they talking about a machine?" At Academic Hospital, I talked to a palliative care physician who worked 25 percent of his time at a medicine unit as a general internist. He found this part of his job unappealing because, as he put it, he did not like to 'look after people's potassium.' At a palliative care meeting in Public Hospital, a physician mocked a cardiologist, who reportedly suggested that 'we [cardiology] can treat [a patient's] medical stuff, and you [palliative care] can talk to [his family] about all the other issues' (the main issue being the family's hesitation to disconnect the patient from life support). And Scott, the palliative care physician I mentioned earlier, frequently warned young physicians of "mistaking the forest for the trees"—of being fixated on solving individual medical problems while overlooking patients' more general disease trajectory.

At the same time, palliative care clinicians applied this integrative perspective to a very particular domain—the end of life. To the extent that they saw forests where others saw trees, their training and day-to-day work made them likely to see very particular forests. Sarah, whom I met during her Hospice and Palliative Care fellowship at Academic Hospital, said that before beginning her fellowship she rarely encountered death.[128] As a palliative care fellow, however, she saw or discussed many of the deaths that took place in the hospital and consulted on dozens of cases of patients who were close to death by varying degrees. The end of life was what she dealt with, every day and nearly all day. Hospitals were full of end-of-life cases for her and her colleagues, just as they were full of cancers for oncologists and failing kidneys for nephrologists. Administrators recruited palliative care physicians to treat dying patients in the same way they hired cardiologists to treat patients with heart diseases. Palliative care work consisted of identifying end-of-life cases and assisting in managing them. "We eat what we kill," one palliative care physician with a particularly controversial sense of humor told me.[129] Such self-deprecating jokes, always prevalent in the medical world, assumed an especially dark tone around the end of life.[130]

This was also how other clinicians perceived palliative care teams: "Oh, the death squad," an infectious diseases specialist cheerfully greeted a palliative care nurse and me as we were walking to see a patient of hers one day. Earlier I mentioned a palliative care doctor whose team preparations for a staff picnic included the suggestion to print on the front of his team's T-shirt "I Work for Obama's Death Panel," and "Ask Me About Your Granny" on its back. His colleague suggested "I See Dead People," whose gruesome double meaning we all found quite witty. This image of palliative care physicians as "death doctors" was something that many of them tried to battle. After all, the main thing that distinguished them from hospice was that they began treating patients earlier in the disease process, before they started dying. "They're not dying," one palliative care physician told me solemnly when I casually referred to the patients on her service as dying. Yet reputation is hard to control: at the end of the day, palliative care carried connotations similar to those the priesthood had carried for many centuries—it was the hospital's harbinger of death.[131]

Beyond any general perception of the specialty, the practices palliative care clinicians exercised specifically targeted the end of life. Take Heidi, a palliative care attending physician, who spent her mornings visiting and examining the patients on the service's list ("rounding") together with a team of medical students, interns, and residents who each joined ("rotated with") the palliative care service for periods of two to four weeks.*

> The seven of us walk into a patient's room. Lying in bed is an old white woman who stares at Heidi with her eyes wide open and jaw dropped. 'Hello, Mrs. Andrews,' Heidi says softly, stroking the woman's shoulder. (Ms. Andrews does not respond.) She takes Ms. Andrews's hand in hers, and then moves farther down to feel her feet. 'She's still warm,' Heidi says to the group. 'We're gonna listen to your

---

* "Residents" are physicians in their first years after medical school (they are called "interns" during the first year of residency). "Attendings" are the senior physicians in charge of them. Specialties vary in the length of residency they require, which can range from three years (internal medicine) to seven or more years (neurosurgery).

lungs,' she says to Ms. Andrews. Heidi and one of the medical residents put their stethoscopes on Ms. Andrew's chest; she still stares at them silently without moving. Heidi turns to the rest of us: 'You see, she's using more of her stomach in breathing, which is something that they sometimes do.' (Heidi moves her hand in circles above Ms. Andrews's stomach.) 'Respiratory distress isn't necessarily forty breaths a minute,' she says. 'They can also be breathing like that.'

Heidi used a person's body as a teaching tool, referring to its temperature, movement, and sounds in the third person—'She's using more of her stomach'—as if the patient was not present. This interaction followed the typical pattern of a case presentation: Heidi spoke *of* the patient far more than *to* her. She focused on biological and physical processes while all but ignoring Ms. Andrews's personality.[132] Medical objectifications are integral to clinical practice. Doctors discussing kidneys, hearts, and lungs treat the physicality of the human body as detached from the people—that is, the subjects—who both *own* and *are* these bodies.[133] But this particular act of objectification reveals the object Heidi trained her team to discern: the end of life. She familiarized the students, interns, and residents with the symptoms that make a human body a dying body in the same way a cardiologist would introduce her students to the symptoms that indicate heart disease.

Minutes later, Heidi's pager beeped, and she and her team rushed to the ICU to respond to a call from one of the interns there:

> Heidi . . . walks straight into the ICU alcove. She stands by the bed, grabs the patient's hand, and touches her face gently. 'We're here to care for you,' she tells the patient and asks if she's in pain. I see no response. I look at the monitor by the bed: it shows a pulse of 38 per minute. I look back at the patient: she stares at Heidi with her jaw dropped underneath an oxygen mask. Heidi turns back to the bedside nurse who stands by the alcove's entrance: 'Can we get OxyContin?' The nurse hesitates for a second, and Heidi repeats in a more urgent and assertive tone: 'OxyContin, morphine, I don't care, whatever you got around!' She asks Katherine, the medical student, to take her place by the bed and walks toward the ICU hallway. An older nurse (perhaps more senior?) approaches her right by the alcove's entrance. Heidi says quickly, 'We're the palliative care team,

we need OxyContin, morphine—any opioid you have!' She speaks calmly, but with clear and great urgency.

Behind me, in the hallway, I hear someone asking, 'Is she actively dying?' Heidi goes back to her place by the patient's bed; on the other side I see Naomi, a young chaplain, holding the patient's hand. Madeline, another student who is rotating with the team, enters her username and password into a computer in the alcove's corner, and I hear Hassan, the other resident, repeating Heidi's orders to the nurses in the hallway: 'We need OxyContin or morphine.' He comes back to the alcove and takes charge of the computer, looking at the possible doses they can administer from the screen: '12.5–25,' he says. 'Yes, make it 25,' Heidi responds quickly and tells Naomi she can be with the patient.

Naomi begins speaking to the patient gently, practically whispering. I hear her saying 'We're all here to help you, there are three women around your bed, and they're all here with you.' Several ICU nurses enter the alcove; I see one male nurse who just stands there watching. Heidi asks them if the patient has any family. One of the nurses responds that she has no family, but there's a friend from her retirement home who is her main contact. Heidi asks them to contact the friend and let her know 'what's happening.'

Naomi and Katherine each take one side of the bed, holding the patient's hands. The monitor indicates a heart rate of 33, then rebounds to 38. I note to myself that the patient is breathing, although the breaths sound more like hiccups. Heidi looks impatient and annoyed with how long it takes the ICU nurses to bring an opioid. . . . Perhaps two or three minutes later, the older nurse comes in, takes the left side of the bed and injects a clear liquid into the patient's IV.

Nothing dramatic happens, but I notice a slightly softer and calmer expression on the patient's face. Her eyes close for a few seconds, then reopen. I look back at the monitor and see her heart rate is now zero. The older nurse is massaging her hand softly. Looking around the alcove, I see a few overwhelmed faces. It takes me a few seconds to realize the patient has just died. The nurse grabs a scanner, leans over the patient, and approaches the plastic bracelet attached to the patient's other arm, which has a barcode on it: a faint beep sounds, similar to what you hear at supermarket registers. The nurse returns the scanner to its place by the computer and continues rubbing the patient's now-dead hand.

The monitor comes back to life a few seconds later. I hear a voice behind me, "She's back," and notice a few breaths. Then the heart monitor goes back to zero. [Breathing stops too.] I follow Heidi's eyes, which shift between the monitor and the patient's face. It goes on for a minute or two. . . . Then I see Heidi rushing out, chasing Madeline, who left the alcove crying. She catches her outside the ICU door and embraces her. Less than a minute later the entire team joins them. . . . Madeline is now smiling, but her eyes are still wet.

Heidi says she's happy we managed to give the patient the Oxy-Contin; somebody asks if she was conscious, and Heidi says she doesn't think we can know. 'We couldn't really prepare for it, because we were really called in the very last minute by an intern, but I'm glad we made it,' she says to the team. 'There was some confusion, because it was an intern who called us, and nobody really knew who we were, so it took them time to follow the order.' She adds that we should contact the ICU team later again and see how they're feeling. She thinks this is one of the roles that palliative care teams should have: not only to care for patients and families, but also for the clinical staff that's taking care of them.

Palliative care was both recognized and practiced as a death expertise in this case. Noticing that a patient was "actively dying," an ICU intern called the experts who handle death. The experts responded: they administered a drug, advised calling the patient's emergency contact person, and provided the patient with other forms of care—the chaplain who whispered in her ear and the doctor and medical students who stroked her hand. These interventions seemed minor and were not very satisfying. As Heidi put it, 'we couldn't quite prepare for it' because the intern had called the team at the very last minute. In this situation, when a team rushes to see a dying patient it has never met before, it has little more to offer than an opioid, soothing whispers, and hand strokes. Just like any other specialist, the palliative care physician wished she had been called earlier, when the patient was approaching "the end of life" and not yet dying "actively." It is, however, oftentimes hard to decide where the end of life begins, and clinicians' judgments may differ.

When I interviewed Eva, an infectious diseases specialist who had no palliative care background, she spoke of such differences in judgment explicitly. As an infectious diseases physician, she saw a relatively wide variety of patients, including oncology patients who developed infections due to their compromised immune systems, patients with acquired immunodeficiency syndrome (AIDS) suffering from opportunistic infections, transplant patients receiving immunosuppressant medications, patients with hospital-acquired infections, and others "from the community" who "presented to the hospital" with infections. Many of her consults she deemed hopeless:

> We call it "Rabbi consults." You know, nobody should die without a Rabbi consult. . . . [134] The patient is in an extreme [condition], they've been in the hospital for a month, there's nowhere else to go, and the family says, "We want everything done," just to make sure that there's no stone left unturned. So they call us in when the chart is yea-thick, there's just no chance in hell it's gonna work [chuckles], and we basically bless the patient and do the Rabbi consult, you know. . . . We joke. It's really too late, we should have been consulted when the chart was yea-thick [indicates a thin gap between her fingers] as opposed to yea-thick [widens it]. Those are the worst.

These would be the *dying* patients, and Eva did not doubt that hospice care (or comfort care in general) would be the most appropriate to them. The end of life, however, is a wider category, which Eva and others described as a "gray area." Here you would find, for example, patients whose infections may be treated but who also suffer from a serious underlying disease that may have caused the infections, such as cancer. "If we get through this [infection]," Eva presented the dilemma, "what's the [patient's] quality of life? Are we doing [him] a favor by bringing him through the infection to live this horrible quality of life? Will they survive? Will they have a meaningful quality of life?" When I asked Eva how *she* made these decisions, she answered,

> It's in the gut. You know, I think it's like pornography—you don't know how to define it, but you know when you see it. . . . You have a gut instinct. . . . I know there was times where I felt that there was hope, that I [wanted] to treat something or do something, and the decision was made not to. And it's never black and white. It's always shades of gray. You know, these are decisions where there's no right, no wrong, and you acknowledge that. You're doing the best you can.

And so, it's like, I feel that we should go on a little further, but I can't totally disagree if everybody wants to stop.

When a group of clinicians discusses a patient's condition, clinicians may have different "gut" instincts and judgments. Compared to other specialists, the judgment of palliative care clinicians tends to lean toward fewer life-prolonging procedures. This, of course, reflects on other specialists as much as it reflects on palliative care. Recall the hammer metaphor that Scott's colleague invoked: "If all you have is a hammer—everything looks like a nail." Specialists would tend to approach patients with their professional toolkit of diagnoses and interventions, and in this sense palliative care clinicians approach patients with their own framework, which tries to counteract other specialists' tendency to prolong life.

> Standing at the nurse station, Scott is reading the patient's chart. Immediately after he opens it, he points at the name of the patient's primary care physician and tells me she's a pain. 'She's this hands-on doctor, she never lets you do anything, really protective of her patients, and she talks a lot but she hardly ever comes to see her patients here.' He continues reading the chart. . . . 'That's a classic example of a patient who shouldn't be here [in the hospital].' I ask why, and he responds quickly, 'Because he's dying. He's demented, and he has problems swallowing. He's malnourished, and he also has terminal stomach cancer.' I ask if he's getting chemo, and he says that oncology haven't even been consulted, and if an oncologist decided to give him chemo it'd only be for the money. . . . He continues reading the chart, says, 'If he's in such condition and not even a chemotherapy candidate and he's having difficulties swallowing, which puts him at a high aspiration risk, and ultimately likely to develop pneumonia, why do you continue screening him for cancer?'

Scott's instincts led him to search for and identify an illogical aspect in the care a patient was receiving. Although the patient was too sick and weak to receive chemotherapy, his physician still had admitted him to the hospital and conducted various screenings and tests on him. In other cases, I heard palliative care clinicians criticize specialists for sheer over-ambition. A palliative care physician told me about a case of a forty-eight-year-old man with colon cancer, which his doctors initially treated with a surgery and chemotherapy. A year and a half of treatment "had done, I think, pretty well," the physician reflected; however, not long after his doctors found a metastasis that reached his liver. The doctors recommended a surgery to resect the metastasis; according to the palliative care physician, in such cases, where the cancer does not spread beyond the liver, "a small number of patients will be cured." But the surgery revealed a very aggressive, incurable cancer, which "you can treat with chemo, but it would always come back, and the remissions would get shorter and shorter until the patient would die." Based on the pathology report, the patient's oncologist predicted a life expectancy of "one or two years." The palliative care physician dissented and identified the patient as dying:

> This guy, very rapidly, went into liver failure. This tumor was growing and infiltrating the liver so fast that his liver failed. That is a terminal condition, [but the oncologist] wanted to treat him. . . . He was responding to one specific bit of information, which was the pathology of the cancer. . . . Knowing that the cancer has a chance to respond to chemo, as opposed to one you know isn't gonna respond, . . . is a useful bit of information, but it's not the *only* bit of information. The patient is *yellow*. Bilirubin is 17 [normal range is 0.1–1.0]. He is *infected*.
>
> There are lots of other contributing bits of information that say this guy isn't gonna make it. He's not a guy who will do well in the ICU. And my point was: Okay, fine. Treat him with chemo. But don't go that far. Don't put him in the ICU, because if he gets that bad—he's not gonna make it. . . . So of course, he gets treated with chemo, and then he continues to decompensate. And the oncologist's point . . . was that this could be a complication of chemotherapy: "He's septic . . . because I gave him chemo that knocked his immune system back." Well, that was partly true. He was septic, he was also going into fulminant liver failure. We have no therapy for that. When the liver shuts down, if you don't have the ability to get a liver transplant—you're dead. . . . You are not eligible for a liver, ergo—this is a terminal situation. Find the false premise! . . .
>
> Anyway, this was my point to the oncologist, who had chemoed this patient, probably inappropriately, and now was going to try to treat him through what he perceived were chemo complications, where it was very clear to me that it was not a complication of chemo. It was a complication of cancer and dying. And we had this fight in the ICU—it was not angry, he's a friend—I said: "Respectfully, I think you're crazy.

I think you decided something on Monday and you're gonna stick with it on Wednesday, no matter what happened on Tuesday." This guy had ammonia of 750—I've never seen ammonia that high. Ever. . . . I mean, this is one dead liver! It can't clean the body's toxins.

I said, "This is the tail wagging the dog. You've given chemo and you're letting that decision determine what the right thing to do is." . . . He disagreed. And what do you think the family wanted? They wanted the optimistic doctor.

The palliative care physician tried to stop what he considered to be bad medical care. Examining the patient and reading his medical file, he saw a patient at the end of his life. The oncologist, who also was relying on some laboratory results that indicated some improvement in liver function (which the palliative care physician did not mention to me in the interview), believed there was a chance the patient would stabilize and be able to continue chemotherapy. (This chemotherapy was not expected to cure the patient but to prolong his life by a year or two.) To this end, the oncologist thought that the many life-sustaining interventions the ICU could offer would be helpful: a ventilator to sustain the patient's breathing, hemodialysis to compensate for his declining kidney function (which had started failing after the liver), and vasopressors to bring the patient's blood pressure to a level that would enable hemodialysis. The possibility of using a continuous hemodialysis treatment (continuous veno-venous hemofiltration, or CVVH) also came up. "It's logically insane," the palliative care physician said passionately when we talked.

Because we have the capability we have a very hard time saying 'no.' All we're doing is dragging like that at the margins. . . . I could march people down a logical game: I could say, 'Okay, well, what are you gonna do when the patient's oxygen starts to drop . . . ? Are you gonna wheel the ECMO* machine over? And they'd be like, 'Of course not.' Well, why not? What's the difference? You know, it's just a step beyond what you were willing to do. Well, a lot of people are uncomfortable when I'm very firm about not intubating somebody. I happen to draw the line before other people.

* ECMO (extracorporeal membrane oxygenation) machines provide both cardiac and respiratory support.

This is the essence of the economizing gaze. Although there are numerous clinicians who would not embrace economization in specific cases, few would doubt it categorically, especially in the contemporary U.S. health care system where the economizing gaze has been substantiated and institutionalized professionally and morally. The presence of palliative care clinicians in the hospital environment means that there are clinicians whose professional predilections lean toward economizing and who would advocate for at least somewhat more moderate and limited medical interventions than those other clinicians offer.

On the other side of the line were clinicians who criticized palliative care services for economizing too easily. A general internist used the last name of a palliative care nurse, Carol Wheeler, as a verb that meant careless economization:

> She Wheelerizes people. She's like, "You are a DNR!" [*Q:* Really?] Oh, yeah. Oh, yeah [laughs]. She is very activist, so we're careful about who we call [from palliative care]. Very careful. . . . She'd come out of those conversations [with patients and families] saying, "Oh, yeah, they're DNR." And she had said [to them] something like, "You don't want all of these tubes and this aggressive stuff at the very end, that's just brutal, and it's not a good thing." [The family] would be like, "Yeah, I know." And she'd [write]: DNR. You know, without necessarily parsing whether they really understand what that means.

An oncologist from another hospital told me that the palliative care service decided too hastily that one of her patients was dying, and when she "looked at the data," she saw something completely different:

> This patient was referred to oncology with no diagnosis, in the presumption by the people that were seeing him that they knew what was going on, that he had far advanced lung cancer. And I looked at the data and said, "Actually, that's probably not what he has at all. And by the way, there's this thing in this guy's liver, and it's growing rapidly, and you haven't biopsied it. You need to do that." And so I sent an e-mail out to hepatology, and eventually they [did] it. [Meanwhile,] the patient is in the hospital, and the house staff in the hospital, they don't have access to all the e-mails that we sent back and forth . . . and they called the palliative care service and had this

long conversation with the patient, assuming he was dying of lung cancer. In fact he has a treatable cancer. . . . So in the last few days, there's all this backtracking.

Away from the bedside, reflecting on their work in an interview, some palliative care clinicians acknowledged they were looking at cases from a very particular angle. One physician told me:

> We [palliative care] see treatment failures. We don't see the treatment successes because we're not called on those patients. The oncologists think in the other direction: they're always going for that 1 percent or 7 percent or whatever [who] do extremely well. And we're biased by the 90 percent that did not. . . . It's hard.

Such differences between clinicians were not just in opinions or intellectual conviction. Differences in how clinicians practice medicine derived from differences in their senses—what they *saw*—which were informed by their daily experiences, what each of them dealt with when they came to work. Everyday experiences created habits, which in turn made clinicians look at and see patients in certain ways. To the average palliative care clinician, the end of life was far more visible than to the average oncologist, infectious disease specialist, or general internist.

Teaching Practical Beliefs

On an early Tuesday morning, Private Hospital's grand rounds* featured two physicians from a local community organization. They spoke about two forms—the Advance Directive and the POLST—that hospital staff used to document patients' end-of-life preferences. The speakers emphasized the importance of filling out these forms and following the orders written in them. They also spoke of the more general social and economic context that made these forms so important in the U.S. health care system. 'The U.S. population is aging, and every day, 10,000 people in the country turn 65,' one speaker said. 'Of the population of 65 and older, 1 out of 8 has

---

* "Grand rounds" are lectures on professional topics that hospitals organize for their staff.

some form of dementia, and by the age of 85, 1 out of 4 people requires full-time care in daily living activities. This is what they call "the silver tsunami," and I think that in medicine we've put it on the backburner for too long.'

The lecture went on to mention several laws that were passed in the area, specifically the relatively recent California Right to Know End of Life Option Act (2009): 'It mandates that physicians who are treating patients with terminal conditions talk to them about their end-of-life options, including the right to refuse treatment, to obtain hospice and palliative care, [and] to refuse food and drink.' One of the speakers cited a World Medical Association 2003 declaration that 'a patient's duly executed directive should be honored, unless there are reasonable grounds to support that it is not valid.' And she also quoted from studies such as SUPPORT, showing that many physicians are not attuned to patients' wishes to suspend invasive and life-prolonging treatment.

The speakers presented POLST and advance directive forms as two ways to remedy these problems and comply with legislation. These forms document patients' wishes formally and make it easier for physicians to ensure that they are respected. Filling out an advance directive, one of the speakers suggested, has multiple benefits for patients and families: they have been shown to improve satisfaction and reduce stress, anxiety, and depression in surviving relatives. In addition, they increase hospice referrals and involvement of palliative care, and lead to 'less aggressive medical care.' This tendency to treat a patient aggressively, she said, may also result from 'biases on the part of the hospital, that are due to our profession, that are due to our own emotional investment in the case, that are due to research biases and other motivations, that we don't carefully consider when we're talking about continuing aggressive care or planning aggressive care for patients who are near the end of life.' Then she invoked potential sanctions: 'Following POLST is *legally mandated*. If you go against a POLST, someone is DNR (Do Not Resuscitate) on their POLST and their surrogate stands by it, and they receive life sustaining resuscitative measures—you can be held accountable.'

After some forty minutes of lecture, the stage opened for questions. I was sitting next to Natalie, a longtime liaison from a hospice affiliated with Private Hospital, who worked closely with the palliative care team. 'Oh, I'm dying to hear what the doctors are going to say!' she told to me quietly, referring to several specialists who were sitting in the auditorium. I had heard palliative care clinicians making similar comments about these specialists, saying that they belong to an old conservative guard who practiced dogmatic medicine and refused to open up to the challenges that palliative medicine highlighted. (Palliative care clinicians often described themselves as a subversive island within an otherwise close-minded and death-denying professional environment.)

But the remarks this "old guard" made were devoid of any antagonism toward palliative care. First stood a senior cardiologist in his 70s who was notorious among the palliative care service for his obstinate resistance to the service. He said that POLST and advance directive forms would not help a person who collapses in the street and does not want to be resuscitated. When that happens, he pointed out, the paramedics would not look for a form in someone's purse before starting resuscitation, so it was important for people to have Do Not Resuscitate (DNR) bracelets or any other sign on them that would be familiar to the paramedics in the city.

Next, an elderly oncologist asked a question in response to the speakers who had mentioned that POLST forms are valid in any place in the state of California so long as patients hold on to them. The oncologist wanted to know what would happen if he filled out a POLST with a patient who then flew to Florida. Natalie snorted and whispered to me, 'Do you know who he is? It's Williams, the shittiest hospice referrer in this hospital. He's notorious for late referrals—sending patients to hospice just a few days before they die. He also doesn't know how to talk to people, so he always leaves the conversation to somebody from palliative care.' (I heard similar observations from several other people in the palliative care team.) Natalie thought the oncologist's question was minor and somewhat beside the point. There were far more cardinal issues to discuss about POLST forms—for example, how to ensure that physicians like himself filled them out in the first place, even for terminal cancer patients who do not travel from California to Florida.

But notice that the oncologist's question—and the question that the cardiologist had asked—*validated* the importance of using instruments such as POLST and advance directive forms and expanding their use to address multiple scenarios. I had a similar experience with an oncologist who a palliative care physician said was doing "crazy shit" to his patients.

His approach, another specialist told me, was that "nobody should die. Ever." In the interview itself, however, the oncologist insisted that he almost always agreed with the palliative care team.

Differences between what people say they do and what they actually do are common and unsurprising. As Jerolmack and Khan put it, "Talk is cheap."[135] But the nature of such differences is revealing. When reasoning theoretically, in interviews or in the hospital's grand rounds, these clinicians could not but acknowledge that economized dying was good medicine. Yet economization was a belief that did not become practical for them. When they were actually treating patients, they did not see them as being in the end of life, so they resisted economizing their death. An interaction that I had with Dr. Lum (an oncologist) and a palliative care physician in Private Hospital's hallway was indicative. The palliative care physician introduced us to each other, saying that I was 'a PhD student from Berkeley who studies the economy of end-of-life care.' Dr. Lum laughed and said, 'Yeah, I'm one of the reasons why the cost in the last days of life is so high.' 'Ever heard of the Lum factor?' the palliative care physician shot back. 'However long he says somebody's going to live, divide it by 10—this would be your best prognosis.' (I heard the same joke from other physicians, too.) The moral of this tongue-in-cheek exchange was clear: Dr. Lum does not economize dying sufficiently— his prognoses are too optimistic, hence he treats too aggressively (and expensively). Both physicians spoke and joked about it openly, but they also seemed to recognize that Dr. Lum was unlikely to change in practice.

Because old habits die hard, most of palliative care's educational efforts focused on the less-formed habits of younger physicians, especially those who were still in training—medical students, interns, and residents. Influencing the young was easier because they were still honing their practical skills. Furthermore, as senior staff, palliative care clinicians could exercise authority on younger physicians more easily and force them to reform their practices.

One morning, I shadowed Scott in an ICU where a large team of doctors—an attending, several residents, and several interns—discussed a patient with advanced cancer. The team stood in a large circle, and a young male intern, who appeared anxious and uncomfortable, talked about the patient's condition. He had reviewed in much detail each of her organ systems and cited dozens of numbers that came back from her laboratory tests. Two more senior residents looked bored and dismissive of this overplayed display of expertise. Somewhat flamboyantly, they opened a laptop and began reviewing a magnetic resonance imaging (MRI) scan of another patient. Scott was also visibly annoyed and impatient. Perhaps in response to these gestures, the ICU attending interrupted the intern, saying, 'You're talking about all the things that are working; maybe you should talk about what's not working?' The rest of the team shared a few smiles, then the intern said quickly that the patient's kidneys were in very bad condition and the left kidney did not function at all. "Oh!" the attending physician exclaimed, drawing laughter from the rest of the team.

Scott took a step forward. "Did you talk about it with the family?" he asked the intern, who said he had not. 'The daughter was focused on helping her get over the infections, so she can continue chemotherapy.' But Scott insisted, 'You may be able to win small battles and improve all sorts of smaller things in the overall picture. But this would be confusing the forest for the trees: the big picture is that she's not going to make it. She has metastases everywhere! Her kidneys don't work! I understand that maybe there's some resistance from her daughter and maybe even from you, but what I'm asking is why didn't you talk to her about her mother's overall condition?' Protective of the intern, a resident joined the exchange, saying that she felt there was 'some level of resistance' that came from the daughter, so it was difficult to talk about it. The daughter came in for only two days, so the team didn't know her well enough to talk about such an enormous topic. 'It doesn't help,' Scott agreed, 'but you've been here for a week—why didn't you talk to her?' The intern who presented the case initially asserted himself again: 'It's a very difficult conversation, and I found that it was hard for me to have it.'

A more senior resident confronted Scott more directly: 'I think that it's hard to come to an ICU intern and ask, "Why did you not have this conversation?" when there's an oncology team involved and when the oncologist is not only an attending [and more senior], but also the person who knows the family for the longest time. Besides, the patient is an oncology patient, and they're the ones who make the clinical decisions about him, so it's hard for an intern to intervene in the relationship between an oncologist and a patient's family.' 'Okay', Scott replied,

> 'But the people who are managing the patient right now [in the ICU] are not oncology—they're you. On the bottom line, when something happens, you're the ones who have to manage it, give her pressors or intubate her. And you should make sure that the family knows how the patient is doing. And you know what the prognosis of patients with metastatic cancer in the ICU is, right? They have a very, very short prognosis [the intern nods]. Calling palliative care whenever you have to convey such news is not enough—you also need to communicate with the family yourself!'

At the end of the exchange, Scott took the telephone and called the patient's daughter to share with her his view of her mother's condition. 'I will talk to the nephrologist, because this may be an issue,' he told me, knowing the patient's kidney specialist was an "aggressive type." The intern and one of the residents who had talked earlier approached Scott by the nurses' station. 'Even when a patient is an oncology patient,' he told them, 'you shouldn't hesitate to make your own diagnosis. Talk to the family, update people about her condition. Tell them that she's not going to make it very long. If you see that she's dying—you can say it. Say the d-word!' They nod. 'You heard how I talked to the daughter on the phone,' he said. 'I was very clear in the fact that she was not going to get more chemo. I made the point that she would not benefit from dialysis, and I also presented the possibility of hospice as the best-case scenario. When you present hospice as the best-case scenario, you make her look at hospice more positively, and then if she does manage to improve so it's safe to discharge her, it'll be easier to transfer her to hospice.'

Such interactions exposed young physicians to the economizing gaze at the bedside. Scott did not lecture about palliative care theoretically, but inserted himself into the practical setting, intervened, and—as far as he saw it—corrected other clinicians' medical practice. Furthermore, instead of asking them to consult him on such cases, he demanded that they internalize the palliative care gaze, talk to families and patients about death, and think when economizing was appropriate on their own.[136] I also found out that Scott made himself available for residents who entered family meetings. He would serve as an invisible observer, who helped residents with practical challenges, monitored their work, and fashioned their economizing gaze at the same time. "I've had family meetings with him outside at the door," one resident told me, "just listening in, to make sure I was okay. He was like 'I'm here if you need me, but it looks like you got it.'"

Residents who hesitated to economize could find themselves confronting Scott. One resident told me that Scott reproached her when he thought she did not properly follow an economizing decision he had reached on a cancer patient. After Scott made the decision, the patient began bleeding from one of his tubes:

> I didn't know what the status of [the patient's] cancer was, I didn't understand that the family knew about the prognosis . . . because I had him that one day. You know, [he] seemed a little short of breath, and so I . . . ordered a blood test . . . because at the time he wasn't full Comfort Care, and I was like, 'well, maybe a blood transfusion might make him feel better.'
> And then I got a call from Dr. Martin[137] [Scott] the next day. . . . And you know, in retrospect. . . . Yeah, I messed up, and I probably shouldn't have ordered that blood test because it wasn't going to change the outcome. I didn't understand at the time, I should've dived into the chart a lot more and tried to figure out what was going on. And I learned from that.

Scott confronted the resident, and she internalized his view that she had made a mistake. Her *mea culpa* was not ideological, but practical: she attributed it to technical, not ideological errors—not looking at the chart closely enough and ordering a test she should not have ordered, despite being generally convinced that economizing was virtuous in such cases. The situation was particularly uncomfortable because this resident was applying for jobs and needed Scott's recommendation letter. Although Scott and his colleagues did not dominate the hospital, their presence meant that their approach had sway, particularly when they interacted with less senior staff.

Perhaps the clearest indication that younger physicians had internalized the economizing gaze was that on rare occasions the senior physicians criticized them for misapplying it. An attending general internist told me,

I had one intern who basically single-handedly made a patient DNR/DNI and comfort care without telling me, and said, "Well, it just seemed like he had a long road ahead of him." I was like, "What?! No-no-no!" This [patient] was a pretty young guy, who was delirious at the time, so he didn't have capacity to make the decision anyway, and I said, "There is no reason why this guy is not going to get through this." . . . I don't know that this particular intern really appreciated that he had just decided to end care that would sustain this man's life. Like, this was a father, and the intern convinced the family that he wasn't gonna get [better]. I found out about it through my resident, who was furious. And it was not a good situation. It actually stuck with me; it was hard for me to trust this intern for the rest of the time we worked together.

This was an example of dysfunction and malpractice—which the attending found jarring not only because of how high the stakes were, but also because the intern completely ignored the professional hierarchy and did not discuss the decision with his superiors. Palliative care was not the reason for malpractice in this case, but it does show how readily available the labels of "dying" and "end of life" are for clinicians today. Within the mixture of professional perspectives and orientations, there exists one that advances a more economizing stance, questions the usefulness of curative, life-prolonging, and life-sustaining medical interventions, and challenges the more ambitious medical specialists.

Conclusion

A June 2016 editorial of *Pallimed*—the main palliative care blog in the United States—invited some of the field's veterans to offer advice to fellows who were joining the specialty. Paul Rousseau, a senior palliative care physician from Stanford, wrote,

Remember the doctors of old, the ones without antibiotics, morphine, and all the other modern medicaments and machines—the ones that sat bedside, held hands, and listened—for they were the true doctors, the ones who were present and shared the anguish of suffering, the ones who understood the burden of fear was too heavy to carry alone; model them, and you'll be fine.[138]

Writing to the young, Rousseau invoked "doctors of old"—a distant and idealized image of medical practitioners, which seems to have been taken from Eugene Smith's iconic photojournalistic essay "Country Doctor." It is by rejecting "modern medicaments and machines" and abandoning modern medicine's technical sophistication that one becomes a "true doctor."

This stance was at the bottom of what I call the medical economization of death: a professional and moral intuition that in end-of-life care, less treatment may be better treatment. This intuition developed in a historical context where medicine became more influential and capable than ever: doctors were able to offer some form of life-prolonging treatment in virtually any situation. When to stop, scale back, or limit medicine was an ever-relevant question: death remained inevitable, yet managing and circumscribing it was now a matter of decision making. The ascent of hospice and palliative care—a specialty whose main focus is managing the end of life—meant that doubts over the course medicine was taking assumed a methodical and professional form: clinicians who were formally or informally trained in the palliative care specialty began following certain frames of thought and patterns of action when treating what they identified as end-of-life cases.

Much of the power of hospice and palliative care lies in its practitioners' professional capabilities. A good palliative care clinician can compile a comprehensive picture of a patient's condition and recommend the appropriate ways to economize this patient's dying. No less important is the *moral* power of hospice and palliative care, namely, its success in defining what people consider as good, benevolent, and virtuous care. The movement for hospice and palliative care very much transformed how laypeople and professionals thought about death and dying. The view that medicine should avoid overtreatment and prioritize "comfort" and "dignity" over life prolongation near the end of life is hardly challenged publically or in medical circles today. Clearly, there are numerous hospitals in the United States that have no palliative care services, and even in those that do, palliative care does not consult on many relevant cases. (See, for example, the case that opens this chapter. Scott was never called to see the patient, and she died without him reviewing her case.) But the expertise's power is growing, and its moral stance on end-of-life care is becoming ever more influential—to the point of pervading clinicians' practical intuitions.

By the mid-2010s, hospice and palliative care became nearly synonymous with end-of-life care. A 2014 Institute of Medicine report, which was commissioned to address "the care for . . . people with a serious illness or medical condition who may be approaching death," focused mainly (if not solely) on palliative care. "Hospice is in the mainstream," the report's authors summarized, "and palliative care is well established in larger hospitals and in the professions of medicine, nursing, social work, and chaplaincy."[139] With the formalization of palliative care knowledge and the growing professional stature of its advocates and practitioners, palliative care experts began exercising power over nonpalliative care clinicians, especially those who were still in training. Younger clinicians were not only more open to new ideas, but also more likely to defer to the authority of senior palliative care staff. Medical socialization in the hospitals—and social control over medical staff in training—now included a component of palliative care medicine, which may discipline or at least question clinicians who did not economize dying properly.

Beyond spreading the palliative care way of dying in health care institutions, the movement for hospice and palliative care also engaged the public and nurtured sentiments that resonated with economized dying. This laid the foundations for the new economy of dying, and the next chapter discusses its financial and organizational aspects.

CHAPTER 2

Financial Economization

I recoiled when Sarah Palin invoked the notion of a "death panel." . . . That was wrong and unfair. But I was left uneasy by her phrase. Had I not been one of a handful of bioethicists over the years who had pushed to bring the need for rationing of health care to public attention and proposed ways to carry it out?

—Daniel Callahan, *Rationing: Theory, Politics, and Passions*

"DEATH AND DYING" and "the end of life" became financial topics shortly after they became medical topics.[1] During this period, numerous social actors explicated *why* the end of life posed a financial problem, *how* to solve this problem, and *who* could solve it. These actors portrayed the end of life as an area of excessive spending, which should be scrutinized, managed, and controlled—economized financially. If the medical economization of dying meant that people took less life-prolonging treatment near the end of life to be better treatment, its financial economization meant that they saw less spending near the end of life as better spending.

In this chapter, my goal is not to rule whether these actors were right or wrong. Instead, I investigate the social conditions that made their financial analyses of the end of life prominent and influential in U.S. end-of-life care. I ask how the end of life became something that people think about and manage as a financial problem.[2] The question is particularly intriguing because on the face of it, it seems improbable that the end of life would become a major financial matter.[3] Life, death, and dying belong to a category of things that have unique symbolic and moral value;

because they are "priceless," people often contest their monetization. Valuating life-and-death decisions monetarily is likely to raise the same antipathy we find around monetizing the value of love and intimacy, children, the environment, or blood and human body parts.[4] And yet by the 1990s and 2000s even those hospice and palliative care clinicians who completely shielded themselves from financial matters were managing an object—"the end of life"—that had become thoroughly financialized.

There are three dimensions to this financialization: organizational, cognitive, and pragmatic.[5] Organizationally, the end of life has become financial because corporations began managing it. The organizations that provide end-of-life care operate as businesses and conduct themselves while considering their financial bottom line. Cognitively, people treat the "end of life" as a financial category. Health economists evaluate expenses of treating patients in the last months of their lives, and policymakers draw on these evaluations when they formulate policy. Lastly, clinicians and advocates have used financial arguments pragmatically as a means of persuasion when they present hospice and palliative care to policymakers as potential cost savers.

My main argument in this chapter is that the financial economization of dying is built upon the hospice and palliative care gaze, which I described in Chapter 1. This does *not* mean that corporate interests and financial thinking replaced the original ideology of hospices. The argument is almost the opposite: some of the very moral principles that hospice and palliative care protagonists championed facilitated financialization because they made cost saving at the end of life appear virtuous, legitimate, and necessary. The further the hospice and palliative care movement went doubting the morality of many life-prolonging procedures, the more questionable spending on these procedures became. Health economists, hospital administrators, and advocates of fiscal austerity— who for various reasons sought ways to cut or cap medical spending— became the unlikely allies of progressive hospice and palliative care advocates.[6]

This chapter follows the very different actors who, intentionally or unintentionally, contributed to this process. The first section focuses on the hospice movement. It outlines the history of U.S. hospice finance, shows how the hospice movement morphed into a corporate industry, and examines how hospice advocates began making financial arguments about death and dying. The second section follows the work of "death economists," who during the 1970s and 1980s began representing the end of life as an area of financial inquiry and argued it could be a target of cost saving. The third section analyzes the agency of hospitals and their attempts to cut spending in general and on patients nearing the end of life in particular. The fourth section tackles the economics of palliative care. I show how in this context of financial uncertainty, as hospitals' ability to strategize became difficult, palliative care advocates redefined hospitals' financial interests and convinced many of them that palliative care would save them money by economizing dying financially.

I'm Not an Economist, but . . . :
Hospices Embrace Finance

Elisabeth Kübler-Ross was not an economist. One has to scrutinize her writings thoroughly, perhaps unfairly so, to find comments that pertain to economics in some way or another. No generalization of the few sporadic and somewhat careless comments she made on financial affairs would do her justice. Kübler-Ross refrained from articulating any programmatic stance on the economics of the U.S. health care system of her time, the very same system she dedicated her life to changing.

A model psychiatrist, Kübler-Ross wrote her magnum opus, *On Death and Dying*, along her discipline's conventional dichotomy: "denial" on the one hand, and "acceptance" on the other. The power of hospice, she argued, was its ability to support terminal patients in passing the five psychological stages necessary for a good and peaceful death: denial, anger, bargaining, depression, and acceptance.[7] In one rare paragraph of financially minded reflection, Kübler-Ross blamed commercial interests for taking advantage of people's fear of death:

> There is no law in this country that prevents business-minded people from making money out of the fear of death, that denies opportunists the right to advertise and sell at high cost a promise for possible life after years of deep-freeze. These organizations exist al-

ready. . . . They actually show the fantastic degrees of denial that some people require in order to avoid facing death as a reality.[8]

It is no coincidence that this criticism of "business-minded people" was directed at cryonics, a relatively exotic and marginal phenomenon that has been uncommon outside U.S. society's wealthiest circles. Kübler-Ross did not seek to challenge the mainstream of the U.S. health care economy and did not suggest, for example, that physicians and hospitals, who treated severely ill patients, profited from these patients' denial and unrealistic hopes to find a cure.[9]

This careful approach characterized Kübler-Ross for the rest of her career. Yet as her life project materialized, and her theory of death, denial, and acceptance was taught in seminars and training sessions with tens of thousands of participants nationwide, her relationship to finance became more complex. Like most of the rest of the hospice movement, Kübler-Ross continued presenting financial questions as secondary to hospices' main goal to change medical and cultural attitudes toward death. But in 1972, when she testified for the first time in a congressional hearing, her tone slightly changed.[10] Senator Frank Church (D-Idaho), the hearing's chairperson, was very supportive of Kübler-Ross's ideas. Only three years after she published her book, he called it a "classic" and quoted from it in length. But Church also steered the conversation in more practical directions and encouraged both witnesses and senators to speak about money.

> It has been said, and I am sure it will be said at these hearings, that Medicare puts entirely too much emphasis upon institutionalization of patients, thereby increasing costs of treatment and anxiety among patients. That criticism is being acknowledged by the Department of Health, Education, and Welfare at least to the extent that many statements are made about the need for alternatives to institutionalization.[11]

This direct reference to costs—so obvious in the context of a congressional hearing—converted Kübler-Ross's medical-ethical criticism into a policy decision to shift federal funds from one type of care to another. "What," asked Senator Church, "in your opinion, has been the effect of Medicare and Medicaid upon the problems that you have discussed this morning?"

Dr. Ross: I am not very good in money matters, but I know that both Medicare and Medicaid tend to enhance institutionalization. The very first response is, "Let's hospitalize the patient." I think many of these patients could be taken care of on an outpatient basis, if the financial and other necessary help would be forthcoming.

Senator Church: In other words, if the program[s] were modified in such a way that the financial help that is now given to pay for the hospitalization, or the nursing care and treatment . . . could be available to promote care in the home, that this would be a great step forward?

Ross: A tremendous step, not only to the patient but also to the family. You see, the patient and the family have to go through the stages of denial: the "no, not me" stage; the anger; the 'why me?' stage; the bargaining "yes me, but" stage; and finally the depression and final acceptance. . . . If the patient and family can reach the stage of acceptance the patient dies very peaceful, and the family who is left has no grief work to do afterwards.[12]

With this promise to eliminate grief work after a close relative's death, Kübler-Ross substantiated the case for transferring money to hospices. Political advocacy converted her ideas into budget decisions, which diverted money from hospitals and nursing homes to hospice care at home. The caveat "I am not very good in money matters" maintained the distinction between the hospice vision and economics, and connected Kübler-Ross to the former rather than the latter.

Many hospice advocates conducted themselves similarly and expressed reluctance to engage with financial affairs, while making arguments that were financial in their consequences. This approach, however, changed as time passed, hospices increased in number, financial evaluations were published, and political circumstances changed. By 1977, as congressional committees and subcommittees contemplated various ways to fund hospices, Kübler-Ross explicitly highlighted the lower cost of hospice compared with hospital care:

When terminal patients are treated in hospitals, costs can run about $300 per day, but at home, using the Brompton cocktail for pain control [as done in hospice], medication materials costs ran about 80 cents per week![13]

This signified the trajectory of Kübler-Ross's financial thinking. At first, it bordered on lack of interest—finance was virtually absent from her doctrine. Then, as abstract thought about reforming the American way of dying became reality, Kübler-Ross advocated funneling federal funds to hospice care at the expense of other health care institutions. Finally, Kübler-Ross explicitly emphasized a financial advantage that hospices had over hospitals: the care they provided was not only morally and medically valuable but also had a financial value. Hospice became an economical way to manage the dying process.

Such a gradual—and always equivocal and ambivalent—adoption of a more financially minded stance characterized the entire hospice movement. Hospice discourse was contemplative, intellectual, and reflective. Philosophical, historical, and sociological observations frequently appeared in hospice literature, and hospice advocates thought of themselves as tackling profound existential questions that concerned the entire human race. Discussions of money, budgets, and finance, however, were virtually absent from this discourse in the beginning.

The first manuscripts that hospice advocates and practitioners published in the 1970s included few explicit mentions of monetary issues. Bibliographical lists of literature on death and dying in the 1970s did not include an "economics" or "costs" section. Books or articles that did focus on "money matters" usually addressed the high cost of funerals and survivors' economic challenges—not the cost of medical care for the dying.[14] Psychologist Herman Feifel's two anthologies, which collected much of the intellectual origins of hospice work, included lengthy discussions of psychology, culture, religion, art, literature, law, education, clinical management, and the history of death in the United States and abroad.[15] Money matters were briefly mentioned only on four pages, which focused on widows' and orphans' financial hardships.[16] No article, let alone section, addressed the cost of medical care near the end of life.

Like analyzing Kübler-Ross's approach to finance, constructing a history of early hospice financial thinking requires a subversive reading of hospice texts, which often goes against the authors' original intentions. One can compile a loose outline of implicit hospice financial philosophies only by collecting brief comments, digressions, and afterthoughts that the advocates added to what they saw as their main contribution: reshaping cultural and medical attitudes toward death.

Partly, this was because of advocates' reluctance to reflect on money matters. Hospice advocates described themselves as staunch and idealistic liberals. "We were as apt to meet at vigils for peace, meetings in the black ghettoes of New Haven on behalf of their civil rights, as we were in corridors, clinics, and meeting rooms of the medical center," reflected Florence Wald.[17] Thinking about money appeared to be foreign to such predilections.[18] Many practitioners declined to approach an emotional and morally sensitive topic such as death and dying in rational business terms.[19] "There are those who would say that a hospice and a director of finance encompass goals which are mutually exclusive," an article in the *American Journal of Hospice Care* stated.[20]

Still, hospices needed resources, and throughout the 1970s most of them operated in acute dearth. In 1979, only two of the nineteen hospices that reported their finances to the Comptroller General received reimbursement from Medicare; only three received income from private insurers and self-paying patients.[21] One hospice reported annual operating expenses of $17,202, which it used to serve as many as 171 patients.[22] The Hospice of Marine declared it did not charge its patients any fees because

> (1) We hoped to be able to establish the practicality of hospice home care without having to focus on reimbursement, (2) we were concerned that if we developed a billing program along conventional lines, hospice care might not be seen as a unique addition to the medical care delivery system.[23]

Despite the little money in their accounts, hospice advocates still aspired to provide care for all.[24] They drew on a volunteer economy, where their small monetary income came from gifts and donations. This economy crystalized spontaneously and in an unplanned fashion, with some hospice figures going so far as to tackle financial difficulties with spirituality and faith; they contended that because the hospice cause was noble enough, money for hospices was bound to appear somehow, miraculously. When the director of a small hospice wondered how to fund its work, a clergyman responded, "This work is vitally necessary, isn't it? Then if you all do your part well, it will succeed."[25]

This economy, however, was limited in size and could not accommodate the ambitions of what became the most central faction within the hospice movement. Hospice, Inc.—which I described as the movement's primary professional hub during the 1970s—was also a center of political and organizational power. In 1973, its board hired Dennis Rezendes, who had worked with New Haven's mayor and Connecticut's governor as a political consultant. A year later, Rezendes became executive director of Hospice, Inc.[26] By 1975, Hospice, Inc., had created a National Advisory Council, whose main goals were to "help the Connecticut leaders build a *market* for hospice" and spread the hospice model throughout the country.[27] The names of the National Advisory Council members reflected the group's professional, intellectual, and political influence as well as its progressive political leanings: Elisabeth Kübler-Ross, Jesse Jackson, Erich Fromm, Hubert Humphrey, and others.[28]

Any lobbyist would pride herself on what Rezendes achieved over the next years. In 1976 he successfully lobbied for liberalizing Connecticut's Medicaid eligibility criteria for home care, which provided Hospice, Inc., with better and more flexible funding opportunities. In 1978, he patented the term "hospice" in Connecticut, and successfully promoted legislation that designated hospice as a distinct form of care.[29] That year, he joined Don Gaetz and Hugh Westbrook, two hospice entrepreneurs from Florida, and founded the National Hospice Organization (NHO). They then organized the first NHO conference in Washington, D.C., where Joseph Califano, the secretary of the Department of Health, Education, and Welfare, declared the government would fund a hospice "demonstration project."[30] A commemorative NHO publication noted that Connecticut Governor Ella Grasso, who knew Rezendes from the time he had worked in her office, lobbied Califano "hard."[31]

The demonstration project, called the National Hospice Study, took place in 1980–1982 and provided the twenty-six participating hospices with a stable, albeit temporary, source of funding.[32] In the meantime, Rezendes continued his efforts to have hospice care approved for

Medicare reimbursement. In 1980, Representative Leon Panetta (D-California) introduced a bill to add a Medicare hospice benefit, which died in committee. NHO members, however, began redrafting the bill, and during 1982 some "two or three dozen committed individuals, most of them from demonstration projects," met monthly in Washington, D.C., for this purpose.[33]

Accounts of participants in those meetings reflect the chasm that emerged within the NHO during those years.[34] A core of entrepreneurial, politically minded people sought to create standards for hospice care, make hospice legally recognized, and provide hospices with a stable source of income from Medicare and Medicaid. But the idealistic grass-roots practitioners argued that bureaucratizing and standardizing hospice would compromise many of its original principles—clinicians' personal commitment to the dying,[35] flexibility in whom and how to treat,[36] and reliance on volunteers.[37] "With all these people rushing to organize," a psychologist who worked with dying patients lamented, "we have to be careful not to wind up with Kentucky Fried Hospices."[38] Smaller home hospice programs were particularly strong in their opposition to standards because maintaining accountability to a federal authority necessitated administrative capacities, which many of them did not have.[39] The tension was so high around the time the Medicare benefit was approved that several groups left the NHO to establish competing associations: the National Association for Home Care and Hospice, the American Society of Hospice Care, and the Hospice Association of America.[40]

But while activists within the hospice movement debated institutionalization—whether they should subject themselves to standard definitions, regulations, restrictions, and audits—the movement was fairly united toward the outside, where debate revolved around another topic. Congress debated a monetary question: whether or not hospice was cheaper than conventional care, and hospice advocates readily agreed that hospice was a better *and* cheaper way to care for the dying. They raised both arguments that Kübler-Ross made in the early 1970s: first, Medicare was biased toward inpatient hospital care; second, hospice was cheaper than hospitals.[41]

This last argument made much intuitive sense: forgoing expensive life-prolonging treatment should reduce the cost of care.[42] But demonstrating this intuition empirically proved difficult. The 1979 Comptroller General report noted that hospices could save costs only if they moved patients to "a lower level of care (home health instead of skilled nursing facility, or skilled nursing facility instead of inpatient hospital)."[43] A year later, a Hospice Project Task Force studied the cost effectiveness of hospice in order to determine whether it should be included in California's Medicaid program (MediCal) but found "no conclusive evidence."[44] The National Hospice Study, which was the largest and most comprehensive demonstration project, was expected to provide a final judgment, and the Health Care Financing Administration (HCFA) recommended waiting for its results. NHO advocates, however, claimed data analysis was too slow, and even without conclusive evidence, argued in every congressional hearing on the topic that hospice would save costs.[45]

Ultimately, the mixed and somewhat anecdotal evidence they presented was sufficient to pass the legislation.[46] The hospice benefit was the only new health care entitlement approved during Reagan's first administration at a time of great fiscal austerity. It passed *because* its advocates convinced legislators that hospice would serve austerity and help to financially economize dying. "Hospice is an effective response to President Reagan's call to American business and industry to fill the gap created by shrinking federal resources," said Reagan's Secretary of Commerce.[47] Representative Panetta defined the passing of the hospice benefit as "nothing less than an organizational and political miracle."[48] Reflecting on the reasons for this miracle, Thomas Hoyer, a Medicare official who participated in drafting the hospice regulations, acknowledged that "the argument for hospice's cost containment had been a masterful sales pitch."[49] Reverend Hugh Westbrook, who advocated for hospices in Congress, said that "the number of cosponsors on the hospice law . . . went up dramatically when the Congressional Budget Office reported that the . . . hospice benefit would save the Medicare system over $1.9 million over a 5-year period."[50]

The "masterful sales pitch" left its mark on regulations. Medicare's hospice reimbursement relied on prospective payment—a model that regulators introduced to the U.S. health care system around the same period. Hospices were paid a fixed rate for every day that they served each patient, regardless of the services provided; if they spent more than this rate, they had to absorb the cost. This was the administration's way to ensure that hospices saved money: it set the rate at 40 percent of the average cost for cancer patients receiving conventional care (cancer patients were the overwhelming majority of hospice patients at the time) and transferred the financial risk to the hospices.[51]

The hospice movement, which initially tended to avoid any type of monetary exchange, established itself as an economical way to care for the dying. American hospices changed in tandem. Annual conferences on hospice care began featuring sessions on "how to market hospice" and trained providers in recruiting more patients.[52] The availability of money also changed hospices' organizational characteristics.[53] Hospice agencies grew in number, and between the mid-1990s and early 2000s there was a sharp increase in their average size. The original vision of hospices as small communities of volunteers gave way to the reality of large organizations that operated as businesses (Figure 2.1). Medicare funneled increasing amounts of money into this economy. In 1998–2008 Medicare's spending on the hospice benefit rose by 509 percent.[54] By 2013 the hospice economy was $17 billion in size.[55]

In the early years of the hospice movement, the desire for hospices to operate as not-for-profit organizations was often too obvious to be spelled out explicitly.[56] But with so much money in this market, caring for the dying became an excellent way to generate profits.[57] The number of for-profit hospices in the United States has risen steadily; in the mid-2000s it surpassed the number of not-for-profit hospices (Figure 2.2). By 2017, 67 percent of the Medicare-certified hospices were for-profit, and only 29 percent held a not-for-profit status.[58] The story of one hospice agency is perhaps most illustrative: Hospice Care, Inc., of Florida, whose leaders were among the founders of the NHO, is today the country's largest hospice agency—as a for-profit, investor-owned corporation called Vitas.[59]

The hospice industry formed a market whose financial rationale was to reduce spending near the end of life, even though its ability to do so was questionable.[60] The steady growth of the hospice market meant an ever-higher number of corporate actors profiting from treating patients defined as "dying."[61] As hospices instituted themselves as a cheaper alternative for end-of-life care, they infused financial significance into the end of life. This was one driver of the end of life's financial economization in the United States.

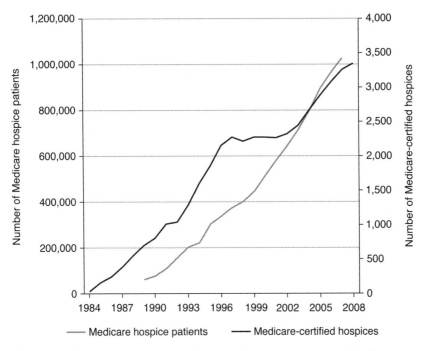

Figure 2.1. Change in the number of Medicare hospice patients and Medicare-certified hospices. Source: Reformatted from Livne (2014).

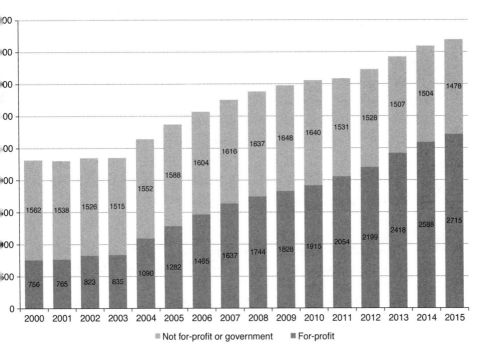

Figure 2.2. Medicare-certified hospice providers by profit status. Data source: Medicare, the National Hospice and Palliative Care Organization, 2012 Facts and Figures.

Economists of Death

The second driver of the end of life's financial economization was "death economists." During the 1970s, a group of health economics scholars began to measure, analyze, and represent the end of life as an object of financial value. These scholars were reacting to three historical developments. First was the passage of the Medicare legislation, which made unprecedented amounts of federal money available for the care of people older than 65, who accounted for some two-thirds of the deaths in the country.[62] (By the mid-2000s, the figure would rise to over 85 percent of deaths.)[63] Second, people began to view the aging of the U.S. population—specifically the growth in the number of elderly people, who need a great deal of health care—as a fiscal threat, which needed to be monitored and addressed. And third, the 1960s and the 1970s were the decades in which the modern intensive care unit (ICU) developed—a site for numerous hyperintensive, highly costly treatments.[64]

Yet the rise in health care spending was not unique to end-of-life care. Since the 1970s, health care spending has risen across the board, and the share of spending on patients in the last year of their life has remained stable (Figure 2.3).[65] Nevertheless, people discussed and represented the end of life as a distinct domain that posed a cardinal moral and financial problem: how much is appropriate to spend toward saving or prolonging the lives of critically ill patients? References to this problem began to appear in the medical literature in the early 1970s, when data on Medicare's expenditures on deceased patients became available. In 1973, a "brief report" in the *Social Security Bulletin* observed that

> Deaths are relatively frequent in the population aged 65 and over and often are preceded by serious illnesses requiring substantial expenditures for medical services. Many of these aged decedents were among Medicare beneficiaries for whom large reimbursements were made under the program. In light of the concern with rising Medicare costs, it is important to examine the size of reimbursements for decedents, as their services and charges represent a relatively inflexible proportion of the total.[66]

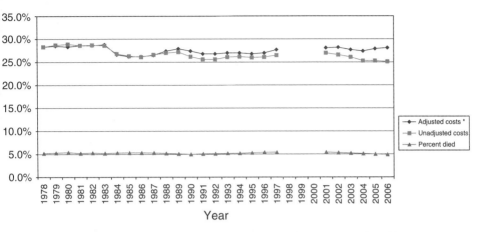

Figure 2.3.   Percentage of Medicare patients dying and percentage of Medicare payments spent in the last twelve months of life, 1978–2006. Adjusted to age, sex, and death rate for 1978. Source: Medicare Continuous History Sample / Centers for Medicare & Medicaid Services / Department of Health and Human Services, as published in Riley and Lubitz (2010), figure 1.

The report presented this observation as a statistical fact and accompanied it with little interpretation. This, however, changed in the following years. The fact that people who ultimately died consumed, on average, more resources than "survivors"—and the fact that a small minority of patients accounted for most health care expenditures in the United States—fascinated researchers, who presented them as problems in need of solutions.

Intensive care units were a prime focus of analysis. Joseph Civetta, for example, analyzed a Massachusetts ICU and showed that, although the average charges for ICU patients who died were only slightly higher than those for survivors ($10,064 versus $9,259), their average daily charge was more than twice as high. Civetta also identified the source of this difference; the hospital he studied billed more than double for a day in the ICU compared with a day in a regular hospital room, and patients who died had longer ICU stays than survivors. "Overall," Civetta noted, "the intensive care costs generated by prolonged utilization of this type of facility seem to be inversely related to the probability of patient survival."[67]

Civetta's evocative statement was not causal. Nobody claimed that higher spending could predict mortality.[68] But given the increase in health care spending and the political interest in controlling it, avoiding expenses for treatment that would be ultimately unsuccessful was very tempting. Doing so would only be possible by predicting accurately who would die and who would survive, which was extremely difficult. Civetta's solution was therefore *not* to withhold treatment from the sickest and most expensive patients, but to identify patients whose severity of illness did not require all the services that ICUs provided and to ensure that they receive only the care that they needed.

> Few patients develop many complications requiring prolonged intensive care and generating huge hospital costs. The mortality in this group is over 50%. Most of the patients who utilize the intensive care facilities, however, recover quickly with few complications and thus require a shorter intensive care stay, which in turn costs far less. It would seem that future efforts should be directed to improve the prophylactic management of such patients to reduce the number of patients who enter the high risk, high cost, low yield group. . . . Specifically defining the patient's risks and severity of illness encouraged proper, efficient, and more economic use of intensive care facilities.[69]

Later on in the 1970s, however, scholars began identifying the most severely ill as a potential source of savings. In a 1976 *New England Journal of Medicine* article, Cullen and colleagues examined 226 critically ill patients who had average hospital charges of $14,204 per patient. Of these patients, 73 percent died within a year, and only about 12 percent reached full recovery. This spending, Cullen and colleagues claimed, could have consequences for other patients because "resources may be diverted from many moderately sick patients to few very sick patients."[70] Spending on the severely ill, they argued, should be reconsidered:

> In the United States, an estimated two million patients die per year. If each patient 'benefited' by a terminal illness averaging $14,000, the charge for final hospitalization, excluding physician fees, would be $28 billion, 69 per cent of the most recent estimate of a year of hospital expenditures. . . . Quite properly, those responsible for advancing medical frontiers do not consider the financial impact of providing increasingly costly, high-quality intensive care on a large scale. Yet, economically, these costs are becoming intolerable and will be self-limiting in yet undetermined ways.[71]

Cost control thus moved to the care of the truly severely ill—not because costs were unsustainable, but because they could become unsustainable if every Medicare patient died in the ICU and fully utilized all possible clinical interventions. Cullen and colleagues clarified that "once a patient is accepted for intensive care, cost considerations should not compromise efforts or be factors in providing less than the best care available." But they still recommended controlling spending either by "not accepting patients for whom intensive care is inappropriate" or by "discontinuing intensive care in patients whose survival to a successful outcome is highly unlikely."[72]

In 1979, Turnbull and colleagues reported on their success in instituting an "informal policy" to reduce ICU admissions. The staff made decisions on acceptance "based on current physiological status, availability of additional therapy, and a subjective appraisal of prognosis."[73] Although the study did not estimate cost savings, its authors cited costs as a main reason to adopt the policy in other hospitals. Aside from fiscal consequences on the national level, they mentioned fears for physicians' professional autonomy. If costs were not contained, "cost benefit analysis by third party payers or government will become an unavoidable, and less satisfactory, alternative."[74] This policy was initially informal because of the staff's resistance to instituting any formal criteria for rejecting critically ill patients from ICU care. Later on, however, it would be formalized.

Notice the trajectory that these studies indicate. Over the course of the 1970s, solutions to the high cost of dying inched toward reducing expenses on care for the most severely ill patients. In 1973 Civetta suggested saving money by ensuring that only patients who were truly critical would be treated in ICUs. The financial savings centered on identifying those whose illness was not acute enough to justify spending. By the end of the decade, researchers contemplated how to save money by identifying patients who were too sick to treat. The subsequent development of the hospice market created an opportunity to save money on these patients. The end of life was economized financially.

There was still a problem, however. Saving costs by withholding or withdrawing acute care from dying patients required accurate and reliable prognosis, which would distinguish the terminal patients from those who could recover.[75] Historically, medicine and medical education have all but ignored the art of prognostication.[76] In the absence of a completely reliable prognostic capacity, defining patients as terminally ill could very well become a self-fulfilling prophecy—doctors would withdraw treatment, and the patients would indeed expire.[77] In the words of health economist Anne Scitovsky, there was a "very real danger of policies being formulated which would relegate very sick patients, and especially very sick elderly patients, to a 'terminal' group before their time to die [had] come."[78]

Scitovsky's cornerstone 1984 article, "'The High Cost of Dying': What Do the Data Show?" challenged many of the intuitive assumptions of scholars who took the end of life as a target for cost reduction. Increasing interest in the high cost of dying, Scitovsky argued, was not a response to an objective growth in expenses near the end of life. The percentage of people dying in acute care hospitals did not rise significantly between 1960 and 1980, and there was no evidence that the intensity of treatment in critically ill patients grew disproportionally to intensity in care in general from 1973 to 1983. Furthermore, from a financial standpoint, only a small proportion of the deceased incurred very high medical expenses, so saving on their care would not make for a transformative saving in Medicare's budget—it would only be about 3.5 percent.

But most troubling were the many cases in which high-cost care was proven to save lives:

> About 5,000 Medicare beneficiaries who did *not* die had Medicare reimbursement of $30,000 or more, and about 25,000 beneficiaries had reimbursements of $20,000 or more, amounting to $652 million, or about 3.6 percent of total Medicare expenditure. In retrospect it is easy to regard these latter expenses as justified and to question the appropriateness of the expenditures for those who died. But it is likely that prospectively the distinction between those who would die and those who would live was not nearly so clearcut. . . . The data available at present . . . do not support the frequently voiced or at least implied assumption that the high medical expenses at the end of life are due largely to aggressive, intensive treatments of patients who are moribund.[79]

This observation remained valid later in the 1980s. In 1988, Scitovsky found that about 73,000 decedents required Medicare payments of $40,000 per year or higher; a similar number of survivors (70,000) belonged to the same expenditure category.[80] No less importantly, Scitovsky and others found that spending near the end of life rose proportionally with the rise of health care costs in general—all areas of health care, not only end-of-life care, have become more expensive.[81] This increase, as the 1997 Institute of Medicine report proclaimed, "is accounted for by population growth, general inflation in the economy, and additional medical inflation."[82]

Because countries vary in how they categorize patient populations and health care budgets, international comparisons of end-of-life spending are difficult to make. But the comparisons that are available show that the relative spending on end-of-life care in the United States is not significantly higher than that of other countries. Medicare's spending on patients in the last year of their life (roughly 27 percent) is comparable to the spending of the Netherlands (26 percent).[83] Medicare spends 25 percent of its hospital expenses on people in the last year of their life, which is lower than the United Kingdom's National Health Service (29 percent).[84]

Yet despite these observations, critical cost evaluations of the end of life continued into the 1990s and 2000s.[85] The mere fact that a small part of the U.S. population accounts for a disproportionate share of national health care spending—an obvious situation in any insurance market—led scholars to declare that high spenders were "an appropriate target for cost containment."[86] Care was particularly expensive in the last months of patients' lives, making researchers wonder whether terminal diagnoses could be made earlier, before the spending peaks.[87]

Perhaps the most explicit and unequivocal statement came from bioethicist Daniel Callahan, who attributed the higher spending near the end of life to fallacies structured into modern medicine: its increased emphasis on curing and its general view that "what can be done medically ought to be done."[88] Callahan radicalized the call to save costs at the end of life; because it was hard to predict who will die, he defined the entire elderly population as a cost-containment target.

> *After a person has lived out a natural life span, medical care should no longer be oriented to resisting death.* No precise chronological age can readily be set for determining when a natural life span had been achieved—biographies vary—but it would normally be expected by the late 70s and 80s.[89]

The challenge of medicine, Callahan claimed, was no longer developing new cures and life-saving treatments but guaranteeing that medical development would be moderate and financially sustainable.[90] Some politicians embraced these statements: "We've got a duty to die and get out of the way with all our machines and artificial hearts and everything else like that and let the other society, our kids, build a reasonable life," declared Colorado Governor Richard Lamm.[91]

This alarming tone might lead one to conclude that the impending bankruptcy of the U.S. health care system would result from physicians insisting on treating elderly, impaired, and extremely sick people with extraordinary measures. Yet the scant data that were collected on the appropriateness of care given at the end of life reflected a far more complex picture. Scitovsky showed that nursing homes, not intensive care, accounted for much of the higher costs of treating older patients, both the dying and surviving.[92] Kelly and Aldridge found that only a small minority (11 percent) of the costliest Medicare patients were at the end of their life.[93] Riley and colleagues found that for most diagnoses, the older a decedent, the lower the amounts spent on his or her care.[94] This implies that physicians and hospitals are already exercising some form of care rationing based on age or medical condition.[95]

The data were highly equivocal, and one can only speculate whether so many economists would have presented the end of life as a cost-containment target with such conviction had the hospice movement not existed. The more hospices grew, the more widespread their critique of categorical life-prolongation became, and the more excessive end-of-life spending seemed. Why should any amount of money be spent on care whose benefit was being doubted by more and more people? The economists of death did not need to recommend that clinicians withhold care to save money—they could simply assert that hospice care, which many considered better anyway, also decreased spending.[96] By providing what Bayer and colleagues called 'humane cost containment,' hospice made end-of-life spending appear redundant and wasteful.[97] Put differently, by suggesting a medical and ethical *solution*, hospice advocates also constructed a financial problem: overspending on end-of-life care.

The Construction of an Uncertain Hospital Market

The third driver of the financial economization of dying was the American hospital, which by the 1990s found itself operating in a precarious, cash-constrained market. Hospital administrations sought ways to avoid caring for potentially costly dying patients, embraced the framing that end-of-life care was overly expensive, and started collaborating with hospice and palliative care to economize dying financially.

There were several sources for hospitals' financial difficulties, though none of them pertained directly to death and dying. First, many of the patients that hospitals treated had lost their insurance coverage. Throughout the 1980s, the Reagan administration attacked organized labor, causing many workers to lose their medical benefits. In tandem, the administration promoted insurance under Preferred Provider Organizations (PPOs), which excluded high-risk patients systematically.[98] By 1992, 37.1 million Americans had no health insurance.[99] This meant hospitals could not trust that their patients would pay for the treatment they received. "Dumping" uninsured patients became common, and public hospitals, which relied on constantly shrinking public funding, had to carry much of the burden of treating them.[100]

Second, the growth of the for-profit hospital sector during those years destabilized the entire hospital economy. In 2008, 19.6 percent of hospital beds in the United States were for-profit, up from 12.4 percent in 1980.[101] For-profit hospitals typically served well-insured populations and narrowed their specialization to diagnoses that brought high return on investment. In effect, they cherry-picked the most profitable patients and diagnoses and left other hospitals with the obligation of treating the rest.[102] With fewer paying patients, those other hospitals increasingly practiced "fee shifting" whereby they billed higher amounts to insured patients to cover the losses incurred from treating the uninsured and poorly insured. Insurance companies, which resented paying the higher fees, used utilization review and negotiated aggressively over hospital rates. Pricing in health care turned obscure: the prices were determined in behind-the-scenes negotiations between insurers and hospitals, and they varied across dozens of contracts that hospitals had with different insurance companies. Medical bills became an exercise in smoke and mirrors; they did not rep-

resent the cost of care, nor did they reflect the actual payments that ultimately changed hands. The impact this pricing chaos had on health care
in general and hospitals' ability to manage themselves financially in particular has yet to be studied in depth. It is clear, however, that it increased
uncertainty in the hospital market.

Third, in 1983 Medicare adopted a prospective payment system called
diagnosis related groups (DRGs). "Rather than simply reimbursing
hospitals for whatever costs they charged," Medicare started paying "a
predetermined, set rate based on patients' diagnosis."[103] Medicare classified diseases into around 500 DRGs and priced them according to the
average cost of treating each diagnosis. The hospitals had to adjust their
expenses to these rates, or, as one figure in the industry put it, "eat the
loss."[104] Combined with the cuts in Medicaid rates during Reagan's tenure
in the White House, the financial pressure on hospitals made them seek
ways to shorten patients' hospital stay. In 1983 the national average
length of a hospital stay was 10 days; by 1995, it had fallen to 7.1 days.[105]
Later DRG-related reforms put further pressure on hospitals. The 2010
Affordable Care Act, for example, sanctioned hospitals that had too many
patient readmissions within 30 days.[106] Hospitals lost money not only on
patients who had prolonged hospitalizations but also on patients they
discharged too soon who came back to the hospital shortly afterward.

Finally, throughout this period physicians remained the ones who
decided whether to hospitalize patients, when to discharge them, what
tests to order, and what treatment to recommend. Most physicians were
still paid on a fee-for-service basis, so they had incentive to treat patients
aggressively and for longer periods. As surgeon and author Atul Gawande
observed, "the most expensive piece of medical equipment . . . is a doctor's pen. And as a rule, hospital executives don't own the pen caps. Doctors
do."[107] Squeezed between the scarce resources available to them on the one
hand, and physicians' uncapped pens on the other, hospitals absorbed
much of the cost of tests, treatments, and hospitalization days that their
physicians prescribed.

These four developments prompted what sociologist Neil Fligstein
called a "transformation of corporate control" in the U.S. hospital market.
According to Fligstein, periods of regulatory changes transform how
organizations perceive their interests, and more fundamentally how they

structure themselves and define their goals.[108] American hospitals tried to adapt to the new market regulations. During the 1980s and 1990s there was a wave of horizontal and vertical mergers in the hospital market.[109] New organizational forms—such as large networks that connected several hospitals, clinics, and physician groups—became common. Hospital administrators pursued such mergers and partnerships in the hopes of achieving economies of scale and securing more insured patient referrals from partnering organizations. The bigger and more diverse the hospital, they assumed, the better it would deal with market uncertainty, and the more immune it would be to future policy changes.[110]

These mergers, however, failed to secure concrete economic benefits.[111] The hospital market remained precarious and unpredictable. Competition over the profitable diagnoses was fierce, and the risks from unprofitable diagnoses and uninsured patients remained high.[112] Hospitals, as the entire U.S. health care market, have remained dependent on always threatened federal and state financing, which has insured the sickest, poorest, and oldest patients and provided badly needed, dependable sources of income (Figure 2.4).[113]

Hospitals have used several strategies to make physicians moderate treatments. For one thing, they have hired physicians as salaried employees. In 2013, 64 percent of the job offers filled through a major U.S. physician placement firm involved hospital employment, compared to only 11 percent in 2004.[114] Similarly, the percentage of physicians working in group practices has grown, from 32.6 percent in 1991 to 62 percent in 2001.[115] When employing physicians directly—or through contracts that they signed with physician groups—hospitals could exercise more control over their decisions. Some managed care organizations (MCOs), for example, underwrote contracts that penalized physicians for providing expensive care and rewarded them for cutting costs.[116] Many of these practices were outlawed during the 1980s and 1990s, yet hospitals continued to encourage medical decisions that would be profitable for them. This was by no means easy; on the one hand, hospitals depended on physicians to supply them with referrals, but on the other hand, hospitals needed to ensure that the cost of treating these patients did not exceed the amounts stipulated in Medicare's DRGs or managed care contracts.

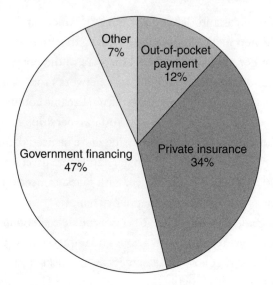

Figure 2.4. National health expenditures (2009). Data source: Centers for Medicare & Medicaid Services, Office of the Actuary, National Health Statistics Group. Martin et al. (2011).

Finding the "sweet spot" in these scenarios was challenging. As Jason, a physician who occupied a senior position at Private Hospital bluntly told me in an interview,

> Jason: Well, I mean, certain doctors, at some point, you gotta talk to. [You] can't leave the patient in the hospital. You just can't. I know you [the doctor] try to do the right thing, I appreciate that you're trying to do the right thing—[but] we need to work on a discharge plan, okay? And ultimately, if you can't work on a discharge plan for a patient who doesn't meet criteria for being in the hospital, then it becomes a disciplinary issue. You can stomp your feet, get upset—I don't want to reach that point. How can I help you come up with a good plan? That's sort of Conflict Resolution 101.
> Roi: How would you discipline [this doctor]?
> Jason: Well, eventually you can lose admission privileges. . . . Meaning, you're not allowed to admit patients to the hospital. I mean, hospitals don't want to do that, because that's what drives their profits. So, you know, somebody who creates a lot of business for the hospital will probably have a bigger hammer to swing in that negotiation than somebody who doesn't admit very often but is a pain in the ass when they do. Because what does it matter to me if you . . . only admit to this hospital three times a year, or [you] only admit your sickest [most] difficult

patients here, and save all your good admissions for [other] competing hospitals. Fuck you. I'm willing to piss you off because you're not doing anything for me. Whereas, when you're a high-volume guy, of course you're gonna get away with more. If you're bringing in good business, it's just kind of the way that it goes. [To me:] I hope I'm not making you upset.

Hospital administrations pressured physicians to discharge patients early, but they had to play a very delicate game. They needed to ensure that physicians would still admit patients so they would not lose business. This was a managerial problem that palliative care claimed it could solve.

The Business Case for Palliative Care

Similarly to hospice advocates, promoters of palliative care were morally driven clinicians, not economists. Yet they too were "not economists, but . . ." Cost savings, their argument went, were not the main goal but an unintended and somewhat fortuitous consequence: "Fortunately, the quality improvements offered by . . . palliative care may also lead to lower total spending on inpatient health care," one article stated.[117]

The financial stances of the palliative care pioneers were more explicit than their hospice predecessors' because they worked in a period when financial thinking on the end of life was already established. The Open Society Institute's Project on Death in America (PDIA) delved deeply into financial discussions from its very beginning. In 1994, at the project's inaugural event, OSI founder and chairperson George Soros asked directly "how much it would cost to deliver appropriate care to 2.2 [million] Americans dying annually?" and he contended, falsely, that half of U.S. medical expenditures were on patients at the end of life.[118] *Approaching Death,* the Institute of Medicine's report that PDIA had pushed to publish (see Chapter 1), included detailed summaries of research on the cost of dying. It presented the end of life as a thoroughly measured, valuated, and monetized object.[119] It also mentioned numerous methods to lower spending on it, whose efficacy still needed proof: advance directive forms, hospice, palliative care services, managed care, and medical futility guidelines in hospitals.[120] Throughout the 2000s, PDIA and other organizations supported research that would provide such proof. PDIA faculty fellow Thomas Smith, for example, found that a palliative care unit reduced the cost of treating cancer patients at the end of their life by two-thirds.[121] Researchers and clinicians from the PDIA-supported Center to Advance Palliative Care (CAPC) and Mount Sinai Hospital in New York found that palliative care saved $1,696 on patients who were discharged alive from the hospital and $4,908 on those who died.[122]

In the realm of finance, however, palliative care advocates went farther than their hospice predecessors. They not only claimed that they could serve financial interests but also explored how financial incentives could serve palliative care. The *Approaching Death* report, for example, invoked the idea of "consumer choice strategies": how to dissuade people from insisting on "marginally beneficial treatments" by charging them for those treatments' costs.[123] A year later, PDIA convened a meeting on the economics and financing of end-of-life care, which among other topics, discussed how to design financial incentives that would "encourage death in one setting or another."[124]

Recall that during that period, the hospice market was already standing on its feet. By then, people recognized the end of life as an expensive area in medicine, and hospitals were facing growing economic pressures as they dealt with diminishing reimbursement rates from Medicare and Medicaid and a growing population of uninsured and underinsured patients. In this historical conjuncture, consistent and hard figures that palliative care could save costs were music to the ears of hospital administrators. Mustering evidence that indicated palliative care could save hospitals money was meant to persuade them to open palliative care services. Advocacy organizations also encouraged foundations, hospital networks, and palliative care clinicians to conduct their own independent research on the topic. A group at Kaiser Permanente in Denver found that their palliative care unit saved a six-month average of $4,855 per patient.[125] Sutter Health in San Francisco reported that palliative care reduced average daily treatment costs by 33 percent.[126]

Palliative care advocacy organizations communicated these data to hospital administrators. A revealing example was a 2007 publication entitled *The Business Case for Hospital-Based Programs*, which had a most ironic lineage.[127] Its sponsor, the California Health Care Foundation, was a charity that Blue Cross / Blue Shield had created after it transformed from a nonprofit to a for-profit corporation.[128] Thus, a nonprofit organization turned for-profit business created a charity, which in turn made a "business case" for palliative care.

The report's target audience was either advocates in need of arguments to present to hospitals administrators, or hospital administrators themselves. Because the United States has numerous types of hospitals—public, private, university affiliated, managed care institutions, and so on—it is hard to think of a cost-saving measure that would work for everyone. The report, however, claimed that palliative care could do exactly that. In the context of an uncertain economy, in which hospitals had difficulty predicting whether their revenue would cover their expenditure on patients, the report claimed palliative care could provide financial certainty. After delivering the traditional not-an-economist-but disclaimer, the report identified its target patient population.[129] In every hospital, the authors argued, there are "high cost beneficiaries . . . with multiple chronic conditions, those with acute care admissions, and those who were in the last year of life."[130] These are "patients who die" [*sic*] and "patients with serious, life-threatening illness" who put a financial burden on hospitals because their care involves "frequent admissions, long lengths of stay, and high costs per case." These patients also have unique needs, which are peculiar to patients at the end of their life: "clarifying treatment goals, expert pain and symptom management, and help accessing care across multiple settings." Palliative care services could address those needs and at the same time "alter the volume and types of resources" that they use—or in more straightforward English, make their treatment cost less.[131]

Palliative care, we learn, is not "designed to attract new-revenue generating business," but instead "contributes to the bottom line by improving the efficacy and efficiency with which complex cases are managed." Unlike specialties such as transplant surgery or neurology, which bring in income because they treat generously paid diagnoses, palliative care helps hospitals avoid the cost of treating particularly expensive patients.[132]

For hospitals operating on "global budgets"—such as Veteran Affairs hospitals or hospitals whose funding comes from a city, county, or state—the financial benefit of palliative care is obvious. The less these hospitals treat, the lower their expenditures and the higher their surplus.[133]

Hospitals whose income is largely fee-for-service are more difficult audiences, however. The report mentioned a "misperception" among these hospitals' administrators, who thought that "cost-avoidance won't work for us because we see lots of fee-for-service patients." However, as the authors explain, since Medicare insures 70 percent of the patients who die in California's hospitals—and because Medicare relies on DRGs (as previously discussed)—providing less "acute care" would shorten a patient's length of stay and be economical.[134] Hospitals wishing to maximize their financial benefit from palliative care should therefore encourage early referrals of patients to palliative care through "marketing and educational efforts" aimed at their physicians—the holders of the pens, who prescribe medications and treatments.[135]

Cost savings, however, was not as visible an outcome as revenue generation. As one hospital's chief financial officer told the report's authors, "I can't spend avoided costs."[136] Thus, advocates needed to develop methods to evaluate palliative care savings and make them visible. The report's appendices explained how accounts of cost savings should be kept, and training seminars organized by groups such as CAPC taught palliative care practitioners how to collect and present financial data to administrators.[137]

The business case for palliative care was not a *representation* of hospitals' financial interests. By putting together numbers, charts, and models and formulating complex economic arguments in a report, these advocates *defined* what hospitals' financial interests were and tried to convince administrators to embrace this definition. In Michel Callon's terms, this work was not descriptive but *performative*—it prescribed what hospitals should and should not do, dismissed certain conceptions as "misconceptions," and validated others.[138]

Unlike what a conventional economic perspective would suggest, hospitals could not adopt rational profit-maximizing strategies spontaneously. For one thing, the hospital market has been too convoluted and uncertain to lend itself to straightforward rational calculations. What explains the financial agency of hospitals in treating severely ill patients were reports such as this one, which pervaded their judgment and informed how they understood their interests. By communicating with hospital administrators, putting together evaluations of palliative care's fiscal impact, and mobilizing clinicians to keep accounts of their work and share these accounts with administrators, palliative care advocates encouraged certain patterns of economic thinking in hospitals.

Targeting hospital administrations also had an organizational benefit. When advocates convinced an administration that starting a palliative care service was beneficial, there was a higher chance that the service would outlive the individual clinicians who promoted it. As one advocate told me,

> Early on, it was much more common for [advocacy] to be the grassroots sort of thing: you had [physicians and nurses] who really felt that it was necessary [and asked] us to explain it to [their administrators], so they agree that it needs to happen. But [top-down support] is much more common than this now, in 2012. And it's also a much more predictable success. I should say—immediate success. If your CEO tells you to do it, and you can't do it—they'll find somebody else who can do it, you know.

Approaching hospital administrations as allies also helped palliative care teams deal with the medical specialists who treated patients more aggressively. The head of Private Hospital's palliative care service once consulted with a colleague who tried to start a service in a neighboring hospital. He recommended that she treat her hospital's vice president as her main ally and ask him for help in reaching out and educating physicians about using palliative care. 'The way health care is changing,' the chair said, 'your hospital is not going to survive if they don't do it, and he [the VP] knows it.'

Similarly to palliative care's professional outlook, its financial outlook also pervaded many physicians' intuitions. Some of them—such as Dr. Lum, whom I mentioned in Chapter 1—disagreed with the palliative care team regularly but still acknowledged that this led to high spending on end-of-life care. Others, who the palliative care service considered to be "allies," invoked finance when I asked them why economizing dying was important. A general internist from Private Hospital told me,

You know, there's always statistics: we spend like, you know, 50, 60, 70 percent of our health care [budget] in the last two years of life, right? And, you know, that's the medical economic side of it, you know, it's just crazy how much we spend. . . . I feel things have to change because, you know, at some point we can't keep on spending this much money on health care. That's a fact. We're spending way too much money on health care and, when I look at it, I just feel like we waste money.

I had a similar exchange at the end of an interview with an ICU physician who worked at both Public Hospital and another private hospital in the area. He emphasized the monetary nature of the problem of end-of-life care:

Q: Thank you so much for your time, I really appreciate it.
A: Yeah! I hope that you fix the problem.
Q: [laughs] What is the problem?
A: What's the problem? The problem is we are burning *so* much money taking care of people who have no chance of recovery, and . . . we don't have a good way to stop them.
Q: Where's the problem? Here?
A: Everywhere. Everywhere. I mean, every ICU I've ever worked in—we were having an eighty-eight-year-old person with a massive stroke, who would never be independent, who would be on life support for reasons that are just, I think are faulty. Primarily because there's pressure from somebody, somewhere, usually a family member, to continue all that kind of treatment. And we don't have a good way of unilaterally stopping it.

Physicians' cognition may therefore be medical and financial at the same time. In certain cases, when physicians looked at their unit they did not only see medical diagnoses and symptoms but also high spending, futility, inefficiency, and an impending national bankruptcy. Some physicians were less comfortable invoking the high cost of treating severely ill patients than the two quoted above. When made at the bedside or in conversation among physicians, arguments for palliative care hardly ever relied on outright financial reasoning; instead they focused on the patients' best interests and preferences (see Chapter 4). Yet institutionally, there was cooperation between palliative care and hospital administrations on efforts to cut spending. Palliative care teams were in hospitals, in part, because they were seen as financially beneficial.

On the other side of the aisle, there were physicians who felt that in some areas of the hospital, people economized financially too carelessly. Unsurprisingly, it was a bioethicist who took the clearest stance:

> The most dangerous person in the hospital is . . . "the lone ranger of justice": the individual physician [who] decides that this treatment is too expensive for this particular patient, outside of any acceptable standards. For instance, . . . you're an alcoholic—therefore you're not going to get antibiotics. . . . I consider [it] unethical. But there are many people that are using personal judgments and coaching . . . [in] costs containments . . . , both individuals and institutions. [*Q:* Did you see it here?] Oh God. [One of the hospital's chief administrators] is known for walking around the ICU saying, "This patient's out of here . . . This patient's not worth it—off to hospice."

Such macabre descriptions of villainous administrators, who sentence patients to death based on how expensive they are to the hospital, showed that the economizing gaze could easily lose its legitimacy once it became financial.

But hospitals could legitimize financial economization by relying on palliative care. Just as in the case of the hospice movement and the actuarial evaluations of death, palliative care clinicians' ability to solve a financial problem in a morally acceptable way has made raising and highlighting the financial problem more morally legitimate. Once a palliative care team existed in the hospital and economized dying medically, it was also possible to point to the financial benefits of the team's work, and to the financial necessity of having this team in the hospital. This was the contribution of palliative care to the financial economization of the end of life.

Conclusion

This chapter followed the role of four drivers of the financial economization of U.S. end-of-life care. First, the corporatization of hospices: hospices were initially averse to any discussion about money, yet starting in the late 1970s they changed and adopted more financial tones. The hospice movement transformed from an iconoclastic anti-institutional group into a largely for-profit corporate industry that generated monetary value from caring for dying patients. Throughout this process, the movement justified its existence on financial as well as moral grounds, claiming that it could lower the cost of treating dying patients while improving their quality of care.

Second, economists of death defined the end of life as a central target for cost containment. These economists were more intentional in the pursuit of financial economization than the hospice proponents were: they constructed explicit, deliberate financial evaluations of care near the end of life. The difficulty of prognosticating and defining accurately who should be considered terminally ill (as opposed to just severely ill) cast a significant shadow over their efforts. But the development of hospices helped remove this shadow. Once an alternative, morally viable, and presumably cheaper care option for the dying was available, it became easier to argue that the cost of end-of-life care was too high.

A third factor was the transformation of the hospital market. Changing regulations and increasing market uncertainty made hospitals eager to find business strategies that would help them remain solvent.

Finally, the movement for palliative care attached itself to the uncertain financial situation of many hospitals and worked to persuade hospital administrations that it could save them money. Similarly to hospice advocates, palliative care advocates promoted a medical and moral solution, and presented it as financially beneficial. Once this solution was available to policymakers, administrators, and practitioners, it was easier to represent the cost of end-of-life care as excessive.

This account offers an alternative to the commonsense economic explanations, which see financial economization as an imperative—resources in the world are finite, hence actors must economize.[139] If we apply this logic to the end of life, the argument would be that care near the end of life is inherently financial: it has a cost, and people and organizations need to think about how to account for it.

Yet, as I have shown, the rise in the cost of end-of-life care has been proportionate to rise in medical spending in general. From a strictly fiscal and monetary perspective, there is no reason why Americans would have targeted conversations on how to save money on end-of-life care. The reason for the financial economization of the end of life is therefore sociological. There were actors who successfully constructed end-of-life care as an area that posed a financial problem.

The four drivers that I have outlined are building blocks of the new economy of dying. They generated monetary valuations of end-of-life care, shaped patterns of exchange between actors, informed how these actors perceived their interests, and defined the regulations that governed the field. They established hierarchies and judgments of value within this field, which predominantly drew on financial power and efficacy.

The palliative care gaze and the financialization of end-of-life care instilled two interrelated notions, which underlie the new economy of dying. First, treating dying patients with *less* life-prolonging procedures means *treating better;* second, *spending less* on such procedures means *spending better.* The next chapters analyze the challenges of applying these notions at the bedside.

CHAPTER 3

What the Dying Want

My friend sought my advice. After talking with his surgeon and another knowledgeable medical colleague, I told my friend that removal of the gall bladder was not mandatory. We then discussed his
two options—removal or non-removal of the gall bladder—and their
consequences. . . . My underlying message was: *The* right decision
was *his* decision. He understood me well.

—Jay Katz, *The Silent World of Doctor and Patient*

W HEN U.S. HOSPICE ADVOCATES BEGAN promoting economized
dying, they invoked two moral justifications to support it. First,
they argued that economizing dying was better medicine because it meant
reflecting honestly and thoroughly on the beneficence of different medical interventions, avoiding futile treatments, and facilitating more dignified deaths. Second, they argued that patients themselves wanted to
economize dying: patients did not want aggressive care at the end of life,
and clinicians had the ethical obligation to respect this.

This chapter examines the second justification critically. This justification is rooted in a pattern of ethical thinking that has become hegemonic
in U.S. medicine. Around the 1960s, U.S. medicine began tackling moral
and ethical qualms by turning to patients. The right way to treat Jay Katz's
friend was following *his* decision.[1] Patients became ethical compasses:
they were the ones who could orient medical practice in ethical directions.[2] The field of bioethics, which developed during this period, har-
bored this orientation. Renée Fox and Judith Swazey dated the origins of

bioethics to the 1950s and 1960s when public and professional discourse filled with discussions of several key issues: experiments on humans, assisted reproduction, euthanasia, and later on organ transplantation and intensive care technologies.[3] The general concern to protect patients' rights, as individuals, from medical institutions and professionals echoed in all these discussions. This concern was at the basis of what bioethicists called *patient autonomy:* an approach that relied "on the principles of 'respect for persons' as well as 'respect for autonomy.'"[4] It identified patients as having an inherent right to participate in decisions about their medical care, refuse treatment they did not want, resist the medical profession's paternalism, and most generally be the ultimate sovereigns of their life.[5]

Ironically, in order to guarantee patients' sovereignty and protect them from professional institutions, autonomy advocates created new institutions. By the mid-1970s, wrote David Rothman, "the authority that an individual physician had once exercised covertly was . . . subject to debate and review by colleagues and laypeople."[6] Institutional review boards, which scrutinized research protocols, hospital ethics committees, which reviewed clinical decisions, and lay cadres of judges, lawyers, community representatives, administrators, and politicians weighed in and influenced medical practice.[7] Sociologist John Evans argued that this transition made ethical discussions thinner—more rational, methodical, and procedural.[8] A significant gap emerged between intuitive moral thinking and the formal casuistry of bioethical reasoning.

Much of the criticism directed at the patient autonomy approach targeted this tension. For one thing, many scholars and practitioners raised concerns that patient autonomy became a formal imperative, which placed the high burden of medical decisions on patients and their families. "Scenarios in which families are offered choice . . . when death is near," wrote Sharon Kaufman, "reveal the dark side of autonomy—full of anguish, guilt, and above all the absence of knowledge about medical outcomes."[9] Giving patients a voice and allowing them to decide what care they would and would not want passed the responsibility to people who did not necessarily want it. As legal scholar Carl Schneider argued, "many patients reject the full burden of decision autonomists would wish upon them."[10]

Beyond that, as ethicist Jodi Halpern pointed out, the practice of patient autonomy became impersonal. Autonomists tended to embrace a negative conception of autonomy, treating autonomy as the absence of external constraints on individuals. The typical application of autonomy involved interrogating what treatments the patients (or families) did or did not want: clinicians studied their patients' preferences and wishes with the same equanimity they adopted when examining hearts and kidneys. They refrained from feeling—let alone doubting or challenging their patients— which ultimately meant that they maintained medicine's traditional attitude of detached concern. They sympathized, but hardly empathized, and thereby they stripped patient autonomy of its most essential humanist characteristic.[11]

This chapter highlights a parallel tension that emerged from the rise of patient autonomy, which had less to do with the burden of making decisions and more with the content of these decisions and the gap between patients' and clinicians' perspectives and expectations for end-of-life care. Historically, advocacy for patient autonomy, like end-of-life care advocacy, emphasized patients' right to refuse treatment. Hospice and palliative care advocates told a blueprint narrative about competent, sovereign, and opinionated patients who resisted the medical staff attempting to prolong their lives. This blueprint appeared regularly in scholarly, public, and policy discussions, leaving the impression that most if not all patients wanted to economize dying.[12] The opposite cases, where patients and families insisted on prolonging their lives despite the clinicians' resistance, were virtually invisible—yet such cases existed.

These cases of resistance virtually disappeared from public consciousness for two reasons. First, they contradicted the narrative that the moral authorities on the topic (mostly, hospice and right-to-die advocates) promoted. Second, they typically involved a high proportion of marginalized and discredited social groups: immigrants, racial and ethnic minorities, and other unprivileged populations. While using a universalist rhetoric and speaking of patients in general, the hospice and palliative care movement mostly gave voice to white, upper- and middle-class, and highly educated people.

In the chapter's first section, I show how the voice of the patients and caregivers who supported economization dominated congressional hearings and research on end-of-life care. As told in Congress, the main story of end-of-life care was about patients (and family members) who refused treatment against their physicians' opinions. The second section presents evidence indicating a different story. I examine files from the archive of a hospital ethics committee and show that during the late 1980s and early 1990s the committee discussed many cases of patients and families who sought *more* life-prolonging treatment than their doctors felt comfortable providing. By 2012, these cases became overwhelmingly common and made up the grand majority of the end-of-life cases that the committee discussed. The voice of autonomous patients, as the committee saw it, had come to collide with economization. The third section raises several potential explanations for this situation and examines the sociological significance of the tension that emerged between economization and the motivation to take patients' wishes into account when making medical decisions.

Representing Ordinary People

Mr. and Mrs. Average Go to Washington

In the early 1970s, the U.S. Congress began to hold hearings on care for the dying. The most prominent witnesses in these hearings were health experts, who came from both academic and clinical backgrounds. Some hearings, however, included ordinary people from various "communities" in the country, who had accepted the invitation to come and tell the committee their personal stories.

In the eyes of congressional committee members, such "ordinary people" carried a great deal of weight. "We have heard from many experts, . . . but I really think the real experts on this subject are the people who have to face the subject very directly," said William Oriol, the majority staff director of the Senate's Special Committee on Aging.[13] Yet these ordinary people came from a very particular range of social backgrounds. Many of them lived in relative proximity to Washington, D.C., most came from middle-class and upper-class backgrounds, and all or almost all of them were white.[14] As one can expect from witnesses in a congressional hearing, they all held relatively clear opinions about the hearing's topic—how policymakers should reform care for the dying. But most importantly, the advocates of hospice, palliative care, and the right-to-die movement, who had central roles in organizing the hearings, had deliberately invited people whose opinions and personal experiences matched their causes. The witnesses all felt that medicine had prolonged the lives of their relatives to a point where it was no longer meaningful. As represented in these hearings, dying patients and their caregivers supported economization very eagerly.

Starting with the first hearing on the topic in 1972, congressional committees heard patients and family caregivers who resented what they saw as medicine's overambition; they preferred "death with dignity" to combating their or their relative's disease, and they favored dying at home to institutionalization in hospitals or nursing homes. The first witness at the first hearing was ninety-four-year-old Arthur Morgan, whom the committee's chairperson presented as "a very distinguished citizen of this country." Morgan was the former president of Antioch College and the first chairperson of the Tennessee Valley Authority—a man of unquestionable stature and credibility. He talked about an essay written by his late wife, Lucy Morgan, "On Drinking the Hemlock," which the *Washington Post* had published in the 1950s and the Hastings Center Report had later reprinted in its first volume.[15] "The average duration of life in America has increased greatly in the past half century," wrote Lucy Morgan.

> This change is usually referred to as an unmixed blessing. But is it? . . . I see as I never did before that one element of the increase in average age is largely a prolongation of senility, and that it must be heavily paid for by the rest of society. . . . I find an almost unanimous feeling that we will never suffer ourselves to be such a burden to our children. . . . None of us [is] afraid of the grave and [has] no feeling of desire for life when usefulness is over. We do not want to give up our present comfort in order that exposure might bring us to a timely end, and we do not want to disgrace our families by anything spectacular.[16]

These words acquired a particularly tragic meaning when decades later Morgan fell, cracked her skull, and suffered a devastating brain injury. "For a good while," testified her tearful husband, the affection between us was enough to give joy and cooperation. . . . Later, her responses were largely ended and life was mostly a burden. . . . She was trying to keep from being fed, and they were prying her mouth open to feed her. I insisted that they should not compel her to eat if she didn't want to eat, and they shouldn't inject medicine into her body.[17]

Two days later, the committee heard a panel of three women who echoed the Morgans's sentiments. "Mrs. William Heine," the wife of an elderly retired painter with advanced prostate cancer who had had a stroke, expressed her feelings for the senators:

We have discussed what life is now to him compared to what life was and what life is for me because the members of the family feel it very strongly. . . . All I can do is express for Mr. Heine and myself how we feel about it. We are scared, scared to death now that he is getting to the point where he is more comfortable lying down than he is being on his feet. . . . He has the feeling, and I agree with him, that everybody has a right, if you have lived with dignity and respect all your life, . . . to decide to die with dignity. Because there is nobody to keep you alive after your mind goes and after everything that really matters is gone. Just to keep you alive on a heart-lung machine and with glucose is not life enough for everybody.[18]

Another panel participant was seventy-nine-year-old Gertrude Clark, a retired Greek Civilization schoolteacher from Silver Spring, Maryland, who recounted how she serendipitously became a euthanasia advocate. After receiving and signing a "living will" that the Euthanasia Educational Fund of New York had sent her, Clark was approached by neighbors in her retirement home who said they wanted to sign the document, too. "At intervals, . . . each time the resident expressed strong support for what the 'living will' attempts to insure," she testified, "until this last week, about 25 persons had approached me quietly with this in mind, and I had become persuaded of how widespread . . . the belief is in this and how general is the desire that a way be provided by which their wishes can be assured." The daily *Washington Star* featured an article on Clark, which led to "a veritable explosion of expressions of approval" from even more neighbors.

Two years before Clark's testimony, 94 percent of the general population and 98 percent of the elderly population (older than seventy) in Silver Spring were white.[19] People like Clark, who could afford a retirement home, also came from a higher class background than average. Clark, however, contended that her retirement home was

> a microcosm of the world of older people in the United States and can be considered a kind of laboratory for testing attitudes of that age group about this idea. . . . I have been telephoned and people have leaned over the table in the dining room and they have met me in the halls, sought me out. It is unanimous from them. I hear that other people have said the same thing and I began to get fan mail yesterday.[20]

The Euthanasia Educational Fund distributed 90,000 copies of the form that Clark, her neighbors, and her fans endorsed so enthusiastically.[21] Its text was a most powerful statement:

> If the time comes where I can no longer take part in decisions for my own future, let this statement stand as the testament of my wishes: if there is no reasonable expectation for my recovery from physical or mental disability, I, _____, request that I be allowed to die and not be kept alive by artificial means or heroic measures. Death is as much a reality as birth, growth, maturity and old age—it is the one certainty. I do not fear death as much as I fear the indignity of deterioration, dependence and hopeless pain. I ask that drugs be mercifully administered to me for terminal suffering even if they hasten the moment of death.
>
> This request is made after careful consideration. Although this document is not legally binding, you who care for me will, I hope, feel morally bound to follow its mandate. I recognize that it places a heavy burden upon you, and it is with the intention of sharing that responsibility and of mitigating any feelings of guilt that this statement is made.[22]

The form summarized myriad experiences, feelings, doubts, and emotions in two poignant paragraphs, which thousands signed: medicine has prolonged my life for longer than I want, and the reader has a moral obligation to stop it. This form was a mass-produced individual plea to economize dying.

The lay witnesses who appeared in later congressional hearings expressed very similar stances. In 1978, Ruth Molendyke, a widow with four children from Pompton Plains, New Jersey, testified, "My mother, too, always said that she did not want to go to a hospital or a nursing home." Don Keating of Maple Heights, Ohio, said that his own eighty-eight-year-old mother "would rather die than be put in a nursing home. Even the best homes in our areas are understaffed. The staffs are not properly qualified and in some instances there is a lack of supervision. Quality of service is not as good as the people could obtain at home."[23] The elderly preferred to die than be treated and viewed home as superior to medical institutions.

By 1984, when Congress debated the proposed payment schemes for hospice care, advocates could summon a new type of ordinary person to testify: family members of hospice patients. Many of the witnesses from the early 1970s, such as Arthur Morgan, identified with right to die ideas and expressed opinions that did not fully correlate with hospice principles. "I do not want to talk about *dying* with dignity, but . . . about *living* with dignity," said Elisabeth Kübler-Ross at her first congressional testimony, trying to distinguish herself from the euthanasia advocates who testified before and after her.[24] Family caregivers of hospice patients, on the other hand, could give testimonies that were far closer to hospice views: they had firsthand experience with hospice care, and hospice influenced their thinking on care for the dying. For one thing, when appearing in congressional hearings, they talked about their deceased relatives as having been unequivocally terminal. They were not people who had rejected life and wished to die, but people who accepted their inevitable, impending death, which physicians had diagnosed without any doubt. In recounting her mother's last weeks, Ann Rosenfield of Bethesda, Maryland, stated,

> The unique care she received [in hospice] was responsive to *her* distinctive physical and emotional needs as a terminal patient. Indeed,

hospice's special understanding of those needs, and of the needs of her family, made the last weeks of her life bearable. She was able to live with dignity until she died.[25]

Rosenfield was either well-versed in hospice rhetoric, or very well-coached by the hospice advocates who invited her to testify. Her statement practically reiterated the fine distinction that Kübler-Ross had drawn between "dying with dignity" and "living with dignity" more than a decade earlier. This remarkable ability to invoke hospice ideas articulately and at the same time speak as an ordinary person was also evident when Rosenfield responded to a challenge from conservative Congressperson Michael Bilirakis (R-Florida):

> Bilirakis: The word "hope" is something that is awfully important to all of us and certainly to a person who is ill and to a person who is terminally ill. I wonder, do they lose hope? . . . I know that the doctor has probably depicted that they are terminally ill but I mean, does hope leave them? What have you seen?

A right-to-die advocate may have responded that when reaching a certain stage of terminal illness, life is worthless and people should be allowed to end their lives. Rosenfield, however, trod carefully and diplomatically, in a way that served hospice advocacy and did not clash with Bilirakis's religious predilections:

> Rosenfield: I know my mother probably lived longer with the hope that when she opened her eyes she would see one of us there. That when she called, someone would come. I know that she would have lost hope if she had opened her eyes at one point in the night and couldn't breathe and had to wait for help. She might have died at that moment. So she had the hope of seeing us, the hope of having what she loved.
> Bilirakis: So you feel that kept her alive longer?
> Rosenfield: Probably. Probably so.
> Bilirakis: But that will to fight, which sometimes, by God's miracle, provides a person with the type of strength that may beat a disease even though supposedly they are terminal. Do you feel that they lose that hope as a result of the program, if you will?

Rosenfield: No, by being able to control the pain and the terrible symptoms
that they are experiencing, they are actually able to have more inner
strength because all of their resources aren't being depleted with the
fear of not being medicated, with the fear of being left alone, with the
constant absolute pain. They are able to have more hope, really, I
think.

Bilirakis: OK. And you have not experienced, I mean from other people,
any instances where they may have lost hope or were losing hope as a
result of, you know, this final type of thing?

Rosenfield: No. It is hard to explain but the family and the patient come to
a gradual acceptance that, yes, you are going to die, that you are all
going to lose each other in the end. It is a question of how that end
occurs. That is the significant thing. And there was hope every day that
she opened her eyes, not that she would recover but that we had more
time together. And that the quality of that time was more bearable for
her, for us.[26]

Rosenfield represented economizing dying as an approach that may
prolong life. Coming prepared for the testimony, she could answer difficult questions by drawing on hospice arguments that others had tried before her. She was a new type of ordinary person—educated, articulate, and
disciplined—who genuinely identified with the hospice ideology, agreed
to come to Congress to represent it, and was able to express it as an advocate. Her voice joined other ordinary voices and infused the discussion with individual patients and their family members' support in
economization.

Being tagged as ordinary, unremarkable, or average is oftentimes
thought of as a weakness. At the same time, much power lies in the social position of the ordinary. For one thing, ordinariness may grant a
person the legitimacy to speak in the name of an entire population.[27]
When recognized as ordinary, one's experiences become common,
and one's views become average and representative. Some witnesses
assumed this role voluntarily: Lucy Morgan and Ms. Heine used plural
pronouns—"none of *us* [is] afraid of the grave"; "just to keep you
alive . . . is not life enough for *everybody*" (emphases mine)—and Gertrude Clark described her Maryland retirement home as a "microcosm
of the world of older people in the United States." At other times, the
committee members pushed the witnesses to make generalizations and

extrapolate from their personal experiences to the experiences of all patients and caregivers. Unlike expert witnesses, lay and ordinary people were not expected to prove these extrapolations' methodological soundness. Their ordinariness vouched for their credibility and the empathy that their moving stories elicited helped advocates garner support.[28]

The power that lies in the average is not distributed equally among all social groups. For one thing, the average does not represent the many experiences and opinions that are on the margins. Even if, on average, U.S. adults say they would not want their life prolonged when facing severe illness, there are still many who would, who are not represented by the average. Moreover, few people get invited to testify in Congress, and those invited tend to come from very particular social backgrounds. The average person is therefore hardly ever in the position of representing the average—the average, rather, represents her. In the cases described here, the lay witnesses who appeared in Congress represented dying patients and their family caregivers as endorsing economized dying univocally.

Patients as Teachers

Much of the period's scholarly work offered very similar representations of patients' wishes. Take Kübler-Ross's bestselling book *On Death and Dying*. Patients' wishes, thoughts, and feelings were major foci of the book, which Kübler-Ross wrote was "simply an account of a new and challenging opportunity to refocus on the patient, . . . to learn from him [*sic*] the strengths and weakness of our hospital management of the patient." Kübler-Ross presented her own expert judgments as secondary to patients' own voices: "We have asked [patients] to be our teachers so that we may learn more about the final stages of life. . . . I am simply telling the stories of my patients who shared their agonies, their expectations, and their frustrations with us."[29]

In line with what ordinary people said in Congress, Kübler-Ross described a fundamental tension between patients' wishes and the care provided in hospitals. Senator Frank Church (D-Idaho), chair of the Senate

Committee on Aging, read her description aloud when he opened the 1972 hearing on the topic:

> Her [Kübler-Ross's] basic point is that the patient may be treated like a thing rather than a person. Decisions are frequently made without his opinion, even on major questions of treatment. He becomes, as the book says, "an object of great concern and great financial investment. He may cry for rest, peace, and dignity, but he will get infusions, transfusions, a heart machine, or tracheotomy if necessary. He may want one single person to stop for one single minute so that he can ask one single question, but he will get a dozen people around the clock, all busily preoccupied with his heart rate, pulse, electrocardiogram, or pulmonary functions, his secretions or excretions, but not with him as a human being. He may wish to fight it all, but it is going to be a useless fight since all this is done in the fight for his life, and if they can save his life they can consider the person afterward. Those who consider the person first may lose precious time to save his life!" . . . To the patient, exhausted and tormented by pain, the will to resist [disease] may seem to be merely a way of prolonging agony. . . . To the physician, the disciplined determination to maintain life may overcome all other judgments.[30]

The book's subtitle summarized its argument on the typical relationship between dying patients and clinicians: "What the Dying Have to Teach Doctors, Nurses, Clergy, and Their Own Families." Dying patients knew something about death, dying, and proper ways to care that the professionals still needed to learn, hence Kübler-Ross and her students asking "terminally ill patients to be our teachers."[31] Kübler-Ross estimated that about 90 percent of the physicians she encountered during her research "reacted with discomfort, annoyance, or overt or covert hostility." They had a "desperate need to deny the existence of terminal patients in their wards."[32] One physician yelled at Kübler-Ross that she should not have talked to a certain patient, who did not know how sick she was; Kübler-Ross responded that the patient *wanted* to talk to her because she *knew* she was dying.[33] Another patient spoke with contempt about "those physicians who can only care for a patient as long as he is well but when it comes to dying, then [the physicians] all shy away." "This was my man!"

Kübler-Ross wrote, adding that the interview with him was "one of the most unforgettable . . . I have ever attended."[34]

"It appeared that the more training a physician had the less he was ready to become involved" in care for the dying, Kübler-Ross observed.[35] Professionalization had made physicians lose an openness to the topic, which they had previously possessed. The same applied to other medical professions. Although compared with physicians, nurses were more open, Kübler-Ross found that "only one out of twelve nurses felt that dying patients, too, needed their care."[36] Even chaplains—the traditional harbingers of death in hospitals—were in acute denial: many of them "felt quite comfortable using a prayer book . . . as the sole communication between them and the patients, thus avoiding listening to their needs."[37]

Contrary to clinicians' overwhelming denial, terminal patients "responded favorably and overwhelmingly positively" to Kübler-Ross's research. Only 2 percent of the people she approached for interviews turned her down, and only one out of more than 200 consistently refused to "talk about the seriousness of her illness, problems resulting from her terminal illness, or fears of dying."[38] This particular patient, she wrote, was in the stage of denial—of which many others spoke to her retrospectively.[39] Like clinicians, terminal patients who wanted to prolong or sustain life were denying death. Acceptance meant embracing economization: understanding that death was near and forgoing "futile" attempts to postpone it was preferable.

Some later research echoed these observations. In 1984, a group of practitioners and researchers from the University of California, San Francisco's medical center surveyed 152 severely ill and healthy patients from the center's General Internal Medicine Group.[40] Of the respondents who reported thinking "a lot" or "a moderate amount" on the topic, large majorities said they would not want to be treated with intensive care (73 percent), resuscitation (71 percent), or feeding tubes (75 percent) if they were demented. A small majority (53 percent) also said they wanted to refuse antibiotics and hospitalization for pneumonia if they reached this condition. The respondents who were older than 65 were almost twice as likely to say they would decline feeding tubes (80 percent) compared with the younger patients (42 percent). The researchers did not report the answers of those who said they thought little or did not think at all about the topic.[41] Seemingly, having few thoughts on the topic made people unqualified to opinionate on whether they would want these procedures. Another study from 1988 found that in its sample of seventy-five elderly patients (aged sixty-five years and older), only 9 percent said cardiopulmonary resuscitation (CPR) should be performed on any person who had cardiac arrest, regardless of her medical condition. A minority said they would want CPR performed on them if they had terminal cancer (28 percent), irreversible heart failure (41 percent), or if they were in an irreversible coma (25 percent).[42]

In the late 1970s and to a greater degree in the 1990s, major public opinion research centers did more comprehensive surveys on the topic. Some of these surveys, which asked people about their end-of-life preferences, yielded even stronger results. In two Gallup polls (1992 and 1996) 9 out of 10 respondents said they would prefer care at home to institutionalization if they met the Medicare hospice criterion of a terminal illness diagnosis of six months or less to live.[43]

Advocates and scholars of end-of-life care cited these and similar figures as testimony that the U.S. public is overall supportive of economized dying.[44] However, there were many alternative ways to frame these findings. For one thing, as in any survey, people's answers depended on how researchers worded the questions.[45] The Gallup polls, which asked *where* people preferred to die, found an overwhelming public preference for home care. Other studies, which confronted people with questions about specific medical procedures, documented lower support for economization. In 1997, researchers compared the end-of-life wishes of people in various age groups and medical conditions. Contrary to the 1984 study, they found that sicker and older patients valued life in severe illness more than healthier ones and were more open to life-sustaining care. For example, among the young and healthy adults surveyed, about two-thirds considered life in a coma worse than death, compared with 57 percent of the older adults and only 44 percent of the terminal cancer patients.[46] Another team of researchers found that 58 percent of the terminal patients they sampled wanted to receive medical treatment even if it could prolong their life only by one week. Similarly to the SUPPORT researchers, they found that these preferences had no significant influence on the treatment the patients received.[47]

These findings aside, and in line with the blueprint that hospice and palliative care advocates have invoked since the 1960s, the most prevalent narrative that researchers told about end-of-life care described physicians who prolonged terminal patients' lives against their wishes.[48] Readers would easily recall cases of people who fought to withdraw life support against legal, medical, religious, political, and organizational dogma—Karen Ann Quinlan and Nancy Cruzan. (A third memorable case was that of Terri Schiavo, whose husband fought to disconnect her from artificial nutrition against her parents' wishes.) These were milestones in the glorious history of patients (or families) fighting for their individual rights and sovereignty, and no account on U.S. end-of-life care is complete without them.

The opposite cases of patients and families who struggled to continue life-prolonging treatments are far less well known. Although such cases appear in media outlets occasionally, at least in mainstream circles, they are usually forgotten and have never added up to a coherent historical narrative.[49] Scholarly discussion of them has also been lacking. In 1990, a case report on clinicians who, against a mother's wishes, refused to prolong the life of a severely ill and incapacitated baby mentioned that "literature on physicians' refusal of patients' demands is sparse."[50] Almost a decade later, there was still "no definitive court ruling on the subject nor a consensus in the bioethics or medical communities" on "physician refusal of ineffective or so-called futile treatment."[51]

The blueprint of patients and families who wanted less aggressive care than clinicians also informed legislation. In 1989, the preface to a bill that eventually became the Patient Self-Determination Act of 1990 stated that "recent advances in medical science and technology have made it possible to prolong dying through the use of artificial, extraordinary, extreme, or radical medical or surgical procedures."[52] Based on this risk, the bill (and, ultimately, law) required health providers to inform patients about their right to make decisions on their care, inquire about whether they have filled out an advance directive, and ensure that such a directive, if it exists, will be followed.[53] The bill's language treated any patient wish—rejection or acceptance of treatment—symmetrically and sought to guarantee patients' right to influence their care regardless of what their wishes were. The rhetoric of the bill's original preface, however, betrayed the scenarios that its authors and sponsors had in mind: describing care with adjectives such as "artificial," "extraordinary," and "radical" was a clear statement against the use of life-sustaining treatments with terminal patients and for patients' right to reject them.

In summary, since the 1970s, medical literature, public discourse, and legislative discussions have emphasized cases where doctors prolonged or sustained patients' lives against their wishes and portrayed these cases as the chief and most quintessential problem that needs to be addressed in end-of-life care. By highlighting physicians' aggressiveness compared with patients' wishes they also made an argument that typically, the patients' wishes resonated with economized dying and therefore that economization was a win-win-win strategy: it provided better care, it provided cheaper care, and it also reflected what patients wanted.

The Changing Nature of Ethical Qualms

Many of the palliative care clinicians that I interviewed embraced the blueprint and described their work as assisting terminally ill patients who rejected life-prolonging treatment. But when I shadowed these clinicians, I saw that they spent most of their time dealing with opposite cases, in which patients (or families) wanted to pursue life-prolonging treatment against the opinion of many if not all physicians. Clearly, I observed very particular parts of the hospitals that I studied. There could be numerous cases of physicians who prolonged patients' lives against their wishes, which the palliative care service did not know about and I did not observe. But as an account of the new economy of dying, this finding is meaningful and important: it helps characterize the relationship between this economy, palliative care, and the agency of patients and families.

Let me substantiate this finding further. With the help of a research assistant, I reviewed 162 files from an archive that belonged to the ethics committee of a California hospital.[54] The archive included documentation of nearly all the cases that the committee had discussed since its beginning. These were situations that clinicians—and in some rare occasions patients and families—had considered ethically challenging enough to refer to a bioethicist. These cases were not representative of all cases in the hospital. In fact, they were exceptional: treating patients in the hospital was usually routine, banal, and instigated few ethical questions or disagreements that could lead somebody to call an ethics consultation.[55] The cases that people did refer to the ethics committee were what Boltanski and Thévenot called "critical moments": unusual situations where "people, involved in ordinary relationships . . . realize that something is going wrong; that they cannot get along any more. . . . Most of the time, [this is] the moment . . . where [people] must . . . express discontent to the other persons."[56] Facing a somewhat controversial case, the clinicians whose notes appeared in the archive's files could not act according to habit. They had to define what was problematic in the case they were managing, then justify their moral and medical views about it and explain why they thought they were right. I was less interested in the committee's recommendations and more in what had made people consult the committee. Specifically, I wanted to see how many of the ethics cases derived from disagreements on end-of-life care, and who (clinicians or patients and families) wanted to economize dying more than the other. The archive also allowed me to examine how these positions have changed over time.

This still left the very likely possibility of a selection bias. First, for various reasons, some controversial end-of-life cases may not have made it to the ethics committee. Second, people's definition of what counts as a problem that merits discussion by the ethics committee may have changed over the years; clinicians could have referred to the committee different types of cases in different periods. For these reasons I do not treat the archive as representative of all controversial end-of-life cases in the hospital but as indicating how clinicians framed what counted as serious ethical problems. Put differently, I wanted to evaluate the selection bias— what cases people singled out as ethically problematic in different periods.

Archives in general, and archives of clinical records in particular, are mediators. They do not document everything, and the documents they do include may omit details that their authors preferred to hide. When talking to the service's ethicists and comparing stories that they told me with the formal notes they left in the files, I saw that their notes often downplayed conflicts and disagreements among the medical staff, perhaps for fear of potential lawsuits or general reluctance to criticize colleagues formally and in writing.[57] Still, the nature of the archive guaranteed that conflicts would show, even if implicitly. The ethics committees typically discussed the disagreements. If everybody agreed on what was right to do, there was no "critical moment" that led them to contact the committee. One way or the other, the files had to acknowledge and characterize these disagreements.

The archive included hundreds of files, each dedicated to one case of one patient. The earliest files were from 1986, the year when the committee began working. Documentation in the 1980s and early 1990s was shorter and less detailed than documentation in the 2010s; the files included few notes from the patients' medical charts, and I had to rely on the minutes from the ethics committee's meetings, where committee members had discussed cases collectively, in order to gather sufficient information. The committee discussed far fewer cases on its first years than it did in the 2010s. To review a comparable number of cases, I read all the files from the years 1986 to 1994 (seventy files), then compared them to the files from June 2011 to December 2012 (ninety-two files). My research assistant and I excluded six cases (8.5 percent) from the first period and seven cases (7.6 percent) from the second period that did not have sufficient information to allow us to analyze them confidently. Of the cases the ethics committee discussed from 1986 to 1994 (with sufficient information in their files), only eleven (17.2 percent) were *not* end-of-life related, compared with twenty-five (29.8 percent) from 2011 to 2012.[58] This reflected how central end-of-life care was to the committee's work.

After reading the files and summarizing them, my assistant and I categorized the stances of patients and families versus those of the clinicians. We then compared our categorizations, reaching agreement on all but one case, which we removed from the sample. Based on these categorizations, we characterized four types of cases that the ethics committee discussed, and I will define each of these types.[59]

The Economizing Patient

In *economizing patient* cases, patients or their families took a more economized stance than the clinical staff. The cases that congresspeople heard in the 1970s, as described earlier, were representative of this category. In the hospital that I studied, most of these cases were of physicians who had viable ways to prolong or sustain a patient's life, yet the patient or her family rejected them. Physicians consulted the ethics committee out of the fear that complying with this rejection and allowing the patient to die was unethical, perhaps even equivalent to assisting suicide.

As an example, Ms. Davenport, an eighty-one-year-old woman, had a severe lung disease and ulcers. A hospital surgeon operated on her ulcer, which led to numerous complications. Ms. Davenport's lungs failed, and the medical staff intubated her. At this point, her husband asked to take her home and continue caring for her there; the attending physician refused the request, stating that "discharging the patient would put her life in severe jeopardy" and referred the case to the ethics committee. The wish to economize was Ms. Davenport's husband's, hence we included the case in the economizing patient category.

In many other economizing patient cases, patients (or families) requested to economize dying, but the medical staff had internal disagreements or showed ambivalence. Mr. Evans, a marginally housed seventy-eight-year-old man, lived in the most devastated neighborhood in the hospital's area. His neighbors had reported not seeing him for several days, which eventually led them to call 911. The paramedics who responded to the call found Mr. Evans sitting in his feces and his room "in total disrepair." When they lifted him, they noticed that some skin fell off his neck, exposing what a hospital physician later diagnosed as a tumor. At the hospital, Mr. Evans told the doctors he had had difficulty getting to the food in his room; he used a mop as a walking stick, which apparently did not give him enough support. He reported treating the tumor, which started bleeding, with Kleenex tissues and said he had never consulted a physician about it. One medical note described the tumor as "quite extensive and dramatic. The floor is extremely friable and bleeding and extends all the way anteriorly to the right side with destruction of the lower two-thirds of his right ear." Still, Mr. Evans "seemed fairly unconcerned by the wound."

The attending physician's note read as a mixture of frustration and puzzlement:

I have recommended biopsy of this lesion for further histopathologic diagnosis. [The] patient has declined. I also recommended imaging of the head and neck to see the extent of [the] disease with a CT Scan as a start. The patient has also declined that. I extensively discussed the possibility of early death; however, the patient is insistent that he does not want treatment for his tumor. I have fully discussed the risks, benefits and alternatives for his plan of action and he understands.

The physician ordered a neuropsychiatry consultation to evaluate whether Mr. Evans could make decisions for himself, an ethics consultation, and a palliative care consultation. The neuropsychiatrist ruled Mr. Evans was competent and could make decisions. The palliative care physician agreed, writing in the chart that Mr. Evans

is very committed to a plan of care that defers medical interventions and hospitalization. He likes being in his apartment, and likes being in control of his [unclear] and surroundings. He agrees with a plan that avoids [hospitalization], focuses on insuring [*sic*] his physical comfort, and allows him to stay at home, even if we do not necessarily agree that it is safe. Having evaluated him along with [other doctors], I agree that he is a poor decision maker, but not an [impaired] one. He does have the ability to articulate the consequences of his actions, including infection, bedsores, and early death if he does not get appropriate help. He agrees with a hospice plan of care fundamentally. He does not want to be re-hospitalized and wants to focus on his comfort when his tumor progresses. . . . Our neuropsychology service as well as our ethic service [found him] to have decisional capacity, even if he is making decisions with which we do not agree.

Based on this assessment, the palliative care physician recommended setting up as many services as possible to assist Mr. Evans at home, including home hospice. He noted, however, that in the long term, because Mr. Evans lived alone, these services would be insufficient.

The attending physician called the ethics consultation because he was ambivalent. He wanted to treat the tumor and at the same time did not want to do it against Mr. Evans's will. His decision to call a neuropsychiatrist to evaluate Mr. Evans reflected his strong doubts about the soundness of Mr. Evans's position. The palliative care physician agreed that the tumor was treatable but thought that because Mr. Evans had a clear, consistent, and competent economized dying preference, they should not pursue curative treatment. Mr. Evans, like Mrs. Davenport's husband, leaned toward economizing dying more than the clinical staff, hence we considered this an economizing patient case.

Economizing Professionals

In *economizing professionals* cases, the clinicians leaned toward economized dying more than the patients and families. In some cases, patients or family members actively resisted economization; in others, they were indecisive, conflicted, or could not communicate because they were unconscious or demented. The clinicians associated resistance to economized dying with patients of very particular social backgrounds. Talking about end-of-life conversations that he regularly had with families and patients, a palliative care physician named Jared said,

> Jared: Well, it's an easy conversation to have with these very literate smart people. [After a good meeting with a family,] I was walking into the fishbowl—the room where all of the nurses and the doctors sit on the unit—and I said, "Gosh, that was what life would be like if all I did was take care of über-literate aristocratic white griffons. You know what I mean? We're horribly politically incorrect in our team. . . . We're just completely bigoted and awful. I take care of a lot of Chinese patients at the hospital. They're hard, man!
> Roi: Russian Jews.[60]
> Jared: [quickly] Russian Jews are BRUTAL. They're fucking hard. I mean, go back far enough, and I'm Russian Jew. I don't know, I think my family told me they're from Russia, Poland, or Ukraine—you know, eastern European ghetto trash, basically. It's embarrassing. They're so hard. . . . The Chinese are VERY hard. The Koreans are BRUTAL. . . . South Asian patients—Indian, Pakistani— . . . of the ten or fifteen cases I probably had, probably seven or eight of them have turned into a HOR-RIBLE . . . mess. . . . I'm speaking totally in generalities, because the individual patient . . . Every once in a while you'll get a Chinese family coming in and saying, "We just don't want mom to suffer. We want her to be hospice." And you're like, "What happened?" You were preparing for the battle of the three dragons, and the next thing you know is like, "Wow, that was easy."

I noticed that many clinicians had similar expectations from African American and Latino families, yet very few of them mentioned them in interviews explicitly. The few who did attributed this resistance to mistrust of the medical establishment, which derived from U.S. medicine's historical relationship with the "African American community." The racialized thinking remained, but references were covered in a thick layer of political correctness, which was absent when it came to immigrants, particularly from relatively privileged backgrounds (e.g. Russia, Korea, China, India, and Pakistan). Some of the clinicians developed quite explicit and elaborate folk theories about "culture" and "ethnicities."

> Larry: Some cultures revere the elderly, and it's sort of like they are the anchor among a family unit, and some cultures or ethnicities tend to stay in the same geographic region because that's their nature, that's what they do. . . . [So] the loss of the patriarch or matriarch can be very destabilizing [to] some family units and ethnic backgrounds . . . [more] than others. . . . You know, I can't really speak to where it comes from, but sometimes I can go into a discussion on end-of-life issues and I'm good at predicting what the outcomes [will] be based on having met family members and knowing a little bit about them and their background. You can kind of predict.
> Roi: What do you have to know about their background to predict?
> Larry: Because of the reasons I just mentioned, some ethnic groups, some religious affiliations.
> Roi: Who for example would they be?
> Larry: Oh, I don't know that I need to get specific, but you'll just have to trust me on that. [Both laugh.]

An illustrative economizing professionals' case was Ms. Poliakova's. When I gave a presentation on this chapter to a team in the hospital, my first slide included only the first sentence from Ms. Poliakova's chart: "Patient is a 96-year-old Russian woman with advanced dementia." I asked the team members how they thought the case unfolded, and got a loud collective laughter in response. They took my question as an ethnic joke. When laughter stopped, I waited an additional five to six seconds and repeated my question without smiling, until one of them said quietly, "They insisted on everything."

Ms. Poliakova's son, who was her representative, was in fact rather ambivalent. Ms. Poliakova was very sick even before her hospitalization. Her chart indicated that she could sit in her wheelchair, "speak a few words, maybe up to about seven at a time"; it also mentioned that "she may or may not understand or recognize people" and listed no fewer than twenty-one medical problems that she suffered from, including congestive heart failure, Parkinson's disease, and coronary artery disease. Over the course of one year, Ms. Poliakova had been hospitalized three times for aspiration pneumonia (pieces of food or liquid got into her lungs and infected them). Clinicians saw this as an indication that she was losing her ability to swallow; eating had become hazardous, and additional life-threatening pneumonia episodes were all but certain. To avoid these episodes, they could start feeding her through a tube; but given Ms. Poliakova's multiple medical problems and what the medical team considered a very poor quality of life, this did not feel right to them.

The team called a palliative care nurse, who met with the son and wrote that she hoped he "will not put a feeding tube in his frail mother." The son deferred to the staff on the issue of feeding tubes, yet requested that in the very likely event of Ms. Poliakova choking on her food to the point of being unable to breathe, the doctors would attempt resuscitation. Considering this a request for "non-beneficial care," the attending physician wanted to refuse. In consultation with the ethics committee, he signed a unilateral Do Not Resuscitate (DNR) order, although intubation and connection to the respirator still remained a possibility. A few days later, her condition stable, Ms. Poliakova returned to her nursing home. But a week after that, she came back to the emergency department. The doctors intubated her, transferred her to the intensive care unit (ICU), and called the palliative care nurse, who commended one of them for drawing a line in the sand:

> Our superb resident, Dan Lee, spoke with [the son] . . . on the
> phone yesterday morning. He stated this is the fourth admission
> for aspiration pneumonia this year and three of those admissions
> have been in the last three weeks. . . . Dan then spoke to him that
> she was critically ill with no realistic chance of survival and that
> when she died, we would not be instituting any further heroic
> measures.

The attending physician told the son there were no "realistic options" for treatment. He also reviewed Ms. Poliakova's advance directive, which said "she would never want to be kept alive artificially if there was no realistic hope of recovery." The son then agreed to transition her to comfort care. "I am very pleased that the son has finally chosen to honor his mother's wish and is acting in her best interest," wrote the palliative care nurse in the chart. Because the clinicians were united in recommending the withdrawal of life-sustaining care and Ms. Poliakova's son persistently resisted the recommendation, we categorized this as an economizing professionals case.

In some other economizing professionals cases, the patient and family's wishes were far less clear. Ms. Armstrong was an elderly woman with severe dementia who had bounced repeatedly between the hospital and a nursing facility where she lived. She had come to the hospital for acute pneumonia, had been discharged, and then returned with a hip fracture and osteonecrosis.* Given her advanced dementia, the orthopedic service recommended comfort care and pain management, discharging her back to the nursing facility. She returned to the hospital shortly after "for altered mental status, poor P.O. [oral] intake, and overall weakness." The physicians who treated her observed that she was malnourished, and a psychiatrist they called to evaluate her mental status wrote that her behavior was "impulsive-combative." Another note that an ethicist left in her chart described her as incapable of having "a meaningful conversation. . . . Currently, she's moaning, but is unable to verbalize if she has pain."

Ms. Armstrong did not have any known relative, and it was clear she could not express her opinions on what treatments she did and did not want. The attending physician who treated her called the ethics committee and palliative care service to consult on the case. After seeing the patient and talking with the staff, the palliative care nurse recommended to "change the code status unilaterally to one that is more medically appropriate, i.e. do not attempt resuscitation with no ICU transfer." She added that "given that challenges in obtaining consent for any services

---

* Osteonecrosis is the loss of bone tissue due to lack of blood supply, which may result from fractures.

outside of the hospital, i.e. hospice, I recommend keeping her within [our hospital] system."

Ms. Armstrong's advanced dementia and the fact she had no known relative who could legally represent her posed two challenges. One was formal: the clinicians could not have her or her legal representative formally consent to hospice care. The other had to do with the clinicians' intuitive moral sense: they seemed clear that treating Ms. Armstrong for a cure would be inappropriate, yet they hesitated to do so unilaterally without calling ethics and palliative care consultations. They leaned toward economizing Ms. Armstrong's dying, and were reluctant to cause an elderly demented woman much suffering, but hesitated to do so without her (or her relatives') approval.

Economizing professionals cases were therefore cases where, for various reasons, the medical staff leaned toward economization more than the patient and the family. This could be because the patient (or family) resisted economization actively, or because they were unable to express any wish, which left clinicians hesitating over whether they could economize legitimately.

Ethical Validation Cases

In *ethical validation* cases, the patients, families, and clinicians agreed to economize dying but were unsure whether this was ethical. They contacted the ethics committee because they needed validation that economizing dying was ethically acceptable.

An example is the case of Baby A., who was born in a "complicated and protracted childbirth." She experienced respiratory distress, and a physician performed an emergency Caesarian section delivery. Baby A had no pulse and regained it only after thirty minutes of resuscitation efforts. She was put on a respirator, and the physicians ordered an electroencephalogram to evaluate her brain function. Having learned that she suffered a severe brain injury due to lack of oxygen supply, Baby A's parents said they did not want to keep her on a respirator. According to the pediatrician's medical note, they were "insistent about taking this approach [withdrawing life support], since they justifiably feared that keeping Baby A on a respirator might leave her in a prolonged vegetative state. The pediatrician concurred, yet called an ethics consultation "to ascertain that there were no ethical problems that he was overlooking." (The ethics committee agreed that withdrawing life support would be appropriate.)

Another case in the category was Ms. Norton's, who one clinician described as "a very odd and unfortunate 88-year-old Caucasian female." Ms. Norton was hospitalized with "dehydration, acute [kidney] failure, sepsis, a-fib [irregular heartbeat], poor mental status, with limited medical h[istory] of hyperlipidemia [elevated levels of lipids in the blood]." She was estranged from her family, except one daughter-in-law who reportedly was not very close to her. The paramedics who brought her to the hospital for "inability to care for herself" found her at home "with multiple ulcers and dry, thick, scaly skin indicating she had not bathed for a long time and extremely long toenails." After her condition stabilized, Ms. Norton was transferred to the hospital's skilled nursing facility. About two months later, many of the clinicians there questioned whether treating her multiple medical problems, which they thought would require surgery, was appropriate and called an ethics consultation.

Initially, Ms. Norton refused to appoint a durable power of attorney who would serve as her surrogate decision maker. After conversation with her case manager, however, she agreed to appoint her only friend. Some two weeks later, a bioethicist, who talked to this friend, reported that the friend fully supported limiting the care Ms. Norton received to comfort measures only.

> The patient was always extremely independent. . . . She has been complaining that people are trying to make her eat. [The friend] thinks that she is probably cognitively impaired for some unknown reason. It may be a rapid acting dementia. She has lost all the things that are valuable to her in life, especially her independence and her family. . . . When I asked about what he was hoping for the patient, he said he hoped that she would have a comfortable dying. He again endorses a comfort care plan and says this is what the patient would want if she could speak for herself. . . . He does not see a point for further surgery or other interventions that prolong what appears to be very miserable existence of not being able to enjoy the things she did like and enjoy in life.

Although the patient's legal representative embraced economiza-tion—and despite Ms. Norton's own resistance to the most basic forms of care (being fed)—the clinical staff still felt they needed validation from the bioethicist. It could be that the absence of an involved blood relative, coupled with Ms. Norton's "odd" character, made them insecure about following their own clinical judgment and limiting care to comfort mea-sures only.

It is worth highlighting an interesting characteristic of ethical valida-tion cases: in all of the cases that we reviewed, clinicians sought ethical validation only when they economized dying. We did not read or ob-serve any case where a clinician asked ethicists to validate decisions to pursue additional curative, life-prolonging, or life-sustaining treatment. Such cases were outside the purview of bioethicists. It was obvious that when everybody agreed and consented, prolonging life and curing or slowing down a disease was ethical. But withdrawing or forgoing such treatment, even when done in a completely consensual manner, could still raise ethical doubts and lead clinicians to call the ethics committee. This asymmetry reflects an important feature in the ethical framing of end-of-life care: clinicians problematize economization far more than life-prolongation.

When analyzing the data, we also used a fourth category for cases where neither clinicians nor patients and families had clear and agreed-upon views on what was right to do, which we called *disorientation*.

The results indicated a significant historical change in the cases the ethics committee discussed. In the first period, there was a fairly even share of economizing patient and economizing professionals cases, whereas the second period included only seven cases (13 percent) of economizing patients (Figure 3.1). The change was statistically significant ($p < .01$).[61]

It is worth examining these seven cases from the second period in greater detail. In four of them, clinicians had doubts over patients' mental status and decision-making capacity. Two of those four cases were of pa-tients who had attempted suicide, and the clinicians thought they were too depressed to think about their condition rationally. In both cases, the ethics committee agreed and recommended that the psychiatry service would treat the depression before any end-of-life consultation took place. A third case was of a patient diagnosed with paranoid schizophrenia,

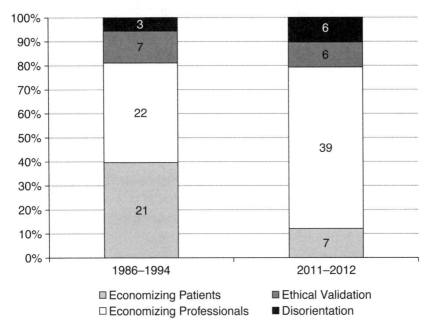

Figure 3.1. The historical change in bioethics consultations (end-of-life cases only).

who categorically refused all forms of care; the medical team hesitated to withdraw life-prolonging treatment from him given what they regarded as a mental state that compromised judgment. The fourth case was Mr. Evans's, which I described previously; the clinicians doubted his ability to make decisions for himself, but after a neuropsychiatrist had ruled he was mentally capable, they concurred with his stated wishes.

Two of the other three economizing patients cases involved physicians who were notorious for their interventionist and aggressive style. In both these cases, palliative care clinicians (a nurse and a physician) as well as other physicians criticized them. Calling the ethics service was a way to condemn the aggressive clinicians. Hence, although compared to the medical staff the patients (and their families) wanted less life-prolonging care, there was still a strong coalition of clinicians who agreed with the patients' position and advocated for it very actively. The seventh case was even more indicative, in this respect: a medical team followed a family's request to transition a severely ill and unconscious elderly patient to comfort care. After the patient passed away, a nurse called the ethics committee and claimed that the hospital was "actively speeding up the dying process . . . [and] hastening death of [patients] using morphine." The ethics committee completely dismissed these claims and recommended "better education of health care staff at [the hospital] re: EOL [end-of-life] issues, pain management, and protocol." Ultimately, none of these cases matched the blueprint that hospice and palliative care advocates have invoked of unquestionably competent and sovereign patients resisting medical staff who uniformly attempt to prolong their lives.

This hospital therefore saw a major transition between the two periods, and some anecdotal evidence suggests a similar transition occurred in other hospitals as well.[62] In 2005, Lachlan Forrow, director of the ethics program at Beth Israel Deaconess Medical Center in Boston, told the *New York Times* that "about 15 years ago, at least 80 percent of the cases were right-to-die kinds of cases" (economizing patient cases), but "today, it's more like at least 80 percent of the cases are the other direction: family members who are pushing for continued or more aggressive life support and doctors and nurses who think that that's wrong."[63] Similarly, Lisa Anderson-Shaw, cochair of the ethics committee at the University of Illinois at Chicago said she consulted on eleven such economizing professionals cases in 2004, up from two in 1998.[64]

What can explain this change?

An Age of Economizing Professionals

Rise in Vitalist Patients

A first explanation for this shift lies in a change in patients' and families' stances on life prolongation. The Pew Research Center surveyed the U.S. adult population in 1990, 2005, and 2013, asking respondents which statement they preferred: "In all circumstances, doctors and nurses should do everything possible to save the life of a patient," or "Sometimes there are circumstances where a patient should be allowed to die."[65] In each of the surveys a significant majority preferred the second and more economizing statement, but this majority has declined from 73 to 66 percent (Figure 3.2).

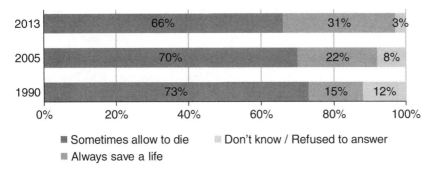

Figure 3.2. General positions on life prolongation. Data source: Pew Research Center, "Views on End-of-Life Medical Treatments," March 21–April 8, 2013.

More significantly, the size of the minority that supports prolonging life in all circumstances more than doubled from 1990 to 2013. This growth occurred in all age groups, education backgrounds, racial identities, and religious affiliations. Even among people who said they dedicated "a great deal of thought to end-of-life wishes"—presumably, a population that engages and reflects on the topic—support for the "always save a life" statement climbed from 9 to 24 percent during the period.

There were, however, significant and important differences in the *levels* of resistance to economization between social groups. In 2013, Latino (59 percent) and African American (52 percent) respondents were far more likely to endorse the "always save a life" statement than white respondents (20 percent).[66] Furthermore, people with no college education were more likely to endorse it (43 percent) than those with some college education (22 percent) and college graduates (18 percent). Finally, respondents who attended worship services weekly endorsed the statement at higher rates (36 percent) than those attending them weekly or monthly (30 percent) and those who seldom or never attended services (25 percent).[67]

At least some of these disparities are attributable to experiences of discrimination in the health care system. There is ample evidence of pervasive biases in the U.S. health care system against patients of socially marginalized backgrounds. African American dialysis patients, for example, are less likely than other patients to receive evaluation for kidney transplantation, be placed on a waitlist for organ transplants, or even be informed about the possibility of receiving a transplant from a donor or a family member.[68] African American men are 20 percent less likely to receive a recommendation for coronary artery bypass grafting compared with white and Hispanic men,[69] and African American children are less likely to receive an acute respiratory tract infection diagnosis and be treated with broad-spectrum antibiotics than their white counterparts.[70] People of color, however, are more likely to be hospitalized involuntarily and be treated with antipsychotic drugs than white people.[71]

Other forms of social marginalization are also common in hospitals. Numerous medical ethnographers have documented how medical teams invested less effort in fighting for the lives of individuals to whom they assigned low social and moral worth.[72] As David Sudnow put it, such patients included "the suicide victim, the dope addict, the known prostitute, the assailant in a crime of violence, the vagrant, the known wife-beater, and, generally, those persons whose moral character are considered reproachable."[73] Some of the clinicians that I studied spoke very openly about taking social worth into consideration when they made life-and-death decisions. An infectious disease specialist said,

> There are a lot of things that sway you. And some of them are medical and some of them are sociological. The age of the patient. I mean, you're always willing to give the benefit of the doubt more to a younger person. You're willing to give the benefit of the doubt more to a person who has a usual lifestyle, has a family, has friends, is employed, is a meaningful member of society than you would be to an addict, or a street person. . . . We'll certainly try less hard for a homeless, family-less, drug-abuser with chronic hepatitis C than we would for a retired school teacher with a family and friends and good quality of life. . . . And part of that is legitimate: you know, who's gonna be there to help them as they recover. . . . But you know, a lot of it is how much you identify with the family, and how much do you like the family, and how much you're gonna be swayed by the family's wishes.

Marginalized populations are particularly vulnerable to such judgments because physicians judge patients of color and of lower socioeconomic status more negatively than they judge white and wealthy patients. As van Ryn and Burke showed, physicians tend to assume that patients of color and patients of lower socioeconomic status lack the social support and character needed to comply with recommended courses of care. Consequently, patients from these social groups receive fewer recommendations for rehabilitation, for example.[74]

It is unsurprising that people who experienced discrimination throughout their life would be suspicious and untrusting of economization when they or their family members face serious illness. Many of the clinicians I studied even expected people they considered "marginalized" to resist recommendations to economize. Quite tragically, acknowledging discrimination only made clinicians see their patients through racial and class lenses and was likely to reproduce experiences of marginalization.[75]

Such discrimination, however, may explain social differences in vitalist stances but not the historical growth in these stances across all social groups. This growth is easier to explain as an outcome of the social and financial changes that apply to the entire U.S. society and economy. Anthropologist Sharon Kaufman argued that in the United States today, "most deaths, regardless of a person's age, have come to be considered premature. . . . For every ambivalent [patient], there is another patient who aggressively pursues treatment in the hope of staying alive, and there are others (though far fewer) who firmly reject treatment."[76] Kaufman attributed this to the dramatic growth of the U.S. medical-industrial complex. The private pharmaceutical and medical device industry's expansion has created an enormous market, which inundates people with information about treatment options for themselves or their family members. Websites targeting health care consumers, Internet forums, billboards, and television commercials that encourage people to "talk to your doctor" about a new device, therapy, medication, or surgery create the impression that miracle cures are out there, waiting for proactive, well-informed patients to find them. Even a person who, in principle, would not like to have her life prolonged in all circumstances, may act differently when facing a serious illness with three or four treatment options. Such "options" are hardly ever curative, but once they are on the table they are very hard to reject.

This is particularly important because declaring one's wish to forgo life-prolonging treatment in an advance directive form is far easier than forgoing it in practice. One of the later cases that I reviewed was of

Ms. North, a ninety-four-year-old woman, who throughout her life had been very clear she would *not* want her life prolonged if she faced a terminal illness. She filled out an advance directive, which her physicians read as unequivocal: one medical note described it as outlining "a clear Do Not Resuscitate order and the hope to avoid a prolonged end of life." Ms. North also talked to her husband about her wishes, who (according to an ethicist) understood them and was determined to represent them properly. After an operation to remove a bowel obstruction, Ms. North had acute kidney failure; the surgery service opined that "while potentially she could be operated on [again], it was unlikely she would return to her former level of independence and quality of life and her risk of mortality was high." The service saw her best case scenario as a "prolonged ICU stay," followed by a "very long" stay at a nursing facility. Three other physicians, including the ICU attending, agreed with this prognosis.

Ms. North's cardiologist, however, dissented, believing that her "abdominal issues should be resolved soon." With this far more optimistic prognosis, the family, who were very involved in Ms. North's care, became interested in treatment options for her kidney failure, specifically dialysis. "Her family is asking good questions," wrote the palliative care physician after talking to them, "but they realize that at this point, . . . the question is whether the current plan for supportive care will lead to a quality of life that she will be happy with, or whether this will only [be] prolonging a state of chronic illness and debility." The family agreed to not "escalate" care, but at the time requested to continue artificial nutrition and antibiotics for two to three additional days, hoping that Ms. North's condition would improve.

'It was a big time team conflict,' one of the people involved in the case told me:

> It's a case of a health care provider, a professional, who lacks understanding about end-of-life care. And then surrogate decision makers knew what the patient wanted but were unable or made to feel guilty for what they were doing. . . . [This attending is] elderly. His privileges have also been restricted because of these kinds of problems. He also doesn't believe in pain medications.

While dismissed as an "elderly" person who "lacks understanding"—some outdated remnant from a distant professional past—the cardiologist's medical opinion was anchored in the present. The hospital where he worked *had* dialysis machines, multiple trained surgery teams, and many other means to prolong life in severe illness. Using them was an option, and once a physician recommended them, even people who were confident and firm about their economized dying preference ended up hesitating. Mr. North, as the palliative care physician described him, "focused mostly on [Ms. North's] kidney function." This case shows how disagreement within the team could quickly turn into doubt among family members. It is very easy to sway families and patients toward vitalism, and much of the U.S. health care system is built to do that.[77]

Another source of vitalist attitudes lies in nonprofessional actors. Sociologist Renée Anspach argued that since the 1980s the field of bioethics has experienced a gradual "hostile takeover" by the conservative Christian right. Conservative figures presented the "right to life" as a mirror image of "the right to die." This conservative advocacy embraced the language and framing of progressive bioethicists, citing ethical arguments about human and civil rights in support of categorical life prolongation.[78] Republican officials' allegations about "death panels" and "government-encouraged euthanasia" further politicized economization and made it controversial. This impacted public opinion significantly (see the introduction) and fed the prevalent antipathy toward the idea of rationing care at the bedside.[79] Several of the ethical consultations that I read mentioned families who resisted economization for religious reasons. As end-of-life decisions became politicized, these families' political and religious identities led them to embrace more vitalist stances.

In summary, part of the significant decline in economizing patient cases derived from changes in the attitudes of patients and families. Today, U.S. clinicians see more patients and families who enter the hospital with vitalist predilections than they saw 20 years ago. Furthermore, in the context of an expanding health care market, where people make decisions while an enormous industry offers them numerous life-prolonging interventions, even the most economizing patients may tilt toward vitalism.

The higher rates of vitalist attitudes among marginalized populations in the United States should be a priority for researchers in the area.

For one thing, at least some of these attitudes are attributable to well-documented discrimination within the health care system. The new economy of dying is no different than the traditional health care system. The dominance of white patients' voices—and the virtual absence of African American and Latino ones—dates back to the first occasions when advocates summoned terminal patients and their families to speak about their experiences. It is of little surprise that forty years later people of color express less economizing stances: they have been marginalized within the new economy of dying since its emergence and have had little to no influence on the shape it has taken.

Although advocates purported to respond to the universal needs of all patients, this economy grew around experiences of upper-class and middle-class white people, which differ from other groups' experiences. Stereotypical stances about inherent "cultural" and "ethnic" dispositions only cement this marginalization. People of color, immigrants, and people of lower socioeconomic status are consequently more likely to find themselves at odds with a medical profession that pressures them to economize dying, then judges them negatively if they resist.

The Rise of Economizing Clinicians

The second driver of the relative decline in economizing patients and the rise in economizing clinicians cases lies in the medical profession. As shown in Chapter 1, since the 1960s, parallel to the growth of the medical-industrial complex and rise in vitalism, some of the U.S. medical profession moved in the opposite direction, toward economized dying. This move has not achieved complete dominance in medical practice. As the case of Ms. North shows, there are physicians whose clinical intuitions are very far from it. But the power of the movement to economize is growing, not only thanks to the rise in the number of palliative care clinicians and services in hospitals but also because of the moral authority they have assumed. Discussions of economization have pervaded even the most acute care environments. A study that compared mortality in two ICUs found that from 1987 to 1988, decisions to withdraw or withhold life support preceded 51 percent of the deaths, compared with 90 percent in 1992 to 1993. Physicians in these ICUs performed CPR in 49 percent of the deaths in 1987 to 1988, compared with only 10 percent of the deaths in 1992 to 1993. In the authors' words, "90% of patients who die in these ICUs now do so following a decision to limit therapy."[80] "Limitation of life support prior to death is the dominant practice in American ICUs," the authors concluded elsewhere.[81]

Patients (and families) who are not interested in life-prolonging treatment are today more likely to find professional allies within the hospital than they were in the past: palliative care and other clinicians who have been exposed to hospice and palliative care. In some cases (such as Ms. North's), these allies would confront and counter their more "aggressive" colleagues; in others, they would call for a palliative care or an ethics consultation, which would often present comfort care as an alternative to life-prolonging treatments.

At the same time, the patients who for various reasons resist economization may find themselves at odds with the professional predilections of a growing number of clinicians and the financial imperatives of a growing number of hospitals. Such disagreements between patients and families who want to continue life-prolonging treatment and clinicians who strongly believe it is inappropriate are therefore a very central challenge in economizing dying in U.S. hospitals.

Conclusion

This chapter describes a historical shift: since the 1980s, the average U.S. patient moved several steps away from economized dying, while the average hospital clinician moved several steps toward it. By consequence, economizing professionals disputes, in which professionals struggle to convince patients and their families to forgo or withdraw life-prolonging care, have become more common. This chapter shows a growing discrepancy between economization and the wishes of many patients and families. Medical scholars and practitioners have treated end-of-life care as both "a method to find out what the patient wants" and "a mechanism to reduce medical care and thereby contain costs."[82] In reality, however, the two often contradict each other. When confronting concrete medical decisions, patients and families may want more life-prolonging treatment than clinicians are willing to give.

There are social inequalities built into this discrepancy between patients' and clinicians' stances on end-of-life care. White, highly educated, and secular people are more likely to identify with economization, and their personal inclinations tend to resonate with the direction medicine has taken. This is no coincidence: socially advantaged groups were the ones who moved medicine toward economization. They had the power to represent patients, speak in Congress, write open editorials, publish memoires, and establish the image of the average dying patient as a person who fights against faceless, heartless, and rational men of science, who seek to prolong life without regard for patient preferences. These people successfully presented their own views and experiences as the average views and experiences—hence, views and experiences that in some way were relevant to the general population. The hospice and palliative care movement embraced and promoted them as credible patient representatives. Patients who supported economizing dying not only provided the movement with moral legitimacy but also with a professional raison d'être. It was these patients for whom hospice and palliative care advocates worked.[83]

Hospice and palliative care advocates have drawn on the assertion that patients themselves would "dis-elect the most aggressive therapy" if allowed to make medical decisions for themselves.[84] The movement's advocates presented economized dying as a win-win-win situation: it provided better care, which patients and families wanted anyway, and which happened to be less expensive. This chapter challenges this view. While at least according to survey data, most U.S. adults support economization to some degree, it appears that the closer people are to the end of life, the more interested they become in life-prolongation. Asking a healthy person whether she would want her life prolonged if she were bedbound and dependent on machines is very different from asking a bedbound and machine-dependent person if she is ready to die. Such patients, even if not the majority of the U.S. population, accounted for an overwhelming majority of the ethical consultations in the hospital I studied. There was clear, significant, and consistent resistance to economized dying.

Hospice and palliative care practitioners tend to portray themselves as professional underdogs, and for many decades this is what they were. Their success in promoting their movement, however, meant that the reality they criticized in the 1970s has changed fundamentally. The movement is now an established medical field, in which economizing dying is the rule. A principal tension has emerged, however: there is a growing population whose inclinations conflict with economization. The further U.S. medicine moves toward economization, the deeper the split between vitalist patients and medical professionals will become, and the more necessary bridging it will be. The next chapter examines this work of bridging between the professional and organizational pressure to economize and patients' inclinations.

CHAPTER 4

Making the Dying Subject

We do not know where death awaits us:
so let us wait for it everywhere.

—Michel de Montaigne

THE TRAGIC DEATH OF Jahi McMath took place about a year after I concluded my fieldwork, in a hospital that I did not study. But it was dramatic and impactful enough to merit a trip back to the field. For over a month, the national media covered an excruciating legal battle over McMath's medical diagnosis. At stake was not whether her illness was terminal or curable but whether she was dead or alive.

In December 2013, thirteen-year-old McMath underwent an elective surgery to treat her sleep apnea. As she was recovering, she suffered massive blood loss, which led to cardiac arrest and hypoxia (interrupted oxygen supply). She stayed at the Oakland Children's Hospital's intensive care unit (ICU), unconscious and connected to a mechanical ventilator. Three days after the surgery, the hospital's neurology team declared her brain-dead. McMath's mother, however, refused to accept the diagnosis. In the weeks that followed, she and a group of supporters launched a legal battle to reverse the diagnosis and force the hospital to "keep Jahi alive." Neurologists from other hospitals came to evaluate McMath's condition as independent experts, and they all concurred that McMath was brain-dead—a diagnosis that the court accepted as well. Yet McMath's mother maintained her position and appealed the decision, demanding that the hospital keep her daughter connected to the ventilator and continue feeding her artificially. After settlement talks, as dozens of supporters (notably, members of the Paradise Baptist Church) held vigils outside the hospital, the hospital administration decided to allow McMath's mother to transfer her to another facility. The local coroner's office issued McMath a death certificate, and she was transferred to an undisclosed location. As of May 2018, she was still connected to a mechanical ventilator and feeding tubes.[1]

Shortly after the court ruling, Academic Hospital organized an event with a panel of experts who discussed the case: two lawyers, a neurosurgeon, and Rick, one of Academic's palliative care physicians. For Rick, McMath's case was familiar. 'These are traumatic and difficult deaths,' he said to the audience. 'If you look at a brain-dead person—these people don't look dead. Their chest goes up and down, their hands and feet are warm. . . . Families tell you that there is meaningful response even though none of us [clinicians] sees it.' This case, Rick said, 'was the tip of the tip of the iceberg.' Underneath that tip were hundreds of other contested cases that did not make it to court or draw national media attention because he and his colleagues resolved them preemptively. Indeed, Academic Hospital's neurologists diagnosed brain death regularly, and Rick has consulted on several very similar cases with families who initially refused to accept these diagnoses. In more common cases—the *economizing professionals* cases, which I discussed in detail in Chapter 3—physicians thought that their patients had poor prognoses and that life-sustaining care would merely prolong their suffering, while their families demanded to keep them alive. 'Most of the conflicts are resolved very quickly, within days,' Rick said. 'These are issues that can be resolved with good communication.'

Listening to Rick, I thought he did not give himself enough credit. He was right that he and his colleagues were superb conflict resolvers, but he did not mention that in most cases they economized dying without even letting conflict emerge. They bridged the gap between families' and patients' expectations and the drive to limit life-prolonging treatment without anyone noticing that such a gap had ever existed. This chapter analyzes the different techniques palliative care teams employ, explains how they economize dying without conflict, and examines how they manage conflict when it does occur. In line with patient autonomy principles, these techniques focus on patients as sovereign subjects. The palliative care practitioners did not prioritize economization over their patients' wishes, but they infused patients' wishes with economizing elements. They engaged patients and families in reflections about themselves, which ultimately increased the probability that these people would embrace economization as their own goal.

The chapter's title—"making the dying subject"—plays on two meanings of the term *subject*. First, a subject means a person—a self-aware being, capable of reflection, judgment, and purposeful action. In the United States, people typically associate subjectivity with individuality: what makes one a subject are the individual choices she makes and the actions she takes.[2] Not all of the patients I observed had the same propensity to choose and act. In the hospital environment, social differences played out as inequalities in what Janet Shim called "cultural health capital."[3] Some patients studied their diagnosis actively, researched the various treatment options they might have, and asserted themselves in meetings with the medical staff; others withdrew, overwhelmed and perplexed by their disease and prognosis, and seemed estranged from the hospital environment and the numerous physicians who visited them. To the medical staff, patients in this latter group appeared reclusive, passive, uninterested, or incompetent. Aging and dying were often associated with such a withdrawal: loss of capacity to reflect, articulate, and act on one's wishes meant that clinicians had difficulty taking the patient as a subject into account when they reached decisions on her or his care.[4] This chapter shows how the clinicians I followed *made dying subjects*—that is, made the dying patients' agency manifest and affect decisions, even when they seemed passive or experienced decline in their mental and physical capacity.

A second meaning of the word *subject* is in its conjugation as a verb: *subjecting* means placing something (or somebody) under the control or influence of something else.[5] Following Michel Foucault, Louis Althusser, and Nikolas Rose I argue that the process of *subjectification*, in which patients became self-aware subjects with intelligible and expressible personalities, combined empowerment with control.[6] For one thing, patients did not only articulate and voice themselves—clinicians *expected* that they would articulate and voice themselves. For another, once patients voiced themselves, clinicians started managing them according to what they said; when palliative care clinicians *made dying subjects*, they also made the dying *subject to* this management and, as I will show, to economization.[7]

The previous chapter discussed final and fairly firm positions that patients, family members, and clinicians took in various cases: their support, ambivalence, or resistance to economization. This chapter analyzes how such positions developed dynamically in interactions between patients and clinicians: how people came to decide and articulate what they thought, felt, and wanted, how clinicians incited them to process and express these thoughts, feelings, and wishes in certain ways, and how clinicians made up their own minds about what was moral to do given what they understood about their patients. I follow the ambivalent, conflicted, and equivocal moments, in which people articulated (or acted on) their support or resistance to economized dying. In these moments, palliative care practice—specifically, how palliative care clinicians consolidated a sense of what patients wanted and who patients were—pushed ambiguity and hesitation toward economization. Methodologically, this chapter goes beyond the formal notes that clinicians left in medical charts and draws on participant observations of interactions between clinicians, patients, and family members as well as reflections clinicians shared in interviews.

The chapter's first section shows that economizing dying was *not* the only consideration that guided clinicians' work near the end of life. I show that acting in line with patients' personalities, preferences, and wishes was no less and, in many cases, far more important to these clinicians. In several instances, they decided to prolong patients' lives against their best medical judgment just because they thought patients wanted them to do so. The second section analyzes how palliative care clinicians made dying subjects—namely, how they constructed a sense of who their patients were, what they thought, and what they wanted in situations where these patients were communicative or uncommunicative, expressive or inarticulate, and active or passive. Finally, in the third section, I show that when making dying subjects, clinicians also tended to *subject* patients *to* economized dying and in effect bridged between the patients and economization. Economization was not an external political, medical, and financial power that clinicians applied to patients. It was a power that operated through the ways patients articulated and defined themselves. This was a most important part of the effort to economize dying: making patients subjects who wanted to economize their own death.

In Their Wishes We Trust

"At Least This Was Her Own Wish"

Leslie Small had advanced liver cancer, which a Public Hospital oncologist diagnosed as terminal. Because of her old age and poor condition, she did not qualify for a liver transplant. In consultation with the medical team, she and her family signed Do Not Resuscitate (DNR) and Do Not Intubate (DNI) forms. They also agreed to have her discharged to hospice, but then changed their mind and left the hospice.[8] She was admitted, discharged, then readmitted to Public Hospital "maybe a good four times since the first time I . . . met her," Dr. Anna Nelson, a general internist who treated Ms. Small, said in an interview about a month after Ms. Small had passed away.

> And each time it was from home, from the family who was taking care of her around the clock. You know, [she was admitted] for various infections, and decompensation of her liver, and in the course of these multiple returns, multiple other medical teams had conversations with [her and her family] about hospice, and [about] going home and not coming back to the hospital.

But Ms. Small and her family insisted that they did not want hospice. Whenever her condition declined, they wanted her to be admitted to the hospital, to be stabilized to the extent that was possible, and then to be discharged back home until the next decline and hospitalization. They knew that the underlying cause of her illness, her cancer, could not be treated, but they also saw that the individual problems that the cancer caused—for example, multiple infections—could be isolated and solved for the short-term if they brought her to the hospital.[9] A palliative care physician from another hospital said this way of caring was equivalent to 'patching patients up, then sending them back home.'

Like other physicians, Dr. Nelson thought Ms. Small would be better off in hospice. "When it's right to advocate for the person to not continue coming back [to the hospital]—I will do so," she told me. Moreover, Dr. Nelson thought that treating Ms. Small in the hospital was "not a great use of our resources." She was working in the scarcely resourced environment of U.S. public medicine, where access to even the most basic medical services was compromised. Providing intensive treatments that had questionable benefit did not feel right to her. Unsure whether she was helping Ms. Small or just prolonging her suffering, Dr. Nelson leaned toward economizing dying. But she still hesitated. For one thing, she thought it would be illegal for her to refuse to provide life-prolonging treatment to Ms. Small:

> I have never signed anything that says, "it's medically futile for this person to continue coming back to the hospital." I've never done that. . . . If the family member, or somebody else says [that they want to be hospitalized] then there's nothing out there for me. I don't say I don't do anything to keep that from happening. I might think that it's not a great thing, but I don't [think] there's anything legal in place that allows me to say, "no, I don't think this person should come back to the hospital."

Not all physicians were as wary of potential legal proceedings. Dr. Nelson was fairly young—in her mid-30s—and she had started working in the hospital only a few months before the case began unfolding. A young physician who makes her first steps at a new hospital is likely to avoid conflict. But I also talked to more senior physicians, and they insisted that hospitals should not shy away from litigation when it was clear that treatments were medically futile. Some of them even doubted that hospitals faced a legal risk; courts rule on compensation based on patients' lost life years and lost earnings, which are both very low for elderly and severely ill people.[10]

Yet Dr. Nelson's reluctance to discharge the patient from the hospital was not simply due to her fear of litigation. She also had *moral* qualms about forcing a hospital discharge because she wanted to respect what she understood were Ms. Small's genuine wishes.[11]

> The patient was very lucid, and she was lucid enough to say, "I want to come back to the hospital." . . . And someone who has the presence

of mind to do so, I think that we're less comfortable telling you, "No, you can't do that." At the end of the day—you're dying. And we like to honor people's dying wishes. . . . So in the case of this woman, even though her coming back to the hospital repeatedly was not a good use of resources, and not a good use of her time or anybody else's—we still allowed that. I don't think anybody felt there was anything wrong with it. . . . Really, we didn't think that coming back [to the hospital] was helping her so much. But I think we were all comforted in knowing that at least this was her own wish. And that the family . . . hadn't forced it on her.

Four things validated Ms. Small's wish to be in the hospital. First, she was "very lucid" and had "the presence of mind" to insist she wanted to be hospitalized. Second, her family did not seem to force the decision upon her. Third, Dr. Nelson found the family credible because they were very dedicated and took care of Ms. Small "around the clock." And finally, Dr. Nelson valued the family's intellect and judgment; she told me they were "actually, a very medically sophisticated family. And they understood—she was DNR [Do Not Resuscitate], DNI [Do Not Intubate] from very early on. They understood that her condition was not reversible." Strong family ties, good communication with the medical staff, and intelligence that impressed her physician endowed Ms. Small with social power. Her wishes were articulated, voiced, and understood, and Dr. Nelson and her colleagues were "comforted" in knowing that whether medically right or wrong, they were fulfilling them. Certainty with regard to Ms. Small's wishes mitigated the moral uncertainty over the soundness of prolonging her life. Having a sense that, dubious as it was, the treatment they were providing corresponded to what Ms. Small wanted was reassuring.

The significance of patients' wishes for clinicians' moral comfort manifested in opposite cases as well. *Uncertainty* over what patients wanted often led to moral doubt and distress. Several clinicians in another hospital shared with me their unease about a case that had been unfolding for about two years, of a patient in a persistent vegetative state whose son insisted on dialyzing twice a week. The patient, I was told, had originally written an advance directive stating that he did not want his life sustained in a vegetative state. Yet his son, whom he listed as a Durable Power of

Attorney,* said that before losing consciousness the patient told him he had changed his mind.

Many clinicians thought the son was not credible. They cited his rare visits to the hospital, which they thought reflected that he was not truly close to his father, and they mentioned that he had a financial interest in keeping his father alive—the father received monthly pension payments from which the son benefited. A general internist who treated the patient told me:

> We brought this up at the ethics meeting . . . got the lawyers involved, got the palliative care [and] ethics team involved. The totally wimpy ethics team said "[the son is] a Durable Power [of Attorney], he says that's what he wants, we haven't gotten a legal stand on it, we're gonna keep dialyzing him." So everybody's so afraid of the death panel, when all that they will have to do will be to meet with this son, say to him, "Bring your lawyer, okay? This has been going on for years, so there's no chance in the world that [the patient] will ever come back [and regain consciousness]." [Fast, impatiently:] But [the son is] hoping for a miracle, that's his point.
>
> The patient was aspirating, [because] we fed him too much through his tube. And I put a long note in the chart, saying, "If we feed him below this level he doesn't aspirate. If he has any sensation, aspiration would be worse than hunger, therefore let's feed him less." And I thought I had a program that would starve him. But somebody turned up the tube feeding, and I guess he's tolerating it, and now his weight stabilized.

This physician openly said in an interview that he had tried indirectly to euthanize his patient. Whether he did so or not—and regardless of how serious his alleged attempt was—sharing this story with me was the physician's way of expressing his deep moral discomfort. He thought the patient was being mistreated and was frustrated with the hospital's reluctance to confront the son. Unlike Ms. Small's family, the son failed to prove his closeness to his father, and the doctors suspected other moti-

---

* Durable Power of Attorney (DPOA) is a person who has a legal right to make decisions on behalf of the patient if she loses decision-making capacity.

vations. Lack of credibility led to disagreement on the patient's wishes and to conflict that threatened to reach the courts.

Perhaps the strongest indication of how important patients' own wishes were for clinicians was that even when clinicians had very strong opinions on a certain case, and the patient (and family) lacked any power to resist, the clinicians still hesitated about what they should do. Mr. Bennett, a white homeless man in his 70s, who clinicians thought suffered from stomach cancer, was hospitalized in Public Hospital in a condition that seemed to his doctors to be terminal. I write "thought" and "seemed" because none of the staff managed to have a significant conversation with him; consequently, his diagnosis was unclear. According to the oncology service, he refused a biopsy, and the clinicians relied on a patchwork of past medical records, which the social worker had worked hard to collect from free clinics and other health and social services he had used. Although Mr. Bennett spoke clearly and heard reasonably well, he rejected every person who tried to communicate with him. His bedside nurse, a gentle young man who had been treating him for a few days when we first met, told me that 'he usually just says "no" to everything.'

The palliative care social worker began looking for people who knew Mr. Bennett in some way or another and could help her and the rest of the team understand his condition and wishes. Over several days of work, she organized a large meeting with hospital clinicians from several services, a social worker from a shelter Mr. Bennett frequented, and a community doctor who had seen him sporadically about a year or two earlier. Also in the meeting was one of the hospital's case managers, who voiced the hospital's financial considerations on the case.

Sitting around a Formica table in a TV room that for one hour served as a conference room, the various doctors, nurses, social workers, and other personnel talked about their repeated failure to engage Mr. Bennett in conversation. A psychiatrist who came to evaluate Mr. Bennett's decision-making capacity explained at length the cognitive tests he used in his work, only to admit at the end of his presentation that Mr. Bennett refused to complete any of the tests, so he was unable to evaluate his capacity. The psychiatrist suggested that because Mr. Bennett refused any biopsy or treatment of his cancer, 'his preference is probably to get discharged home.'

Mr. Bennett posed an organizational problem. On the one hand, the clinicians could not treat him in the hospital because he rejected even being talked to or touched. On the other hand, he was badly ill, utterly destitute, had no home or known family who could take care of him, and thus could not be discharged safely from the hospital. The community physician, who had seen Mr. Bennett in the past, said that his impression was that he had a very short time to live, so they had three treatment options: they could keep him in the hospital; they could send him back to a shelter—which, given his condition, he noted, was not a good idea; or they could find him a nursing home. The case manager immediately dismissed the first option, arguing that there was no justification to keep him hospitalized: Mr. Bennett refused care and was occupying a hospital bed unnecessarily, which was a waste of resources. Yet without being able to communicate with Mr. Bennett in any way, the clinicians found it hard to decide to admit him to hospice, even if a bed at a public inpatient hospice facility, which served the county's uninsured patients, became available.

Two weeks later, Mr. Bennett was still in the hospital. Two palliative care nurses who tried to visit him agreed that 'he was clearly distressed just from our presence by his bed and was relieved when we left.' This prolonged hospitalization seemed to torment him, and it was difficult for the staff as well. The problem of how to care for a severely ill patient who refused to convey any type of preference except for the wish to be left alone seemed unsolvable. A long life in social isolation and extreme poverty had made him virtually asocial—he did not engage in conversation and did not express any wishes that clinicians could follow or acknowledge. The medical staff began a long, slow process of conservatorship, which meant that a court-appointed individual would take on the responsibility of representing him in medical decision making.

Days later, however, the palliative care social worker reported at a team meeting that she had found a distant relative of Mr. Bennett's. The team rejoiced:

Physician: Did anyone see Mr. Bennett yesterday?
Chaplain: Yeah, he kicked me out of the room [laughs].
Social worker: You know, I talked to a second cousin of his in Minnesota,
    [Physician: Really?]—and he described him as being very guarded, but

a very nice human being and a quiet person. He told me a lot about him, that he likes walking in parks, and that he was born in this area. And the cousin is visiting California this week for a family event, so he's going to come to the hospital.

Physician: Great! Ohh, wonderful! So we're going to have a meeting with him.

Social worker: I didn't get a sense that they were very close. They talked to each other a few times a year, and I started asking about what [Mr. Bennett] valued in his life, but I didn't get a sense that he had a good sense of it. But he did want to help, he sounds very nice. . . .

Physician: It's great, it's great. Such good news, really. I think what we're hoping from [the cousin] is not a ton. If he's visiting him—it's great. But I think that just, if we can have someone who can say . . . [Mr. Bennett] is in agreement with being discharged, but I think we're uncomfortable because he doesn't have an insight into his condition. The reality is that there's not a lot of options, it's just kind of [saying], this is what we're thinking. Does that sound okay to you, and are you willing to sign him in and be an emergency contact for him if the [hospice] doctors have any question? If he's cool with that then. . . . Phew! We can get out of the conservatorship.

Nurse [to the social worker]: How did you manage to get a hold of [this cousin]? Do you have a private investigator or what? . . .

Physician: You saved the county *so* much money! You should get a little commission!

Finding a distant cousin who could help make medical decisions for Mr. Bennett provided the team with some moral relief. Although, as the physician noted, Mr. Bennett was clearly dying and there was not much to decide about anyway, the clinicians were still somewhat 'uncomfortable because he doesn't have an insight into his condition.' A cousin who knew him, as distant as he was, could remedy this situation by giving his own consent to the transfer.

As the physician's last comment shows, this moral challenge had financial implications. Mr. Bennett was uninsured, and although the social worker applied for Medicaid coverage for him, this would never cover the cost of his prolonged hospital stay. But it is worth noting how strong the clinicians' moral motivation was in this case. Mr. Bennett's ability to resist transfer was very limited: he was physically impaired, extremely unlikely to sue, and had no friend or relation who could push back against the medical staff and the hospital. Nevertheless—and despite the hospital's financial interest, staff members' wish to rid themselves of a frustrating patient, and the clinicians' best medical judgment that hospice would be the most appropriate to him—they hesitated to move forward without clearer guidance from a relative. The detective work done to find a cousin on the other side of the country shows how important it was for the staff to find solutions that they felt were morally acceptable.

Clinicians treated patients' wishes as an important moral compass. Knowing that a patient wanted a certain treatment was orienting, and this orientation was crucial in cases where the boundary between beneficence and maleficence was murky. At the same time, concluding what patients' wishes were was often difficult. The more doubtful and obscure these wishes were, the more strenuous and ambivalent making decisions became. The clearer and more trusted the wishes were, the more certain and confident the involved parties were in economizing dying or prolonging life. The patients with stronger social ties and with intellect that impressed clinicians were far more likely to present clear and undisputed wishes that the clinicians would follow.

Solving a Practical Problem

The clinicians' interest in patients' and families' views also had a practical dimension: it helped avoid conflict and streamline the patients' care. Several palliative care clinicians told me that being attentive and showing interest in people's experiences was important for "building trust" with them. When people felt heard, they were more likely to be satisfied with the conversation's outcome, agree to leave the hospital when recommended, and be more receptive to economization. One palliative care physician said,

> Oftentimes, when I meet someone for the first time, I will just sit and listen and say very little. People can talk for forty minutes straight, which feels like a really long time, but it makes it actually faster, because they've told the whole story, they know that you kind of

understand where they're coming from, so I think that builds a lot of trust. . . . It's mostly a trust issue. I spend a lot of time listening, trying to understand what's important to people.

In a conversation at a palliative care meeting, a fellow physician from the same service said that listening to patients and families made them more likely to forgo resuscitation and intubation:

> It's important to let families talk. . . . I actually got the sense that when you come in[to a meeting] with your list of things that you want to say, and you just go through them, and come out of the meeting and think to yourself, "Great, I covered everything that I wanted," eventually it turns out that these patients stay Full Code.*

Listening to patients and families was also informative to clinicians. One of the palliative care clinicians' main goals was reaching a "safe-discharge plan" from the hospital—bringing patients to a condition that allows them to continue their treatment elsewhere, which usually meant home (with or without home hospice) or a nursing home. A good discharge plan has to meet the needs and life circumstances of all those involved. That is, a daughter or son who works full-time cannot be the only care-giver for a parent who needs around-the-clock care; a terminally ill patient who lives alone needs to move to an inpatient facility at some point. "Bad plans" are likely to result in readmissions to the hospital, which may incur penalties from Medicare and Medicaid.[12] The hospital staff was thus dependent on the family members who cared for the patients after discharge—they had to understand what those members needed to keep the patient out of the hospital.[13]

But there was another challenge. Even if a discharge plan met every-one's work schedule, housing situation, and care needs, patients could still return to the hospital because they wanted more curative care. When meeting patients and their family members, palliative care clinicians tried to intuit "where they are" so that they could match a care plan to their predilections and increase the chances the patients would stay wherever

---

* A Full Code status means that physicians will attempt resuscitation (and, if needed, intubation) if a patient's heart stops.

they are placed. About a month into my fieldwork at Academic Hospital, I heard of an elderly patient who had a combination of heart and kidney failure. Her son and daughter-in-law had been nursing her very closely; a resident who had met them the day before mentioned that they were both chemists who thought of illness in very rational and technical terms. 'They document everything,' he said to the palliative care team. The son 'was able to tell me that she [the patient] coughed nine times since the morning, and also in exactly how many of them she had bloody product.'

That afternoon, I joined the palliative care social worker to meet with the patient and her son. The meeting, I wrote in my notes, went very slowly: the patient did not talk at all, and the son's attention was mostly dedicated to nursing her. The conversation between the son and the social worker was constantly interrupted: "He [the son] feeds her, puts ice in her mouth, suctions liquids from her mouth whenever she coughs (and she's coughing several times as we speak), changes her position in bed." The social worker validated the son's style of caring, saying, 'It's okay, she's the most important person in the room.' In between this laborious bedside care, the social worker talked to the son about palliative care. She emphasized that palliative care was not necessarily hospice and that most of the patients they consulted were not discharged to hospice. She explained about the different types of nursing homes and home-care services the patient could use after being discharged from the hospital. At the son's request, the social worker provided her contact information for future reference.

Noting to herself how intensely the son was caring for his mother, the social worker ruled out the possibility that he would be interested in anything close to hospice care. Outside the patient's room she told me,

> 'It's crazy. I've seen many families like that, you've been here for a month and a half and you've already seen two, so imagine how many I've seen. They're just so detail-oriented, so intense in the care that they're giving her, that it's impossible to satisfy them. When you look at the patient, she's just full of fluids: in her mouth, in her body [the patient's legs were swollen]—she's full of fluids that she just spits out because she can't absorb them [hence the need to suction her frequently]. And she's still connected to the IV fluids and the blood transfusions because the son insists on giving them to her.' She laughs. 'No chance I'm going to send them to hospice. It's just not going to work.'

Neither the son nor the patient expressed an explicit wish to not go to hospice; the social worker concluded that this was their wish from the son's behavior. Beyond her wanting to respect this wish, the social worker simply thought she would not be able to convince the son otherwise; she believed he would either dig his heels and insist on keeping his mother in the hospital, or capitulate, move her to hospice, but then change his mind and return to the emergency department. Following the son's presumed wish was a practical solution: the social worker tried to economize dying by other, more moderate means that had a higher likelihood of success, such as moving the patient to a nursing home instead of keeping her hospitalized.

I have so far outlined the significance of what can be called *patients' own wishes* for medical practitioners working near the end of life. First, patients' own wishes provided guidance to clinicians, serving as a moral compass. Second, listening to patients and family members and considering their wishes had a practical importance: it helped consolidate care plans that they were more likely to accept. I have also shown that patients and families who were expressive, reflective, and talkative—and whom clinicians deemed credible—were far easier to treat and manage. They voiced wishes that clinicians could discuss, process, and follow.

Subjectifying Patients

The Subjective Ontology

Given the practical and moral importance of patients' *wishes*, much of the clinicians' attention was directed at understanding what patients wanted. Palliative care work, however, targeted a deeper personality layer than simple wishes. It sought to consolidate an intelligible and agreed-upon sense of what palliative care clinicians called the patients' *goals and values*. These goals and values had to connect to what I call patients' *subjectivity*.

It is important to distinguish between these three concepts: wishes, goals and values, and subjectivity. In the palliative care context, *wishes* are specific desires or requests that patients or their family members voice. A patient may wish, for example, to get morphine, to have another cycle of chemotherapy, or to never be admitted to the ICU. Wishes may be realistic or unrealistic; a patient may wish to be cured of a cancer that is incurable, or to die in the hospital despite the fact that, by her insurance company's standards, her condition and treatment make her ineligible for hospitalization.

Goals and values, on the other hand, pertain to one's more fundamental personality traits. As Charles Taylor observed, in order "to be a person in the full sense you have to be an agent with a sense of yourself as an agent, a being which can thus make plans for your life, one who also holds values in virtue of which such different plans seem better or worse, and who is capable of choosing between them."[14] Accordingly, palliative care clinicians were more interested in patients' selfhood, personality, and values. A patient, for example, could value independence, staying alive at all costs, or interacting with her family.[15] Values could not be deemed realistic or unrealistic because they were taken as features of patients' personality. Clinicians could doubt that a patient's personality was well understood or represented, but they could not claim that a personality was invalid.[16] *Goals* marked out the long-term and ultimate purpose of a certain treatment. Legitimate goals had to be connected to the patients' values. For example, when a patient expressed how important his relationship with his daughters was to him (a value), clinicians could suggest that his goal of care was moving closer to them. When deciding on the appropriateness of various treatments, they would ask themselves whether these treatments served this goal.

The term *subjectivity* highlights an ontological assumption that lies beneath palliative care work. Subjectivity, as sociologists Bernard Lahire and Nikolas Rose put it, is an abstraction; it is the assumption that people possess "a natural locus of beliefs and desires," which is the origin of their "actions and decisions." People are supposed to have an "inside": personality traits that represent them, guide their behavior, and summarize their entirety as human beings. This inside should be at least somewhat consistent and coherent—and it can be worked on, actualized, processed, and improved through conversation and guided reflection.[17] Palliative care clinicians aimed their practices toward a *subject* (or self) that they assumed existed inside patients. They assumed the integrity and solidity of patients' personality, which included features that were inherent to the individual and characterized her or his entire being.[18] In their work, they tried to consolidate a sense of this ontology by talking to patients and families and mapping out their "goals and values." Although they assumed that there was a real *subject* that existed inside the patient, clinicians did not take this subject as an inalterable reality that they should passively and unquestionably accept.[19] Interactions between clinicians, patients, and families were recursive processes through which they fleshed out the patients' subjectivity. The goal was to make the patients themselves—and the family members who accompanied them—clearer about who they were and what they wanted, which would render them more manageable from a clinical and organizational standpoint. These were interactions that interpellated patients' subjectivity.[20]

The basic question that drove palliative care clinicians' work was, "Who is the patient?" They addressed it by subjectifying patients. This involved several practices and techniques. First, clinicians elicited patients' illness experience and gained an understanding of their personhood. Second, when the patients were uncommunicative, the clinicians turned to family members (and at times friends and other people who knew the person) and solicited their insights about who the patients were. Third, clinicians used what I call "assistive conversational devices," which "helped" patients verbalize their goals and values. Fourth, clinicians drew on written evidence—such as advance directive forms—to draw conclusions about what patients wanted and who they were. Finally, clinicians intuited the patients' wishes from unconscious bodily movements and gestures.

Let Them Speak

The first move in subjectifying patients was to solicit their *illness experience*. Palliative care clinicians asked questions about patients' personal and subjective perception of their condition: "Most of the times I let them talk," one palliative care physician told me. "This [interview] is probably the most talking I'll do all day. A lot of time, my job is to listen." This approach deliberately reverses the common structure of medical interviews. As Elliot Mishler observed, in a typical interview, doctors control the conversation. They ask questions, assess the adequacy of the patient's response, and filter out information that they deem irrelevant, such as personal histories and how the illness's symptoms have affected the patient's life more generally. Physicians, Mishler argued, direct their attention "solely to physical-medical signs that might be associated with [patients'] primary symptoms"; their professional and technical orientation suppresses accounts of the patient's "life world."[21]

The palliative care clinicians, however, wanted to discuss this very life world. They shifted clinical attention from the physical condition of the sick body to people's subjective perceptions, feelings, and experiences of this condition. When I asked one palliative care physician how he started conversations with patients, he said,

> We just go to the patient, and we get to the subjective side of things immediately. So it's not, "Hey, Roi, Dr. X said this and that, and whether you know it or not—you're in heart failure and here's what you need to do." [If we do that,] you're almost like a player in your own life: we're telling you what [to do], it's devoid of your experiences, devoid of your personality, it's all based on your [physical] heart. [In palliative care] we go immediately to your experience: "Roi, tell us what it's like to live with a dysfunctional heart—it must be really hard. How do you cope with that?" [These are] questions that we use, so we get to the subjective immediately. . . . So you're not just a patient in a bed having shit done to you.

By asking such questions, palliative care clinicians infused technical medical work—diagnosis, prognosis, and the formulation of care plans—with the patients' reflections on their illness experiences. Palliative care clinicians *wanted* to hear stories of suffering, pain, frustration, and discomfort from illness, from the medical system, from the hospital, and also from the clinicians—so much so that these clinicians felt challenged by patients and families who were not very verbal or talkative, who acted timid or seemed reluctant to share personal stories, or who focused on the technicalities of their disease and its treatment rather than their feelings and personal experiences. Even in such cases, good clinicians could notice and react to underlying feelings and subjective experiences. During a nurse-training lecture on end-of-life care, a palliative care physician said,

> Patients often communicate both on an emotional level and on the technical level. For example, a person yells at a doctor, "Dammit, I want my IV, and I want it now!" There is a lot of emotion and anger communicated through that statement, a lot you can learn about how the patient feels from that. But there's also something technical here: he wants an IV. Mostly, doctors—but nurses too—we are really good at the technical, and we don't pay enough attention to the relationships. So we take only the technical elements from the message that this person gives us and address them. We'll just go and give that person an IV, while this is only one part of what this person is communicating to us.

As the physician described it, the palliative care skill was to hear and understand beyond what patients said explicitly, to sense their emotions from their tone of voice, behavior, and body language, and to address their more fundamental problems instead of fulfilling their immediate, technical, and superficial wishes.

In the process of inviting patients to share their illness experiences, palliative care clinicians also assessed patients' understanding of their disease.[22] They evaluated whether and how much patients knew about their diagnosis, what information the medical staff had already given them, and how patients understood and interpreted this information. A palliative care nurse told me,

> Another question [that I ask when talking to patients] is, "What do you understand about what's going on?" Your illness, or your disease, or whatever. You phrase open-ended questions, designed to elicit the person's understanding of what's wrong. And sometimes there are more probing questions: "Hmmm. . . . So, you told me what the doctor told you. What does it mean to *you?*" I'm trying to assess understanding.

Beyond the trust-building component that such conversations had, the clinicians made use of how the patients answered these questions. First, they treated the answers as signals for how careful they should be when talking to the patient. For example, when patients mentioned that their condition was terminal, the clinicians would talk about death more directly and openly. Second, by asking patients to talk about their condition, the clinicians learned whether the patients had heard and understood the medical information shared with them in earlier meetings. As an example, a palliative care nurse from Public Hospital was happy to hear that a patient told me he was "terminal," because the day before he had had a long meeting with the physician who informed him about this condition.[23] Third, palliative care clinicians judged patients' medical literacy and ability to contribute to decision making based on how reflective and detailed they were when they talked about their experiences. Recall how Dr. Nelson referred to a patient and a family as "medically sophisticated" when she explained why she trusted their decision-making capacity. Opposite cases existed, too: physicians described some patients as "lacking insight" into their conditions, and they felt compelled to temper the patients' preferences with more clinical judgment.

The main purpose of asking personal questions, however, was to gain insight into who patients were. The palliative care clinicians went deep and aimed to gauge the patients' innermost personalities. They honed their conversational skills and worked on identifying opportunities to ask probing questions, which would go beyond immediate wishes and force the patients to reflect and verbalize how they thought about their life and their medical condition. When one patient told a palliative care physician at Academic Hospital that she wanted to live, the physician asked what a meaningful life would be for her. The patient responded she would want to go back home and be independent, and the physician suggested this as the patient's definition of a life worth living, which could inform future medical decisions on her care. Because her own definition of a meaningful life involved being independent, life in the hospital or a nursing home, let alone in the ICU connected to a ventilator, would contradict her goals and values.

When patients and families insisted that they wanted to wait for a miracle and pursue more treatment in order to fully recover, the prescribed palliative care response, which I heard in all of the teams that I shadowed, was to acknowledge that hope and suggest that they should "hope for the best, prepare for the worst." (One physician was more careful in his choice of words and said, "Hope for the best, prepare for everything.")

I noticed that palliative care clinicians repeated this rubric verbatim in different family meetings. Typically this directed conversations toward more pessimistic scenarios, which were discussed as hypotheticals, and the medical staff took what the patients said as indicating their goals and values.

When a patient was unable to participate in decision making, when their ability to do so seemed compromised, or when they seemed harder to communicate with than their family members, the palliative care clinicians treated the family members as the "best proxy" for the patient. In an interview, a nurse who spoke about the questions she asked people in meetings moved quickly between the questions she directed at patients and the questions she asked family members:

> I start [the conversation] with either, "the doctor asked me to see you, and before we get to the medical part, maybe you can tell me something about yourself, and who you are, and who you are when you're not a patient, and who your loved one is, not the sick person in bed, but [the person] you see and know."

Both conversations—with family members and with the patient—helped the nurse sense the patient as a person. The questions' generality could lift some of the heavy burden of making decisions at the end of life from the family.[24] Reflecting on the patient's personality and life history was far easier than deciding, say, whether to keep her on life support.

Such concrete decisions, however, were still looming. One common strategy to make the conversation easier for family members was assigning them a role of passive *reporters*, who merely described the patient, her personality, and her values to the medical staff, as opposed to surrogates who had to make decisions for the patient. In all three hospitals I studied, I documented cases of families of patients in persistent vegetative states, who spent weeks hesitating about whether to disconnect them from life support. In three specific cases, the neurology teams involved were confident in saying that meaningful recovery was very unlikely—which still left the families hesitating. In two of the cases, palliative care clinicians told the families that their role was not to make decisions for the patient, but to provide the staff with information about what the patient would have wanted had they been able to speak. They suggested a division of labor between the family and the clinicians: the family would provide information about the patient's goals and values, and the clinicians would make the appropriate medical decision, given this information. "Did she ever say anything about what she would want if she were in this condition?" was a typical question that palliative care clinicians asked in such situations, which was at times followed by stories about things the patient had said or positions she or he had taken when another family member was dying. Yet for many family members involved in those cases, who knew that their answer could mean that the patient would be allowed to die, this made little difference. In both cases, which occurred in two different hospitals and were managed by two different teams, the family members expressed the desperate wish that the patient would wake up and instruct them on what to do.

This reveals the key paradox of subjectification: the clinicians' efforts to hear patients and recognize them as subjects also meant that they *expected* patients to be and act like subjects—to express their values and goals, and possess sufficiently clear personality traits that would be evident in conversation. When the patients were unconscious or uncommunicative, the expectation was that family members (or friends, when no known family relations existed) would be able to report on such personality traits. Subjectification was an opportunity as well as an expectation, an invitation as well as a demand, which in many cases burdened people as much as it empowered them.

Go Wish

The bulk of palliative care work involved talking, communicating, and reflecting existentially on what one found important and valuable, specifically near the end of life. These practices were sensitive to sociological factors. For one thing, patients who did not feel comfortable and confident interacting with doctors found it harder to express themselves in palliative care meetings than those who felt at ease. Moreover, quasi-psychotherapeutic existential reflections, while common and naturalized among highly educated middle- and upper-class people, are not something that all people embrace spontaneously. As one palliative care physician told me,

> We have a lot of people in this hospital who have not planned in advance for anything. Ever. And that's why they're in the situations that they're in. And they may have used substances, or things that are not healthy that they don't have access to now in the hospital to cope with them. I mean, someone who has been drunk, kind of perpetually, for years and years and years, who now is in the hospital, totally sober, and is facing down this decision. . . . [Physicians] want to come in and say, "What do you want your final days to look like?" And [the patient is] just a total deer in the headlights. . . . I think that we have some mechanisms to try to get at what's important to people.

One "mechanism" that I saw being used on several occasions was a pack of cards (branded as a "game") called "Go Wish," which Coda Alliance, a Silicon Valley nonprofit, has produced and distributed.[25] Go Wish included dozens of cards with printed statements that qualified as legitimate goals and values. Palliative care clinicians asked patients to sort these cards into three categories: "very important," "sort of important," and "not so important or unimportant to me." If the "very important" category included many statements, clinicians asked patients to choose the most important statements from it and rank them. Among other statements, the cards included "to maintain my dignity," "to be kept clean," "to say goodbye to people in my life," "not dying alone," "to be mentally aware," "to have my family with me," "to be at home," and "not being connected to machines." These statements drew from a survey of patients, family members, and clinicians that was published in the *Journal of the American Medical Association* in 2000.[26] The game's outcome—three ordinal categories of various statements—were taken as indications of the patient's goals and values.

In an interview, a palliative care physician told me

> Things like this [the Go Wish activity] can spark ideas. You know, not everyone is really able to fully engage and do this, but we do

this on a fairly regular basis. We sit down with people and try to go through these, and get a better sense. . . . [27] A lot of times, it's not even just the sorting, it's the conversation that happens while they're reading it. You know, you just learn a lot more. And the nice thing is that they're at a fairly accessible level for different people. . . . I actually have a printout of this. I put it on a piece of paper that you could leave with a patient, and then the patient can circle it to say what's important to them. Because sometimes this is a little bit overwhelming.

Go Wish had three practical advantages. First, it catalyzed choice: the cards made some patients, who otherwise would not engage in such deliberations, sort out, rank, and choose between statements, which clinicians could treat as goals and values. It was far easier to make people sort and rank statements than it was to make them reflect on what they found meaningful in life, then ponder life-and-death decisions. Second, because the cards included prearticulated statements, they contained and controlled what "wishes" patients could express. Go Wish cards (or written printouts based on them) were mediators that oriented interactions in directions that palliative care clinicians deemed productive.[28] They excluded unrealistic expectations (such as "I want to be cured") and only included wishes that clinicians saw as indicating meaningful goals and values. Notably, the Go Wish pack included a blank card, which allowed patients to fill in their own wish. In some cases, clinicians skipped that card; when they did not, by the time they got to the blank card the patients were already trained in thinking about wishes that qualified as reflecting goals and values. The blank card was an opportunity for already tame patients to articulate palliative care statements on their own. Finally, the Go Wish activity produced written records of these goals and values, which clinicians and patients could keep and refer to at later decision points.

This was how a nurse reported to a palliative care team about a Go Wish conversation she had had with a patient:

'Being free of pain was clearly the number-one important thing for him, and he said he was okay with that even if it'd make him drowsy. He would be okay with being kept on machines, as long as he can speak with his mom. If he's in a situation in which he cannot speak with his mom, he wouldn't want to be kept on machines. He's been really reflective and pensive about his history with HIV; so the HIV unit would be a good place for him.'

Still, Go Wish did not solve all problems. Ultimately, it was most popular among people who were likely to reflect on their life, condition, and end-of-life plans anyway.

> There's a cancer support group here, at the hospital. So I did this game with them on a piece of paper, and they said, "Well, this is actually a really great way for you to go to your family and say, 'Hey, this is what we talked about in our group tonight.'" And that has been demonstrated in studies, that when people act as surrogate decision makers, the best way for there to be concordance between what the patient wants and what the surrogate thinks the patient wants is that they actually have the conversation about it.

People who attend a support group tend to be talkative and expressive with or without a card game. Yet other patients, who were often Go Wish's chief target population, found it less appealing. In Academic Hospital, I shadowed palliative care clinicians who were visiting an ICU patient whose condition was improving. The medical team planned to discharge the patient to a nursing home. One medical student who rounded with the palliative care team had had a "Go Wish" conversation with him, in anticipation of a future decline in his condition.

> The med[ical] student asks him if he remembers that they played that card game together, about wishes, and says that she printed out his wishes. She shows him a few printed pages, and asks him if he would like her to put it here, maybe in his bag. He says that anything here would disappear, so maybe not. She suggests putting it in his bag [again], then says that she could always print out more copies, if he wants.

The medical student was, in fact, far more eager than the patient to have his goals and values printed and documented. She, not the patient, initiated the Go Wish conversation and tried to ensure that its outcomes would be kept, known, and followed. I observed a similar situation in Public Hospital:

> Denise [social worker] and I go to do the Go Wish together. . . . As it turns out, Dr. Evans asked Denise to do it with the patient a few days ago, and she did—but then the patient lost [the form]. . . . As we walk, I tell Denise that I'm surprised she managed to do the Go Wish with him. I saw the patient a few days earlier, and he wasn't extremely communicative. She agrees and says, 'Yes, I also think that he forgets a lot. It's possible that the Go Wish form that we filled out together is in the trash. He doesn't really remember what he did with it.'
>
> We go to his room. [The patient] doesn't seem alert, hardly engages in conversation, and eventually Denise decides not to repeat the Go Wish activity with him.

The Go Wish activity is an example of a structured way to produce written records of patients' goals and values. It induced the patients to make explicit statements, which the clinicians took to represent the patients as subjects. Some patients not only participated in this activity but also enjoyed it and embraced its outcomes. They were willingly subjectified, becoming people with clear views that defined them, who wanted to document these views and have them respected. Others did not—in their cases, not being subjectified meant not having clearly expressed and communicated positions on their medical condition and treatment, which posed significant difficulties for the medical staff.

Forms That (May) Speak

When trying to gauge the subjectivity of unconscious or uncommunicative patients, one of the first things the palliative care clinicians did was check to find out whether they had filled out an advance directive. This formal document, which comes in various formats, levels of detail, and lengths, asks people about the treatment they would want to receive if they reached various degrees of physical and mental disability. The objective of advance directives is to have people make medical decisions before their condition declines and they become uncommunicative. After filling out the directive, the patient and two witnesses sign it, then the patient keeps it.[29]

Advance directive forms have become a gold standard of U.S. medicine. Physicians are encouraged to fill them out with patients, regardless of the patients' age and medical condition. Progressive health care reforms such as the Affordable Care Act have worked to make advance directives routine and universal.[30] In a 2000–2006 survey, the relatives of 67.6 percent of deceased patients who had required decision making but lacked the capacity to participate reported they had filled out an advance directive.[31] By contrast, an ethnographic study in an Illinois ICU found that only 35 percent of the unit's patients had at least a partly completed advance directive. From a sociological standpoint even this far lower figure is notable. Any piece of paper that one third of the relevant population uses indicates a significant and fairly powerful social institution.[32]

The clinicians that I studied used advance directives as indicators of the patients' goals and values. They treated advance directives as anticipatory instructions, which the patient left when she or he was still communicative. Supposedly the directives spoke for patients whom disease had muted; in reality, however, there were many intervening factors and circumstances that could weaken an advance directive's credibility.[33] First, in several cases, when patients' conditions had declined such that they lost the ability to express themselves, the physical copy (or electronic record) of the advance directive could not be located and used. The Illinois ICU study found that "despite continual prodding of family members to bring in copies of these advance directives" only about a quarter of the directives that family members (or patients) said existed made it to the medical record.[34]

Second, even the advance directives that were found were often disputed. Family members questioned the circumstances in which the patient filled out the form or suspected that the patients did not fully understand the form and its meaning, and they insinuated that the physicians who had helped complete the form had misdirected or biased the patient. Ms. Chang, an elderly Chinese American woman who was hit by a car on her way to the grocery store, was hospitalized unconscious and connected to the respirator in one of Public Hospital's ICUs. One attending physician told me that nearly every bone in her body was broken. Her primary care physician sent the hospital an advance directive, which she said she had filled out with Ms. Chang three years earlier. The form indicated that Ms. Chang would not want to have her life sustained for longer than five days if she reached a similar condition, and the clinicians involved in the case thought that it clarified Ms. Chang's goals of care and were ready to remove her from the respirator. Her daughters, however, who were not aware that the advance directive existed, doubted its validity. They said Ms. Chang only spoke Mandarin, so it was impossible she could have read the form, filled it out, or fully understood the consequences it would have for her care. Three years after the form was filled out and signed, her primary care physician had no recollection of the exact circumstances in which Ms. Chang had signed the form, which cast a significant shadow on its validity.[35]

Third, advance directives have been challenged over their temporality. Individuals fill out advance directives before the decline in their condition, sometimes years before they are opened and used. Yet people evolve—and so do their views on end-of-life care. In many cases, family members have intuitively sensed changes in patients' inclinations, in ways that were not represented in the directives' short, written texts and checked boxes.[36] Ethicists also have raised doubts about whether advance directive forms do not lead to situations where "former selves . . . bind later selves."[37] The "disability paradox"—the fact that people with serious disabilities report experiencing a high quality of life—further complicates the picture.[38] It is always possible that a healthy person who did not want to be hospitalized would change her mind when her condition declined and hospitalization was needed. Clinicians who unquestioningly treated advance directives as genuine representations of patients' goals and values assumed that these goals and values were stable and consistent; they bracketed off the inherent changeability and unpredictability of human agency. The bureaucratic imperative to create consistent documentation for things as capricious and dynamic as human feelings, fears, and values can create perceived discrepancies between people and the forms that are used to represent them.

Finally, it is impossible to follow advance directives verbatim. These forms outline general scenarios; by definition, there will be gaps between these scenarios and a patient's actual condition.[39] A patient, for example, could check a box next to this statement:

> I do not want my life to be prolonged if (1) I have an incurable and irreversible condition that will result in my death within a relatively short time, (2) I become unconscious and, to a reasonable degree of medical certainty, I will not regain consciousness, or (3) the likely risks and burdens of treatment would outweigh the expected benefits.[40]

Even families who trust such forms still had much to decide on. Should the time left indeed be considered "relatively short"? Has "a reasonable degree of medical certainty" that the patient will not regain consciousness been reached? And at what point could they confidently say that the "risks and burdens of treatment" outweigh the expected benefits? No checked box or written text could cover all possible disease trajectories and treatment possibilities. How advance directive forms play out in actual decision making is circumstantial. It would depend on how people interpreted these forms, how they filled the gaps that the forms' text left, and in what emotional state the surrogate decision makers read them.

An advance directive "success story" that a palliative care social worker shared with me illustrated this point. The patient, the social worker said, was an elderly woman with a very large family, who had sustained a major stroke.[41] The palliative care team was consulted when the patient was in the ICU, and after a conversation with several of the patient's children they decided to transfer her to comfort care. At that point, many other people from the family, who had not participated in the original conversation, "rushed down here" and said, as the social worker recounted, "She's a fighter, maybe we should start tube feeds, maybe we should start antibiotics again." The social worker asked if she had an advance directive, and "they said, 'Well, she is a really organized person, why don't we go and look?'"

At home, the family found a letter where, remarkably, the patient guessed that her relatives would characterize her as a "fighter" and would hesitate to transition her to comfort care. "It was two pages; it was the most beautiful document I've ever read," the social worker told me. In those two pages, the woman clarified that she would be fine living in a wheelchair, but she would want to be able to transfer to the wheelchair on her own, and be able to enjoy food, and to have conversations with people. "But if it's not going to be like that," the social worker recalled her writing, "DO NOT give me tube feeds, DO NOT extend my life, DO NOT let me stay in the ICU more than five days. And it was all documented with each condition." "And so the family read this," the social worker said, "and they let her go. . . . At the end of this *beautiful* two-page document, she told them what she hoped for them. . . . It was beautiful. That's what I'm talking about. That's thinking through your values ahead of time."

The social worker spelled out the intended moral of this story at its end: people should think through and document what they value. Between the lines, however, the story shows that the power of documents lies in the social circumstances where families and clinicians open and read them. The exemplary success story that the social worker used to illustrate the importance of advance directives to an interviewer (she also told me that she used it in a class that she taught) is about a two-page letter that had little formal legal credence. The letter bore the patient's signature, but there were no witnesses who guaranteed that it was genuine. A Durable Power of Attorney could legally ignore it. But the letter's power lay elsewhere, in its personal and nonstandard character, which gave it maximum strength in the circumstances that developed: a family confronts an agonizing decision, they find a hidden letter, the letter successfully predicts how they would feel and react, and it ends with a touching note about the woman's wishes for her descendants. It was possible to challenge this letter on formal-legal grounds, but it was virtually impossible to challenge it in the social situation that developed.

More than everything, the letter, in its striking informality, left a clear impression of the patient's personality, values, and goals on the family and the clinical staff. Subjectification—in this case, the clinical effort to consolidate a sense of a mute patient's subjectivity—felt genuine. The success of this subjectification, manifested in the uncontested recognition of the patient's own values, led to a morally satisfying closure. The patient was transitioned to comfort care, extubated, and passed away shortly after.

It is unclear to what extent clinicians follow advance directives. In the 1990s, there was overwhelming evidence that advance directives and living wills had limited impact on how clinicians treated patients.[42] However, more recent surveys have shown that advance directives now have significant influence.[43] The cases I have discussed show that, given the inherent unpredictability of the courses of illness and the instability of people's goals and values, deciding whether an advance directive form was followed or not is always open to interpretation. Recognizing these inherent uncertainties, palliative care physician Rebecca Sudore and geriatrician Terri Fried have called for revising the traditional objective of advance directives—having "patients make treatment decisions in advance of serious illness." Instead, they suggested using advance directives to prepare patients and families for making decisions in real time, by starting a conversation on end-of-life care early.[44] Similarly, advocates of advance directive forms have emphasized that filling out a form should only be the beginning of a conversation between the form's "owner" and the surrogate decision maker on end-of-life decisions.

These recommendations recognize that, in and of themselves, advance directive forms have limited influence. They become influential only when people recognize them as valid representations of the patient, or alternatively when people use them similarly to Go Wish cards, as an assistive tool in sparking a reflection on one's views on end-of-life care. When used in this way, the forms provide scenarios that *train* people in thinking and reflecting, in preparation for the decision making that awaits them in the future. They coach people in certain ways to achieve self-knowledge, behave as subjects, and reflect on the subjectivity of people whom they know.[45]

Advance directives are therefore important parts of the effort to subjectify patients. They epitomize an expectation that people would reflect and communicate about their views on end-of-life care so that they can later present coherent and consistent goals and values to their clinicians. Ideally, people should prepare detailed orders, which explain exactly what type of care they would and would not want. They should talk to their family members and family doctor, spell out their goals and values clearly, and remain consistent about them.

The fact that I did not have an advance directive of my own reflected very badly on me in the field. When I casually mentioned it at one point, people reacted with a deafening silence. Like any person, I was one car accident away from a coma, and without an advance directive I could find myself treated against my will. This made me appear irresponsible and uninformed, which was rather embarrassing for a person who purported to be a sociologist studying end-of-life care.

Respect for patients' self-sovereignty was therefore not simply respect for subjects, but respect for subjects who held clearly ordered preferences and values, which they expressed and documented. In Carol Heimer and Lisa Staffen's terms, palliative care clinicians "responsibilized" patients: they made patients responsible for formulating and communicating their goals and values. By consequence, people who did not meet this expectation (myself included) were considered irresponsible.[46]

There are numerous reasons why a person would not have an advance directive. Many patients that I saw lacked appropriate and stable access to a health care provider who would encourage them to fill out an advance directive. Furthermore, there is evidence that in many cases refraining from filling out advance directives "is a deliberate, if not an explicit, refusal to participate in the advance directives process."[47] The expectation to fill out an advance directive is, after all, not obvious. "Even patients making contemporary decisions about contemporary illnesses are regularly daunted by the decisions' difficulty," wrote Fagerlin and Schneider. "How much harder, then, is it to conjure up preferences for an unspecifiable future confronted with unidentifiable maladies with unpredictable treatments?"[48] Very hard for all and even harder for some: patients from unprivileged backgrounds—who did not have a doctor they trusted and were suspicious of the medical profession, the hospital, and the health care establishment in general—were less likely to have a directive. These were also the patients who were historically underrepresented in the hospice and palliative care movement. These people, who had comparably little social power, were the most difficult for clinicians to subjectify, and therefore were most likely to find themselves at odds with the ideas and practice of palliative care.

Bodies That (May) Speak

Another way in which clinicians subjectified unconscious patients was by following their bodily gestures. Most commonly, clinicians relied on unconscious patients' facial expressions to conclude whether they were in pain. Deep wrinkles on an unconscious patient's forehead were signs that the patient was in pain; a patient who looked "peaceful" was presumed to be free of pain. Clinicians also interpreted certain bodily postures, specifically the fetal position, as signaling that the patient was in pain. When they already felt ambivalent about a course of treatment, identifying the patient as being in pain added to their doubt.

Interestingly, there were also many cases where clinicians went further and attributed *intention* to unconscious patients' movements, especially when there were other indications that they did not want to have their life prolonged. As a former palliative care physician told me,

> Very seldom I've butted heads with families and patients, who demanded certain things that I thought were really not right.[49] In particular, one was a young patient who had made it very, very, very clear— there's no question, he had verbalized it, he had indicated it, his actions had completely been consistent—that he did not want to be intubated. . . . [After he became unconscious,] the family decided that they wanted him intubated, transferred to the ICU and all this, and I said no. This is not what he wants. . . . This goes completely against his wishes. And in fact, when we compromised and decided to do something called CPAP,* he just ripped the mask off, because it was so uncomfortable. So I went to them and I said, "Do you get it now? Do you see that this is not what he wanted?" And it was such a hard . . . Normally, it would be so easy to just give in and do it, but I knew so well that this guy . . . There was just no part of me that could accept that, because I knew *so* well what he had wanted. . . . This was kind of an idealistic decision that he would never be uncomfortable or whatever. He was in deep trouble, and he felt like crap, and he was barely gasping . . . so he knew that he was progressing and dying. So for me, the decision that he had made was absolutely his decision. But his family was completely trying to reverse his decision, because they

---

* CPAP (continuous positive airway pressure) is a mask that maintains the airway open with moderate air pressure.

were having a tough time with him dying. . . . [I think it was a cousin who said,] "Oh, but I think that he's making a decision that he doesn't quite understand," and I said, "He fully [understands]."

A palliative care social worker described a similar case, where she interpreted an unconscious self-extubation as validating a patient's previous statements about not wanting life-prolonging treatment:

> We got right now, in the ICU, an African American guy. A lot of drugs, alcohol, noncompliance. Family never came up to multiple hospitalizations. This guy defied, but *very clearly* [in an] advance directive and [said] to his doctors who know him very well, please don't ever intubate me. Please don't ever give me a trach.* Please don't ever give me tube feeds. It's clearly documented, [there were] conversations. He's now in the ICU, can't make his own decisions, a son who hasn't been involved—a very dysfunctional family—has now showed up and said, I want everything done. [So now] he's intubated, he's on tube feeds. He's pulled the tube feeds out twice. They [the ICU staff] put them back in. He extubated himself—he pulled out his ventilator. He actually pulled it out. . . . Unbelievable. But it tells you, you see, that in there, he still doesn't want this, but he can't talk anymore.

Patients who pulled out intravenous lines, feeding tubes, or respirators were very difficult to watch. For one thing, their actions often caused noticeable injuries, which involved bleeding and, one could imagine, much suffering to those who still felt pain. Moreover, it created a caregiving problem: patients who self-extubated still needed a respirator to survive. After the staff reintubated them, there still remained a chance that the patient would self-extubate again. The only way to eliminate this risk was either to have a person sitting next to the patient at all times (a "sitter") or to restrain the patient to the bed. Due to staffing constraints, the second solution was much more common in the three hospitals that I studied.

---

* A trach (tracheostomy) is an airway opening in the neck (into the trachea) that physicians create via a surgical procedure (tracheotomy). In palliative care consultations, the question of whether to perform a tracheotomy often comes up when a patient has used a mechanical ventilator for a long period. Mechanical ventilation through the mouth makes patients susceptible to infections. When patients need more than two to three weeks of ventilation, physicians open a tracheostomy to continue ventilating them safely.

Few situations created more moral qualms than having a bleeding, severely ill patient restrained while nurses worked to reinsert the intravenous lines he had pulled out. In all of the cases that I documented, when such a situation persisted, unless the family agreed to not reinsert the intravenous lines or reintubate the patient, the hospital staff called an ethics consultation and confronted the family very directly.

The source of the moral distress in these cases is worth exploring. Would clinicians have been so distraught about reinserting intravenous lines and reintubating a patient had they not felt the patient was trying to communicate otherwise by pulling out the lines and ventilator tube? In one remarkable case, a patient who had sustained a stroke and was hospitalized for several months in Public Hospital pulled out his trach twice. The internist who treated him said that the patient, who still had some limited capacity to communicate, responded affirmatively when his daughter asked him if he wanted to be Full Code and have the trach. There was a discrepancy between what the patient *said* and what the patient *did* unconsciously. Trachs and ventilators are, after all, physically uncomfortable; even people who want their life prolonged can try to remove them when in delirium. In this case, the palliative care team was ready to call an ethics consultation, but the physicians on the floor "felt comfortable" that the patient wanted the ventilator and called off the consultation.

In the more common cases, when the patients who pulled out IV lines or self-extubated could not convey a sufficiently clear verbal message that they were actually interested in the treatments given to them, clinicians took their actions as statements against life prolongation—or at least as indications that they could not "appreciate" the treatment they received.

In summary, I outlined five subjectification practices that palliative care clinicians used in their work. First, when patients were communicative, palliative care clinicians worked to make them express sufficiently coherent goals and values by talking with them about themselves, their lives, their understanding of their illness, and their hopes. Second, clinicians turned to families, as the people who knew the patient the best, and asked them to reflect and share who the patient was and what her or his goals and values were. Third, palliative care clinicians used assistive conversational devices, such as Go Wish cards or forms that summarized them, to spark conversations about these topics. Fourth, clinicians used forms such as advance directives as expressing the values of unconscious patients and as voicing subjectivities that were mute. And finally, clinicians read preferences and inclinations in the patients' bodies, and treated them as demonstrating the patients' wishes.

Subjectifying patients was a process of empowerment, in which patients' subjectivities—or selfhoods—were consolidated. By empowerment I do not mean that characteristics that had already existed in patients were given the faculty to surface and influence decisions. Empowerment is not an excavation of an already formed self, but an enactment and articulation of self, which clarifies to patients, families, and clinicians who the patient is. A successfully subjectified patient was one whose subjectivity was not in doubt. Family members, the patient, and the clinicians agreed on who the patient was, what they wanted, and what they would want. Ideally, they were also aware and accepting of each other's perspectives.

Translating and Hooking: Bridging between Subjects and Economization

Once the patient's goals and values were established, clinicians connected them to concrete decisions on medical care. They made this connection through two practices, which I call "translation" and "hooking." Translation is restating a patient or a family member's statement and transforming it into a concrete medical goal.[50] Hooking involves attaching a specific end-of-life decision to this goal. This section presents two cases to illustrate how palliative care clinicians employed these practices.

"My Father Loves Life"

Mr. Becker was an eighty-one-year-old white man, who lived about a two-hour drive from Academic Hospital. In the months that preceded his meeting with the palliative care team, he was hospitalized three times for recurrent pneumonia, and effectively became a "revolving door" patient, who was rotating in and out of the hospital, with his hospitalizations becoming longer and more intensive.[51] I met Mr. Becker during a particularly traumatic hospitalization: he got sick and became very short of breath, literally gasping for air, until his daughter Lynn decided to drive him to the hospital. Lynn later said she was not sure if they would make it to the hospital on time.

But they did. The emergency department physicians intubated Mr. Becker, put him on intravenous antibiotics, and transferred him to the ICU. Several days later, his pneumonia was under control, and the ICU physicians extubated him successfully. Given his recurrent hospitalizations, they decided to call a palliative care consultation to discuss how to plan his care for the longer term. I accompanied three members of the palliative care team—a fellow, a social worker, and a medical student who rotated with the team for two weeks as part of his training. The four of us walked into Mr. Becker's ICU alcove, where we found him sleeping in his bed in front of a television showing highlights from a recent LA Dodgers game. Dr. Ashley, the palliative care fellow, touched his right arm gently, and he immediately opened his eyes and smiled at her. We introduced ourselves, and when Dr. Ashley asked Mr. Becker how he was doing, he looked her in the eyes and said flirtatiously that he was always okay when she was around.

A short conversation ensued, in which Dr. Ashley asked him if he was in pain (he said he was not) and 'What are you hoping for?' (he said he was hoping to get better). Mr. Becker said he had a bakery that he wanted to get back to, and then mumbled something I did not fully understand. After several minutes of small talk, Dr. Ashley said she enjoyed talking to him and would let him rest; she added that she was going to meet with his daughter Lynn, and asked if he would be okay with that. 'Of course,' Mr. Becker answered. We shook hands with him and left for the conference room, where the ICU attending physician joined us. Lynn came in a few minutes later, apologizing for making us wait. Mike, the medical student who ran the meeting as part of his training, said it was not a problem: 'We spend our days in our windowless office, so sitting in a sunlit conference room is always nice.' We introduced ourselves, one after the other, and then Mike began.

> Mike: We just met your father, but wanted to start by learning more about him. So could you tell us more about what he's like as a person when he's not here?
>
> Lynn: My father loves life. He's always loved life, even though he has had a very difficult life. He was born in the same house where he's living today, and his brother was very sick when he was young and eventually died. He still talks about his death, says that it's such a shame he died when he was so young, such a loss. They had a family business, a bakery, which still exists. And it's been very difficult to keep it. We've been trying to convince him to sell it for a long time, but he has always insisted that as long as he is alive, the bakery will keep going.
>
> Mike: And how has he been recently, in terms of health?
>
> Lynn: Well, he's been getting short of breath when we were coming down to see the bakery, and you know, sometimes he gets upset about how things look like there, and then he gets more short of breath, so I've been trying not to do those trips too often.
>
> Social worker: Tell me something, how is he when he's at home? How much time does he usually spend in bed or in his chair?
>
> Lynn: I'd say that quite a lot, I think he spends most of his day in the chair, reading the paper.
> [Conversation about how the daughter treats him at home and the mattress they bought to avoid bedsores.]

The meeting began with a general narrative about Mr. Becker's character and life story, which the medical student elicited from the daughter. Very talkative and friendly, the daughter responded at length and appeared to appreciate Mike's interest. The social worker, who was the most senior palliative care team member in the room, asked a more pointed question about the patient's medical condition and life at home. After some fifteen minutes of conversation, the social worker turned the focus of the conversation to the daughter's feelings.

> Social worker: What would you like to ask him right now?
>
> Lynn: [Moved by the question, she seems to be close to tears.] Mainly, I would really want to see him back in his house. This house has really

been important for him, he's always been so connected to it, and all of
his memories are from there.

[Lynn tells about financial problems they've been having with the
bakery.]

Social worker: And what worries you the most?

Lynn: Look, I know that at some point he can decline, and I'm just really
worried about the moment we wouldn't be able to take him home and he
wouldn't be able to live there. [People nod.] You know, it's not the first
time that this happens: he had pneumonia in the past and was hospitalized, and he came back. And he spent some time in nursing homes after
each hospitalization, and he really didn't like it. [Talks about the
experience of going to the hospital with her father this time.]

Lynn's engagement in the conversation and her emotional connection to
her father were evident by her tears. She shared her worries about him and
expressed their illness experiences articulately and with considerable detail. Mr. Becker's subjectivity was now on the table: Lynn did not list any
concrete wish of his, yet she spoke very clearly about his character and
their fears for the future. At this point, the social worker started to prepare
the ground for hooking. At first, she summarized what Lynn had told her,
showing that she had heard and understood what she said. Importantly,
this summary was not a simple reiteration of what Lynn said. The social
worker *translated* Lynn's story into concrete and concise goals.

> Social worker: You know, *what I hear from you* is that he's not really a
> person who wants to be in a facility. He's not going to live well
> there—he's happy at home, and this is where he'll be the happiest—
> sitting in his chair and reading his paper. . . . [People smile, Lynn
> nods and chuckles.] (emphasis mine)

Once Lynn approved of the translation by nodding and chuckling,
the social worker began hooking. She mentioned the possibility of admitting Mr. Becker to hospice and tried to connect it to the goals she has
just stated.

> Social worker: And if this is our goal—to bring him back home—it's
> important to remember that there is this thing called "hospice." I'm not
> even saying that this is a place where you are in right now, at this

moment. But it's good to remember that this is a possibility for the future. We just want to put this idea out there, on the table.

Lynn: [Her tone of voice seems to change slightly.] I don't know, my understanding has always been that hospice basically means not to treat him anymore, and in case he gets pneumonia and needs antibiotics, this will not be a great solution.

Social worker: So first of all, if you're on hospice and for any reason you're unhappy—you can always sign off, and it's not a problem at all. And second, although in principle hospices are not going to give him IV antibiotics, you can also get him antibiotics in pills. He doesn't have trouble swallowing.

Lynn: So this is something that I didn't know.

Social worker: Again, it's not that I'm saying that you're there yet. But if you want to keep him at home, this is a type of support that will help you do that. [Lynn nods.]

Like many other people, Mr. Becker's daughter recoiled at the mention of hospice. Indeed, Mr. Becker was not discharged to hospice at the end of this hospitalization. At the same time, the palliative care social worker successfully presented hospice services as something that matched Mr. Becker's goals of care, and in that way, increased the probability that his daughter would admit him to hospice at some point in the future. Throughout the exchange, the social worker maintained the focus of the conversation on Mr. Becker's goals of care as his daughter understood them. She did not *tell* the daughter that her father's medical condition meant he should be admitted to hospice. Rather, she and the medical student elicited Mr. Becker's subjectivity from his daughter's stories and hooked hospice care to it. Consequently, if and when Mr. Becker would be admitted to hospice, it would not be because the social worker told him to do so, but because it would match *his* (or his daughter's) own will. Mr. Becker was successfully subjectified; his daughter, the main decision maker in the case, recognized and endorsed certain personality traits that represented him as aligned with hospice care.

The related practice of *unhooking*—detaching a patient's subjectivity from a certain course of treatment—was done in a similar way: clinicians used certain details or themes in narratives of patients' subjectivity to highlight how certain treatments contradicted their goals of care. One patient's daughter, for example, told a palliative care team about her father's terrible experience at the nursing home where he lives. She explained that her father had been suffering from a lot of pain and that the nurses, who were badly understaffed, never managed to treat this pain properly. A palliative care physician responded

> It sounds like *your* biggest concern right now is that your father has been through too much, and you want to make his life as peaceful and as comfortable as possible. So it's actually not a question of should he have surgery [or not], it's a question of does a surgery accomplish what his goals are. (emphasis mine)

The possessive form "your" was of prime importance. The physician did not refer to his own medical opinion, but to the daughter's and the patient's subjectivity. It was the daughter who was concerned about her father's pain, and it was the daughter's own goal to make her father as comfortable as possible. The physician translated the daughter's experiences into a concrete goal of care, then *unhooked* a surgery from this goal. The logical outcome was that surgery did not correspond to the patient's goals of care.

These subjectification techniques allowed palliative care clinicians to navigate around more difficult questions. They asked families and patients about patients' character, life story, feelings, illness experience, and attitude toward medicine—not about whether to relinquish resuscitation, ICU admissions, or surgeries and succumb to death. No less important, these conversations were participatory: clinicians did not impose medical decisions on families and patients, but elicited patients' subjectivities through the conversations then hooked their care plans onto them. This process established patients' and families' *consent* to end-of-life decisions. It bridged between the clinicians' inclination to respect patients' wishes and the clinicians' own wish to avoid "aggressive" treatment and economize dying.

"Did He Say No?"

I did not have to know Mr. Emery's exact diagnosis to see that he was extremely sick. When I met him, a white man in his mid-50s, he was bedbound and had multiple organ failures. Despite not having eaten for six months (he was nourished intravenously by TPN*), he was badly over-weight. He had been hospitalized for more than eight months, he had a tracheotomy opening in his neck, and he had just been transferred back from the ICU to a step-down unit,[†] after having been resuscitated and in-tubated. That morning, the palliative care attending physician thought the team should give up on this case: they had discussed the matter with Mr. Emery before the resuscitation but could not get him to consent to a less aggressive course of treatment. The team's nurse, social worker, and chaplain, however, thought there was still a chance that he would recon-sider his position.

In the team's morning meeting, the attending physician raised his arms in exasperation and conceded, 'I've been here only for one day, so I'm not really updated. If the team likes him, and you want to keep him on the service. . . .' The chaplain, nurse, and social worker agreed they would go to see him together, and the chaplain declared that 'the doctors are released from this task.'

Hours later, outside Mr. Emery's room, the three of them, a medical student, and I congregated. Mr. Emery had two daughters who lived far away, did not come to see him, and were disengaged from the decision-making process. The consolidation of his goals and values and their translation into concrete treatment decisions involved him and the med-ical staff only. As we were waiting outside his room, Dr. Estefan, a young resident from the step-down unit who was in charge of Mr. Emery's case, joined us. Rebecca, the palliative care nurse, told him she did not think Mr. Emery should go to the ICU again if things got worse, and the resi-dent, surrounded by the five of us, seemed to nod. "He [Dr. Estefan] doesn't argue back," I wrote in my notes, "doesn't express opinions that are different from theirs. Possibly because he agrees with them, but very likely because he doesn't have a clear opinion of his own."

Laura, the chaplain, said that her impression from their last conversa-tion was that Mr. Emery tended to change the topic whenever it was inconvenient for him. When she asked him about DNR/DNI, he did not

---

* Total parenteral nutrition (TPN) provides nutrition through the bloodstream.

† A step-down unit is an intermediate level of care between ICUs and regular medicine units.

respond and instead asked her to bring him some ice. Rebecca laughed and said, 'Then I'll bring some ice to the meeting, and we can have it ready, right next to us.' A few minutes later she came back with a disposable plastic cup full of ice chips. As we walked into the room, two technicians were covering a bloody dialysis machine and wheeling it out. Mr. Emery was lying on his side. Whenever he wanted to talk, Dr. Estefan had to remove a tube from his trach and seal it with a cap, which allowed air to flow back through his voice box. This allowed Mr. Emery to utter short sentences; after each one he had to stop for twenty seconds or so to catch his breath.

Rebecca, the palliative care nurse, was Mr. Emery's favorite. She had been treating him for four months, first for a pressure wound that refused to heal, then as a member of the palliative care team. "We brought you your favorite people here," Dr. Estefan started the conversation, "Rebecca and Laura." The rest of us introduced ourselves to him, then he signaled to Rebecca to come closer to him. "You're making me crazy," he whispered.[52] I felt uncomfortable, but Rebecca did not show any sign of discomfort: 'I like you too,' she responded with a patient smile. He said that the day before, one doctor came in and made him feel like he was in the "losers' club." 'Who was that?' Rebecca asked, but Mr. Emery could not remember. He apologized and said that he forgot to take his card, and we all laughed. Laura said 'it doesn't matter now. We shouldn't care about whatever he said. We came to talk about how *you* feel,' she told him, 'and what *you* want.' Laura asked him if he wanted some ice. He did, and she handed him the plastic cup. He took one ice chip from the cup and put it in his mouth.

> Dr. Estefan: We're here to talk about your goals, Adam. And we want to ask what are you goals? What are you expecting? [covers his trach opening]
> Mr. Emery: [quietly, with some effort] I want to go to Tennessee to live near my daughters.
> Dr. Estefan: We made a big step forward when you got out of the ICU, you know. But right now your condition is not good enough to go to Tennessee. You would need a long-term acute care facility to stay in. [Mr. Emery moves his hand, seems to signal that he wants to say something. Dr. Estefan covers the trach.]

Mr. Emery: There's a facility right next to where my daughter lives.

Dr. Estefan: It's true, but it'll be difficult right now to move you there because your condition is not good enough.

[Mr. Emery sobs voicelessly; tears roll down his cheeks.]

Laura: [to Dr. Estefan] Just a second.

One could say that Mr. Emery's wishes were clear: he wanted his condition to improve and to move to a facility near his daughters. Yet his doctor thought it was impossible to follow this plan. Mr. Emery had just returned from the ICU, and his condition was still unstable. Transferring him from California to Tennessee was very risky, and since Mr. Emery was poor and only covered by Medicaid, he could not afford to pay for an air ambulance. There was no way to follow his wish, given the circumstances. His disappointment made him very emotional, which, at least for me, was devastating.

Such situations, however, are the bread and butter of palliative care work. Mr. Emery was showing intense emotions, which could be used to further explore his experience of his suffering and be *translated* into other goals of care.

Laura: [a few seconds later] Adam, it's really difficult. You've had a really difficult time in the ICU, I know. And you've been here for a long time. Tell me something: what's keeping you through that? What makes you fight so hard?

[Dr. Estefan places the cap on the trach, so Mr. Emery can speak.]

Mr. Emery: My children. [mumbles something unclear] They're important for me.

Laura: I can see that.

Dr. Estefan: Were hoping that you will go there. Getting out of the ICU is a big step forward. You could go to a facility here, and then if your condition improves, go to Tennessee. That would be a big step forward. And we're working hard with you to get you there. We know you've been working hard. Now, given all that, Adam, I want to ask you: if we see that you have to go to the ICU, and we know that this is a step backward, would you like to go back to the ICU? [He puts the cap back on the trach.]

Mr. Emery: If I know that there's no chance I'll get out of there. . . . Then what for?

Dr. Estefan: So you're basically agreeing that if you go backward, the doctors here will decide what are the chances that you'll get out of the ICU?

[Mr. Emery twists his wrist several times, perhaps signaling "kind of" or "I'm not sure." Dr. Estefan puts back the cap.]

Mr. Emery: More ice.

[Rebecca gives him another ice chip.]

Laura: Let's talk about what we're understanding from you so far, Adam. Your main goal is to go to Tennessee and live in a long-term acute care facility by your daughters. Until then, if it's not possible, we want to move you to an acute care center here, and hope that your condition will improve and you'll be able to move there. And if things go backward, and you have to go to the ICU, then you don't want that.

[Mr. Emery seems to nod.]

Laura: Yes.

Mr. Emery: [Signals he wants to speak, and Dr. Estefan covers the trach.] The ICU was really bad. They let me eat some fried chicken there, and I didn't like that.

Rebecca: [chuckles] That must have been a great dream. . . . Tell me something, what can we do for you to make you feel better?

Mr. Emery: Beer.

[People chuckle.]

Rebecca: You know, maybe it will be possible. We'll see. [Dr. Estefan looks puzzled.] Maybe just a little bit of beer, just to feel the taste, especially since he swallows so well. [He had a good swallowing test earlier in the day.]

[Dr. Estefan now nods.]

Rebecca: What else would you like?

Mr. Emery: Spaghetti. [Says something unclear about how much he misses eating. He's very short of breath when he speaks.]

Rebecca: [nods] You know, I feel it's been enough for today. We've probably made you tired. You've been through a lot, and you worked hard to get out of the ICU, which is great. And you know, it was your hard work—not ours.

Mr. Emery: You think I didn't work hard?

Rebecca: No, this is what I'm saying—that you did work harder than us.

As the conversation went on, Mr. Emery's responses got shorter; he struggled to catch his breath when he spoke, and interaction became difficult. Before we left, however, he insisted on having his trach covered again, thanked me and the medical student—the two observers who joined the meeting—for coming to see him, and wished us luck.

How did the palliative care clinicians consolidate Mr. Emery's goals and values? At first, Mr. Emery said that if he had no chance of getting out of the ICU, he would not want to be transferred there in the first place. In the rest of the conversation he voiced concrete wishes—such as drinking beer and eating spaghetti—both understandable wishes coming from a man who has been fed intravenously without eating anything for nearly six months. Dr. Estefan tried to translate his words and suggested that "you're basically agreeing that if you go backward, the doctors here will decide what are the chances that you'll get out of the ICU." This translation emphasized the agency doctors would assume in determining the severity of his condition, and by consequence whether his life would be sustained. Yet Dr. Estefan did not get Mr. Emery's endorsement for this translation. Mr. Emery only made an unclear signal with his hand and asked for more ice.

Laura, the chaplain, made a second attempt. She translated Mr. Emery's words into an ordinal description of his goals and values: first, moving to Tennessee; second, transferring to a nearby facility in California; and third, not being transferred to the ICU if his condition declines. This map was devoid of doctors' agency: Laura did not mention that doctors would determine whether his condition was irreversible but simply mentioned that he would not be transferred to the ICU if his condition declined. Furthermore, this translation included Mr. Emery's original wish to live in proximity to his daughters and gave a more central expression to his agency. Whether Laura's translation received Mr. Emery's endorsement or not is open to interpretation. Mr. Emery appeared to nod, Laura said "yes," and he did not challenge her but instead asked for ice, beer, and spaghetti. When the conversation ended, and the meeting's participants left the room, they had to decide what to make of it. Dr. Redcliff, a senior resident, joined them in the hallway.

[Dr. Redcliff] is a tall white man in his late 20s, acts and looks much more confident than Dr. Estefan. Rebecca says that we talked to Mr. Emery and he said he wouldn't want to go back to the ICU. Dr. Redcliff looks a bit doubtful, asks her a couple of times "did he say *no*?" Laura says that he was very clear, and Dr. Estefan agrees with her. Dr. Redcliff says, 'What does it mean? I guess, DNI?' He chuckles, seems uncomfortable, looks at Dr. Estefan.

Rebecca says 'I think you should feel totally comfortable making him DNI.' Dr. Estefan nods, says 'I think this is what I understood too.' Laura says, 'My impression was that he's much better, he knew what he was talking about, and he understood the decision.' Rebecca says, 'He got his sarcasm back, which is important.' They talk about whether to give him beer and laugh about it together. 'I don't think it'll be a problem, since we're not talking about large quantities anyway. He could have half a cup a week or so. And since he keeps talking about eating, we could give him a little bit of food too.' Laura agrees with her; 'from a palliative care perspective, it's not a problem even if he aspirates and gets pneumonia.'

This conversation converted the rather ambivalent, inconsistent, and uncertain interaction between Mr. Emery, Dr. Estefan, Laura, and Rebecca into an unequivocal and formal order written on a standard printed piece of paper not to intubate Mr. Emery if he stopped breathing. The form did not capture much of the conversation that had taken place, nor did it reflect qualifiers that clinicians used before signing the form, such as 'my impression,' 'I think,' or 'I guess.' The DNI form did not cite Mr. Emery's twist of his wrist, nor did it mention the ambivalence and equivocation that appeared throughout the conversation. Finally, the term "DNI" was not mentioned even once in the original conversation; when talking to Mr. Emery, clinicians spoke of the "ICU," where he had difficult experiences, and not of a form that would mean he would not be intubated if he stopped breathing.

The next day, Mr. Emery stopped breathing. His doctors followed the DNI order, did not intubate him, and he passed away. About a month later, in an interview with Laura, she reflected on the difficulty of reaching this decision:

> I think [doctors] need to feel like, you know, a hundred percent certain that they're doing the right thing, which is often not a possibility. I think they need support. And that's why this collaborative decision-making model—it has many pitfalls—I think it's partly to serve, you know, the needs of the clinicians so that they don't feel

guilt. You know, I think that the nurses who are actually doing the extubation, who are doing the administration of medicine, they think 'it's causing suffering,' and they also need a lot of support. But they're not in the decision-making level. Their distress is different. They have to do things that they maybe have moral compunctions about. But the doctors . . . I think they just often fight it off till the next one, because they don't want it hanging over them.

[With Mr. Emery], . . . you were there when he decided not to have the. . . . And then the next day, he had this condition, the circumstance that led to him dying. . . . Because he was saying no, he didn't go back to the ICU and he died. The doctors involved in that were like, "Hmm. I hope he [Mr. Emery] made the right call." They would have been a lot happier if they had had some [time], there had been a few days that have gone by, where they could keep asking him, and he could keep telling them. It was virtually instantaneous after that conversation. And I felt like, ouch. That's a little heavy. You know? I don't know. If it could have been: "this is gonna happen, we know this is gonna happen, are you sure?" Because every time in the past when it had happened, he had wanted to go [to the ICU]. You know? You just don't know. You don't know. And I actually wrote that doc [Dr. Estefan] [an e-mail], 'How ya doing?' Are you doing okay? And he wrote back and said, 'I'm doing okay, yeah.'

Laura acknowledged the moral difficulty in reaching decisions to let patients die. She argued that in practice, physicians involved patients and families in making end-of-life decisions because of their own moral needs: doing so took some of the burden off of them. In fact, Laura's reflections on Mr. Emery's case illustrated this very mechanism: she completely erased her agency from her account of the decision-making process. At no point did she mention how central she was in the conversation with Mr. Emery. She kept referring to the decision to not be intubated as a decision that Mr. Emery himself made.

At first blush, Laura's reflection seems paradoxical. If Mr. Emery was the one who made the decision against an ICU transfer, why should the clinicians feel responsible for it? Yet after observing the entire working process in which clinicians elicited goals and values, translated, and hooked, this paradox is clarified. The patients' subjectivity was invested in the agency of clinicians. While clinicians did not construct patients' subjectivity singlehandedly, and while clinicians could not read anything they wanted into what patients told them, they were the ones who carried out subjectification, and consequently they had much impact on what they eventually documented as patients' goals and values.

Conclusion

Decisions to stop artificial nutrition, withhold ventilation, and forgo future hospitalizations pose some of the most difficult ethical predicaments in modern medical practice. In many cases, these decisions have morally unsettling outcomes; people hesitate before making them and have doubts after. In this context, the clinicians who treated patients near the end of their lives sought after any indication that the patients approved of the care they were giving.

Such approval, however, was hard to garner. One obstacle was incapacity: many severely ill patients could not think clearly, let alone communicate their thoughts, when their condition declined. But no less importantly, many patients (and families) were, quite simply, undecided. Anthropologist Sharon Kaufman, who studied end-of-life care, noted how she began her research "holding the common, negative opinion about 'being attached to machines'" and against "artificially prolonged death." After two years in the field, however, equivocation replaced her certainty: "I *think* I know what I would want or what I would do, how long I would ask for life-sustaining procedures, and how long I would maintain hope—but I learned that I cannot be sure."[53] Subjectifying patients meant transforming such equivocation into more solid sets of preferences. The process, as I showed, involved delving into people's biographies, values, and personalities and harnessing them to the economization effort.

Palliative care clinicians empowered and controlled patients at the same time. On the one hand, they brought patients into the decision-making process, making them active and opinionated agents who held an inalienable right to be the authors of their life's last chapter. The idea was not to present their uncertainty as certainty, but to produce certainty— make patients more certain, clearer about how they wanted to be treated. On the other hand, being such active agents, who had personalities, opinions, values, and preferences that could guide medical decisions, was an expectation. Clinicians *needed* patients to have intelligible personalities and sufficient insight. The palliative way of care prompted patients to become agents in the decision-making process. Furthermore, teasing out and processing patients' goals and values also meant controlling them: patients (or families) voiced feelings, thoughts, and reflections in response to premeditated questions that palliative care clinicians were trained to ask. What patients wanted—and more strongly, who patients *were*—was often an outcome of these conversations rather than their point of departure.

Sociologist Pierre Bourdieu observed that administering a questionnaire is a situation where "opinions are made to exist which did not pre-exist the questions, and which otherwise would not have been expressed."[54] Much of this observation applies to interviews. Interviews are unique social situations: they confront people with questions they may otherwise never contemplate, forcing them to provide answers. The palliative care clinical interview demands that people stop and think about who they (or their family member) are and what they wish. How patients and families express themselves and what they say partly depends on palliative care practice—what Bourdieu called "the modes of production" of personal opinions. Patients would have said different things had clinicians asked them different questions in different ways. Regardless, in many cases patients' positions would have "had little chance of being formulated spontaneously" without clinical intervention.[55]

Unlike interviews that pollsters conduct, the outcomes of palliative care interviews quickly turn back on patients. What a patient says to a palliative care clinician, writes into an advance directive form, or places in the "very important" pile when playing Go Wish comes to represent her. The practice of palliative care essentializes personhood: it transforms volatile and possibly momentary feelings that people have and statements that they make into a fixed and solid set of personalized traits. This was the essence of subjectification: the written forms where people declared their wishes, values, and preferences—and the conversations with palliative care clinicians where they uttered them—were what held patients' "personhood, identity, selfhood, autonomy, and individuality in place."[56]

Advocates of patient autonomy may take pride in how diligently palliative care clinicians work to make patients speak. They are, however, somewhat less reflective about the fact that once patients speak, their speech and the forms that they filled come to control them and dictate how they would be treated.

The interactions between palliative care clinicians, patients, and families depended on the patients' social and economic power. For some people, subjectification began prior to hospitalization: patients who had good health insurance and a stable relationship with a primary care physician were more likely to have thought about end-of-life care ahead of time, filled out an advance directive, and talked to their relatives about the topic. Those with stable family relations were also likely to have a close relative who would represent them confidently in the hospital. Other patients, those who did not have the economic, social, and cultural capital that made them more receptive to subjectification, very often left clinicians uncertain and frustrated.

Unsubjectifiable patients did not necessarily *disagree* with the medical staff, but they were closer to what Bourdieu referred to as unopinionated people, who respond "I don't know" when asked questions in social surveys. Bourdieu attributed such responses to several causes: self-censorship (i.e., reluctance or discomfort engaging a certain question), social perception of incompetence (feeling unable to formulate an opinion on a certain topic), or lack of interest.[57] All these causes are distributed unequally; they usually apply to marginalized and undervalued populations, and end-of-life care is one among many realms where this inequality shows.

Even when such inequalities did not influence the *content* of end-of-life decisions directly, they had an impact on people's experience of their illness, on their understanding of their illness, and on how their clinicians understood them. When I asked a former palliative care physician from Academic Hospital how social differences mattered in end-of-life care he answered,

> I don't know about a quantifiable difference, in terms of survival benefit or something like that. In terms of [people's] experience, in terms of their acceptance of what happens to them—it's much better.

[People with whom I have good connection] will generally have a better experience with their disease no matter how good or how bad the outcome is. . . . They'll have, generally, a better death, if there is such a thing.

People's social background impacts whether they get to articulate themselves, spell out their goals and values, and pursue them successfully. Ultimately, the patients who had the opportunity to think through and formulate their positions on end-of-life care, who were comfortable and capable of engaging in conversations on the topic, who were assertive when talking to medical staff, and whose agency the medical staff validated were the ones who became the authors of their own lives and died in a way that represented the goals and values that they had articulated.

CHAPTER 5

Goat Taming

[If] a true effort went into helping them make that decision and they
didn't, then the other arm comes in.

—A palliative care physician

PHYSICAL DECLINE IS HARDLY EVER STEADY, and oftentimes it involves short-term improvements. Even undoubtedly terminal illnesses
may progress unpredictably. A terminal cancer patient may recuperate for
a few days and start eating; an end-stage Alzheimer's disease patient may
recover from pneumonia and be slightly more responsive; and a patient
with an end-stage liver disease may regain consciousness for a few hours
or days. Such developments do not change the bigger picture—these patients would still have terminal cancer, Alzheimer's disease, and liver disease—but they may give people the hope that they can buy more time.

The modern hospital is a fertile ground for such hopes. Numerous
specialty services, each offering innumerable treatment options and diagnostic tests, are available to those wishing to pursue every trace of op-
timism. Frequent changes in treatment decisions are likely: the cancer
patient's family may want to try another chemotherapy once she perks up;
the Alzheimer patient's family may reconsider his Do Not Resuscitate / Do
Not Intubate (DNR/DNI) form and ask for dialysis; the family of the liver
disease patient may ask to give him full life-sustaining care in the intensive care unit (ICU), betting on an improbable scenario that he would
enter the transplant candidate list.

One palliative care doctor called such situations "goat rodeos," and although he never defined them to me explicitly, the meaning was clear from the context. Goat rodeos were erratic, untamed, and unpredictable medical decision-making processes that changed course capriciously according to people's immediate wishes and mercurial moods. Every sign of improvement, as temporary and uncertain as it was, led to consulting new specialists, trying new medications, requesting diagnostic tests, and reopening economized decisions that had seemed closed.

Subjectification, which I discussed in Chapter 4, was one way to avoid goat rodeos. It replaced immediate wishes and caprices with a more solid abstraction—the patient's self and personality, which clinicians could better manage, control, and economize. This chapter focuses on what the palliative care clinicians did when subjectification failed, or when it was insufficient to stabilize the families' and patients' wishes and expectations. I analyze techniques that palliative care clinicians used to contain, constrain, and manage specific wishes that threatened to develop into full-blown goat rodeos.

When controlling wishes more directly, palliative care clinicians walked a thin line between two models of decision making: "consent" and "assent." As sociologist Renée Anspach put it, in the model of informed consent, patients and their families "are treated as the principal participants in the life-and-death decision," whereas in the "assent" model they only give their formal approval to a decision that the medical staff have already made. Studying two intensive care nurseries in the 1980s, Anspach found that the latter model dominated. Clinicians presented their professional views to parents as unequivocal and objective facts, they concealed their professional disagreements, they framed neonates' medical conditions in ways that directed their parents to agree with clinicians' recommendations, and they neutralized the parents' resistance by psychologizing it. As Anspach put it, the clinicians focused on producing parents' assent and diffusing their dissent.[1]

All the practices that Anspach observed appeared in my field sites, but I also found an important difference, which requires refining the dichotomy between "consent" and "assent." Even when palliative care clinicians deliberately tried to influence patients (or families), they were aware, reflective, and self-critical. Knowing how much power they possessed as professionals and being genuinely interested in allowing the patients and families to affect decisions, the palliative care clinicians often constrained their own efforts to constrain patients and families.[2] Constraining patients and families was a delicate art, and those practicing it were mindful of not completely overwhelming their patients' agency and depleting consent of all meaning.

'Every physician goes to the bedside and lets the patient drive decisions,' said Andy, a senior organ transplant surgeon. 'But patients [depend] . . . on the presentation that you give them.' Andy felt that he could sway patients' wishes in any direction he wanted.

> You can drive them to the fountain: I can say, "Mrs. Smith, grandma is eighty-five and it'll only make her suffer if we operate on her, and it's not going to cure her." Or I can say, "Mrs. Johnson, you know, I think I can get the cancer out of you." And what do you think they'll want to do? Of course that if I tell her that I can cure her, she'll go with me, no matter what other people are telling her.[3] As a doctor, you come to talk to patients with your biases. If your experience is that you've done transplants in eighty year olds and they turned out fine, then you're biased toward that.

This is what scholars of medical practice have called "the illusion of choice." Medicine may hail patient autonomy and informed consent rhetorically, but in reality professionals (such as physicians) and institutions (such as hospitals and insurance companies) heavily control patients.[4] If a physician or a hospital does not present a patient with the option of having a surgery (or conversely, of transitioning to hospice care), the option will most likely remain outside of the patient's realm of possibility.[5] Notice, however, that Andy recognized and reflected on the influence he had on patients. He alluded to his "bias" as a transplant surgeon—not unlike palliative care physicians, who, as I mentioned in Chapter 1, admitted that they drew the line before other physicians because they were more exposed to treatment failures. Clinicians were aware of their power and thought about it critically. The impact they had on patients as experts was inevitable, and they thought about how to use it methodically and fairly. While clinicians deliberately influenced patients and families, they did not want to manipulate, completely dominate, or dictate their decisions.

This chapter examines several basic tricks of the trade that palliative care clinicians used to navigate the fine line between consulting and manipulating, as they worked to economize dying. The chapter's first section outlines the chief "don'ts" of palliative care: common patterns in doctor–patient interactions that palliative care clinicians criticized for being restrictive to the point of manipulation, or unrestrictive to the point of risking "goat rodeos." In the second section, I summarize several examples of practices that palliative care practitioners encouraged and advocated. The third section examines how palliative care clinicians dealt with situations in which, despite their best efforts, patients and families resisted economizing dying and insisted on continuing life-prolonging and life-sustaining treatment. In these cases as in others, the effort to economize dying and influence the patient (or family) was methodical. Clinicians clearly constrained patients but avoided dominating them completely.

The Don'ts

Disfavored Formulae: "Do Everything" and "Laundry Lists"

Mark was an attending nephrologist, a senior kidney specialist, who worked as a partner in a private practice and saw patients at Private Hospital. As a nephrologist, he regularly consulted on the treatment of ICU patients whose kidney function had declined. One intervention that he and his colleagues regularly offered was dialysis. Yet the acute condition of many of his ICU patients made him doubt the appropriateness of dialysis in their cases. When I interviewed him, he criticized interns and residents who worked in the ICU and blamed them for not interacting with families properly.

> Nothing irritates me more than when I'm called onto a case and the house doctors* say, "Well, we asked the patient if they wanted

---

* "House doctors" (usually referred to as "house staff") included interns and residents—physicians in their first years after medical school.

everything"—"everything" is the term they usually use . . . —and [the patient] said "Yes." Or, we asked the wife, "Do you want us to do everything?" and she said yes. . . . I don't think that's an appropriate question or appropriate wording. [*Q:* Why?] . . . It puts family members and decision makers in a real uncomfortable and precarious place, where they feel pressured to say, "What do we want . . . to do? Of course, we want them to be healthy, we want them to be alive, we want them to regain their health, so of course—do everything, because that's the only way we're going to achieve that."

Words matter. In end-of-life care, the intuitive phrase "do everything" has become a red flag because it prompts very particular reactions from patients and families. Textbooks and seminars on end-of-life care present the use of "do everything" as a common clinical mistake, which can and should be corrected. In a 2012 article, pediatricians Chris Feudtner and Wynne Morrison cited several circumstances in which "do everything" came up at the bedside:

> The physician may offer this up as a pledge: "We are going to do everything." Or asks the question: "Do you want us to do everything?" Alternatively, a family member may utter the phrase as a request or demand: "We want you to do everything." Heads nod in silent agreement. We will do everything.[6]

Feudtner and Morrison found the term "do everything" to be misleading. First, it is logically impossible to do everything because any treatment necessarily comes at the expense of something else. One cannot "hold a loved one's hand while they are dying at the same moment that a code team yells 'clear' and attempts to defibrillate the patient's heart."[7] Second, by "do everything," families and clinicians may mean different things: a family's demand to do everything may be a simple cry for help and support, but clinicians typically perceive it as a concrete request for aggressive medical interventions.[8] Finally, "do everything" confronts families, patients, and clinicians with a binary choice: either *everything is done* or *not everything is done*. This fosters "an adversarial air in conversations": families and patients "may be more likely to fear that care is being rationed for some reason other than the patient's best interests." The "do everything" phrase is therefore "dangerous nonsense. A moratorium is warranted, halting all medical personnel from further casual utterances of 'do everything.'"[9]

The palliative care clinicians that I studied criticized the "do everything" phrase on lexical as well as indexical grounds. They not only took issue with the phrase's dictionary meaning but also with the effect it had on interactions at the bedside. Other phrases and expressions that had similar effects attracted similar criticisms. Laura, a palliative care chaplain renowned for her superb communication skills, told me,

> If you ask people, "Do you want to live?"—99.9 percent of them are gonna say, "Yeah, I want to live." If you ask them, "What do you hope for?"—99.9 percent of them are going to say, "I hope to live."[10] When you ask a question—you influence the answer. . . . [You ask,] "What are your goals?" [and they answer,] "My goal is a cure." It's sort of a formulaic question, "What are your goals?"

As I described in Chapter 4, the term "goals" has a very central place in palliative care vocabulary. But as Laura said, when clinicians used it to ask a patient or a family a direct question about their wishes, it became an invitation to request more curative treatments, which stifled the introspective reflections that economization required. A palliative care social worker told me that the wording of some advance directive forms had a similarly problematic effect:

> If somebody, at some point in their life, doesn't want to be in an ICU intubated—that can be recorded in [an] advance directive. [But only] in a really good advance directive—not these crappy pieces of shit that we have here. I don't know if you've seen them, but it's awful. They say, "Do you want to be intubated?"—of course you're gonna say "yes." You don't know what that means; you could have pneumonia, and you'd be intubated for five days and recover and go back to your life. They're just very black-and-white, and they're very . . . It says, "Do you want to prolong your life?"—of course people would want to prolong their life! Why would people say no?

We can notice several palliative care don'ts. First is the "do everything" phrase. Second are the general, open-ended questions about patients' "hopes" or "goals," which are likely to elicit unequivocal "I want to be cured and live" answers. And third is any phrasing of yes-or-no questions about the use of specific medical procedures. Similarly to "everything done," asking patients and families whether they do or do not want to be intubated, resuscitated, or transferred to the ICU if their condition declines is far too narrow, too "black-and-white" to capture the unpredictability of scenarios and the nuanced preferences that patients and families may have. Making the term "everything done" more concrete by listing all of the medical procedures under discussion does not solve the problem. Pointed yes-or-no questions still set families to respond "yes" to any medical procedure that clinicians mention.

Learning these conversational skills is a slow process, and new palliative care clinicians were certain to make mistakes. A nurse who began working with Public Hospital's palliative care service joined the rest of the team to meet the family of a severely ill elderly woman. The morning after the meeting, the team sat to debrief, and the nurse admitted she had made a conversational mistake.

Physician: It was a tough meeting yesterday.

Nurse: [smiles] Yes, it was.

Physician: The [medicine team] doctor there was frustrated that the family couldn't understand that we can't fix [the patient's] aspiration. Just to keep you in the loop [addressed another nurse, who wasn't in the meeting], she had a brainstem stroke . . . and she was at [a nursing home] where she kept getting fever from infections . . . because she's having problems with aspiration. The family is very medically focused, they're constantly talking about the small details. . . .

Chaplain: I actually felt that they were a little bit open to talking about the situation in general. They were clear in saying that they have to say "yes" to everything, but at the same time the sister said that she didn't want [the patient] to suffer.

Nurse: Right, and I did notice this small crack open, when the sister said she wanted to do everything, but at the same time she didn't want [the patient] to suffer, so I immediately tried to jump in and try to open this little crack . . . I'm sorry.

[Physician nods without saying anything.]

Nurse: And I asked her what does she mean when she says she doesn't want [the patient] to suffer—would she want [the patient] to be intubated?

> And she said yes. Would she want [the patient] to be admitted to the
> ICU? And she again said yes. And then at the same time she says that
> she doesn't want [the patient] to suffer . . .

The nurse's brief apology ("I'm sorry"), followed by the physician's silent nod, showed that they both recognized and agreed the nurse had made a mistake. The nurse was right to notice a "little crack" but wrong in how she tried to "open" it—asking yes-or-no questions about specific interventions, which triggered unequivocal affirmative answers. Asking such questions would be a mistake in any conversation with any family, let alone with a family that, as the chaplain mentioned, was "clear in saying that they have to say 'yes' to everything." Palliative care clinicians, as the chaplain implied, prefer to keep the conversation on the "general" level. At this general level, the family's stance would have still been open to interpretation and could still have been negotiated.

In another hospital, for example, a palliative care social worker who talked to the children of a severely ill patient interpreted a similar request differently. When they said "we'll have to say 'yes' to everything," the children implicitly requested that doctors would *not* ask them what life-prolonging treatments to provide—because they felt obliged to say "yes" even to procedures that made their mother suffer. Public Hospital's nurse, by contrast, made the family specify all the concrete life-sustaining interventions they would "have to say 'yes' to." The general statement quickly solidified into a set of demands and expectations from the medical team. Although these demands could still be discussed and perhaps even changed, the process would require a lot of work and time.

Many nonpalliative care clinicians, however, felt they could not comfortably withhold life-sustaining treatment without hearing an explicit request from the patient (or family). Presenting direct questions to them was the most intuitive thing to do—what could be more straightforward than asking whether they would want a certain procedure done? Scott, the palliative care physician I had mentioned, criticized this tendency to me:

> [These doctors] reason in a way that . . . pisses me off. Everything that
> is not prohibited is mandatory. . . . It's the idea of a medical provider . . .
> being a cafeteria worker, throwing stuff on people's plates [and asking],

"Would you like some pressors* with that?" Seriously—no! . . . The
incentive for the team for the moment is to say, 'Do you want prunes?'
It's easier for them to give [patients and families a] choice.

On one of the days I shadowed him, Scott took the opportunity to
engage a resident who rotated with him. The two of them debriefed
after a meeting with the son of a ninety-eight-year-old woman who had
terminal metastatic cancer. In previous conversations with the internal
medicine unit's physicians, the son was very eager to prolong his
mother's life in any way possible, and the internists decided to call the
palliative care team, thinking that their superior communication skills
could help nudge the son in a more economized direction. But during
the meeting, the son consented to DNR/DNI orders very quickly, which
left Scott with little to do. Scott was happy, but he still had some reservations about how the internist had interacted with the son. 'You did great,
thank you,' he told the physician, but then added, 'feel comfortable not
to check off all that laundry list of interventions when you talk to families.'[11] After the internist left, Scott turned to a resident (Kara) who shadowed him that day:

> Scott: So what did you think about how the code status conversation
> went? I think we saw the pattern, the laundry list that they went
> through.
> Kara: I think it was already established when [the son] said, "Don't do chest
> compressions, and I don't want to intubate her." You didn't necessarily
> need to ask him again.
> Scott: [nods] Well, it's all a personal call, right? It all depends on the
> physician's confidence. What would you, as a physician, need to hear to
> feel comfortable putting that order in? So it can range all the way from,
> "Listen, dude, I'm not gonna code[†] a ninety-eight year old with metastatic
> cancer—I'm not asking you." You can say it [more] nicely, but you *can* say
> it. I don't *need* [the son] to tell me that in order to do that. . . . I might say,
> "Let me propose this to you: we're going to treat her urinary tract
> infection, in hope that she improves enough to eat and drink. If she does
> not, and there are signs that she is dying, we will *not* do things to her that

---

* (Vaso)pressors are drugs that sustain blood pressure when it drops.
† The verb "to code" means to perform cardiopulmonary resuscitation (CPR).

will only hurt her. By which I mean: we will not put her on life support, we will not put her on dialysis, we will not give her a ventilator, or do CPR." . . . Do you need to spell that out? Or do you need to be comfortable just with the general concept, and not go through the laundry list . . . just say, "We will do the things that will help, and not do things that have no chance of helping her, or will only hurt her." There are all sorts of ways to approach it. The question is, Kara, What do *you* need to get in order to put that order in?

Kara: I thought what the son said was enough.

Scott: But let's take it from the specific case to the general case. How would you handle that, if the son hadn't said it that explicitly? What would you have done?

Kara: [She hesitates and smiles uncomfortably.]

Scott: Do you need to hear it spelled out? [Kara is still quiet.] "No, I don't want dialysis; no, I don't want a ventilator?" Do you *need* to hear those words in order to put that order in? Or do you just need to hear the general concept? Or do you not even need to hear that?[12]
[Silence. I start feeling awkward myself.]

Kara: I think. . . . The general concept. I think . . . given the fact that he doesn't have a medical background, most people, if you put too many details of possible scenarios . . . I think it's confusing . . .

Scott: I agree with you. But that means that you're comfortable describing a general concept, meaning as soon as they say things like, "I don't really want them to go through a lot of interventions"—[you will sign a DNR/DNI]?
[Kara is quiet again.]

Scott: Because I think it's going to come up a lot, especially if you want to be a hospitalist, eh? You're going to have to figure out what you need to hear to feel okay putting in an order.
[She smiles, nods, but doesn't say anything.]

Scott: It's not my usual approach, but [what] I want to first clarify, beyond the goals, is the general understanding. Then on the more specific level of what to do—some of these are doctor decisions, not family decisions. One of the things that [I try] to avoid is that laundry list: . . . "Yeah, have a little bit of dialysis, maybe a ventilator, hold the pressors and the CPR"—these mixed plans don't make any sense, right? [Kara nods, smiles silently.] That's how that happens. Because if you, as a physician, need to have a written contract with every potential intervention ruled out . . . I remember one time—I'll never forget it: a really good resident told me about his patient, "He didn't say no to blood transfusions!" And I remember saying, "Is everything not prohibited mandatory?" Think about this for a second: if a patient doesn't specifically say "don't do it"—then you're obliged to do it? In other words, let's say we check her hemoglobin and it went down to 8 or 9. Will you have to transfuse her, because we didn't talk about it in that conversation?

[Kara hesitates. A few seconds of silence ensue, Scott continues looking at her, waiting for an answer.]

Kara: I feel like the son would want it.

Scott: Um-hm. There isn't a right or wrong answer. But I think that one of our struggles is this idea that every single decision is turned over to a family, and then our critical thinking [as physicians] disappears. So this is a case where I would feel very comfortable saying that we can't do this. We're not going to put hemoglobin. We'll do our best, but we're not going to do things that would hurt her. Just so you know, as a physician, me, personally, I feel comfortable to say "no." You need to develop your own style and the level of comfort you need to do what is medically right. And my recommendation to you is not to go through a laundry list, but to elicit a general understanding of the medical situation and the goals of care. . . . Because you know what will happen [in this case]—right? She'll get either dehydrated or infected, because that's what happens when people have terminal cancer. . . . Does that make sense? How do you feel about that? [Kara nods, still with an awkward smile.]

Scott presented to Kara his method: he avoided asking pointed questions about specific treatments and instead focused on the general gist—"the general concept"—of what patients and families told him. When economizing dying by relying on such a gist, clinicians could interpret general statements much more flexibly than specific requests for pressors, ventilation, antibiotics, or dialysis. Recall Laura's observation from Chapter 4 that physicians "need to feel . . . a hundred percent certain that they're doing the right thing." This observation certainly applied to Kara, who carefully acknowledged that she would need to hear from the son an explicit request before withholding a treatment from his mother. As a resident who was talking to a senior physician in what felt like an educational interaction, she was quite careful and uncomfortable expressing disagreement.

In general, palliative care clinicians flagged certain vocabulary and interaction patterns as flawed and sought to eliminate them from interactions with families and patients. When junior clinicians made such "mistakes" in meetings, palliative care people approached them after meetings ended and explained why avoiding these words and phrases was preferable. They defined variants of the "everything done" phrase as overly vague and prone to creating conflicts and misunderstandings, and they criticized direct yes-or-no questions—"Would you like us to readmit her to the ICU?," "Would you like him to be resuscitated?," or "Would you like her to be intubated?"—as presenting families and patients with counterproductive "laundry lists."

What patients (and families) did and did not want was of prime interest to palliative care clinicians. Yet they pursued this interest through very particular methods. They did not take patients' agency as unalterable. Knowing that how they asked questions affected people's answers, palliative care clinicians chose their words and phrased questions carefully and deliberately. In this way, while maintaining the focus on the patient, they contained the range of possible reactions and preferences that patients and families could express: they *tamed* patients' and families' agencies.

Futile Interactions: Manipulations and Altercations

In part, palliative care clinicians criticized "do everything" and "laundry list" formulae because they passed too much responsibility to patients and family members. The opposite tendency—of completely opposing the patients' and families' preferences and trying to dictate what they should do—drew much criticism as well. Knowing how to back off and let the patients and families have the last word, even if it completely contradicted the clinicians' medical and moral intuitions, was an important skill, which many clinicians found very hard to practice in real time. This is what made economization a process that draws on patients' own reflections and calculations, instead of a project that imposes external limits on people.

The palliative care team at Academic Hospital met to talk about a meeting they had had a day earlier, which Dr. Robbins, a senior general internist and one of the hospital's most accomplished physicians, had managed. Perhaps because of Dr. Robbins's status, the team's younger physicians enjoyed parodying his somewhat limited conversational skills.

Fellow: Dr. Robbins—he was the attending—kept telling [the family] that CPR is "violent." He always says this word, "violent," I don't know why . . .

[Another member of the team emulates how Dr. Robbins presented CPR to the family, improvising aggressive chest compressions. People laugh loudly.]

Fellow: He kept asking them if we should do this "violent" thing to [the patient], and the family kept saying "yes." So he asked again and again, and there was this back and forth for a while. "Are you sure you want us to do this violent thing?" [emulates chest compressions, pushing an invisible chest down with both hands]—"Yes"—"Are you sure?"—"Yes"—"But are you?"—"Yes."

Dr. Robbins had made a mistake—asking a direct yes-and-no question—and at the same time he refused to accept an answer he did not want to hear. The team found it grotesque and clumsy, if not outright manipulative. For one thing, Dr. Robbins had exposed the fact that he already held a clear opinion about the case and left the impression that his interest in the families' and patients' opinions was a mere attempt to validate his own inclinations with an appearance of shared decision making (that is, he sought to produce assent).[13] For another, his attitude led to a very awkward exchange, in which he asked the same question and received the same answer several times.

A month later, the team's clinicians confronted a very similar situation, when they consulted on the case of a seventy-two-year-old woman who had had a major stroke and lay unconscious in the ICU in stable condition. The neurology team was very pessimistic about her chances of regaining meaningful cognitive abilities, but her husband, a devout Catholic, was reluctant to disconnect her from the ventilator. The following exchange occurred during the staff meeting:

> Nancy [a nurse] talks about the patient, says that it's a Catholic family and they are not willing to disconnect [the patient] from the respirator. One of the sons also has severe medical problems, and the experience with him has made them somewhat less willing to go in this direction. She says that Sarah [a palliative care fellow physician] had a conversation with them last week. . . . The husband did say . . . that [the patient] wouldn't want to be in a vegetative state, but at the same time he felt that taking her off the respirator would be murder. [I was present in that meeting, and heard him use the word "sin."] Sarah also talked to the son, who said that he understood that 'a decision has to be made.'

Anna [a palliative care fellow] asks if there was any discussion about the fact that there is no real choice here, since [the patient] is never going to be able to live out of the ICU. She *has* to be taken off of the respirator.

John [the attending physician] agrees: he thinks that it's really a false decision. We know that we have to disconnect her from the respirator, and this is a *medical* decision. He says that maybe we should just inform the family that we have reached this medical decision, and it will take the burden off of them. He says that he talked about it a lot with Sarah [the palliative care fellow] and Dan [the ICU physician treating the patient], and this was what he told them. Although they were talking about a family making a decision, from his point of view this was just a false choice.

Anna says she talked to the son, who seemed to be more in line with the palliative care team's approach. The son said that knowing his father, he's the type of person who would become a lot tougher if you told him that extubating her was your own professional decision. But if you let him feel that this was a decision that he was making, he would be more likely to agree.

John says that he's concerned about what would happen if he . . . asked the husband what he would want to do, and the husband said he wanted to make a trach [tracheostomy] and keep her in the ICU. In this situation, John says, he'd have to tell the husband, 'Well, no, actually this is not really your decision, and we have decided to take her off the respirator.'

By emphasizing that the team should ask questions only when it is willing to hear several different answers, John substantiated families' agency and acknowledged that he did not fully control what they said. Discussions with families should not be a manipulative pretension that their preferences mattered but a genuine invitation to participate in the conversation and influence medical decisions. When a clinician knows she or he would not be able to accept certain requests, she should not present them as possibilities. Taking patients' and families' agency seriously necessitated constraining it.

Similar cases of unconscious and ventilator-dependent patients occurred in ICUs regularly and often led to complex decision-making processes. In some circumstances, medical teams presented continued ventilation and artificial nutrition as possibilities; in others, they refused to offer them and gave families the time to look for other institutions that would. Confronting families directly was, however, something that palliative care clinicians tried to avoid. They considered outright altercations with families to be as futile as manipulation, and they criticized the physicians who became involved in them.

> Around 1:00 p.m., I see two big men in suits and ties near the [ICU] nurses station, and in the meanwhile—a heated exchange between Carol [a palliative care nurse] and one of the ICU residents. The ICU resident tells Carol, 'It was written in the chart,' and Carol, more than a foot shorter than him, looks up straight into his eyes and asks a rhetorical question assertively: 'So what do you want to do?' I learn from the ICU social worker that . . . the son of Mr. Levinsky, a ventilator-dependent ICU patient, told somebody on the phone, 'Somebody will get hurt here,' so the ICU team called security, apparently by protocol. The social worker says that the son is on his way, and 'It's going to be a mess.'
>
> By the time the son arrives, only one security guard stands at the ICU entrance. He is probably about 6'7" and 240 lbs. . . . But the son turns out to be far less intimidating than he apparently sounded on the phone: he's maybe 5'7" and seems very shy. The senior resident, a tall and assertive young man, does everything short of yelling at him. He speaks loudly, dramatically, asking him pointed and confrontational questions very bluntly: 'Would you do anything like that to yourself?' 'You can see how he's doing. Would he want to be like that? Do you want him to suffer?'
>
> The son answers in a much lower tone of voice, with a strong Russian accent. He says that *he* [his father] is not suffering anymore. 'It's we, the people who are here that are suffering.'

A few days later, when I asked Carol how the case turned out, she answered in a cheerfully sarcastic tone, "Yes, trach 'n' PEG!"—referring to tracheotomy and percutaneous endoscopic gastrostomy, the two surgical procedures required to keep ventilator-dependent patients on life support for the long term. An outright confrontation—which had involved a security guard and a direct, aggressive series of questions from an emotional ICU physician—had made the son dig in his heels and keep his father ventilator-dependent and artificially nourished in a long-term acute care (LTAC) facility.

Not all practitioners avoided the *don'ts* of question phrasing—employing disfavored vocabulary, phrasing yes-or-no questions, or manipulating and confronting patients. Yet these don'ts marked out a general approach to communication. Looking at this approach, we can see that, first, palliative care clinicians valued the opinions of patients and families and relied on them when engaging in end-of-life decisions. They saw economization as a process that drew on deliberations of individual patients. Second, clinicians were aware that how they asked questions—the vocabulary they used, the question formulae they employed, and their general approach to interaction—had a great deal of influence on these deliberations and, consequently, on the preferences of the patients and families. Third, palliative care clinicians encouraged their colleagues to methodically control how they phrased questions and what vocabulary they used. And finally, neither palliative care clinicians nor their colleagues saw patients and families as completely amenable to how they phrased questions. The irreducibility of the wishes of families and patients to the clinicians' speech acts was what validated and substantiated their impact on medical decisions. At least to some degree, economization had to come from the patients themselves.

Embedded Agency

Having discussed the vocabulary and formulae that palliative care clinicians criticized, we should look at the conversational techniques that they endorsed and practiced. When applied properly, these techniques struck a fine balance between passing decisions to patients (or families) and dictating the decisions to them; the key to striking this balance was treating the patients' agency as embedded in the clinicians' agency. I will outline three categories of techniques: first, question phrasing; second, presenting palliative care as an active way of caring; and third, contextualizing and interpreting the diseases and treatments provided.

Phrasing Questions the Palliative Care Way

On my first day in Academic Hospital, I shadowed Ben—a medical resident who rotated with the palliative care team as part of his training. Ben was highly regarded by the palliative care staff, who appreciated his efforts to learn from them, his interest in palliative care, and his general sensitivity and insightfulness. (Three years later, he would decide to specialize in palliative care.) Abigail, a medical student in her fourth year, was also shadowing the palliative care team. Because she was at an earlier stage of her training, Abigail was not working as independently as Ben.

> Ben and I walk into the office. Abigail is there too, writing [medical] notes. They talk about the experience of rotating [with the palliative care team]. Ben says that he actually feels he misses a lot this month, because since he's a resident, they sort of tell him, "Okay, you're a resident, go do your thing" [i.e., talk to patients and families and manage cases on your own]. But he feels that he gets the most from shadowing [the palliative care staff] because then he can see people from the palliative care team like Hanna, or Laura, or Zach in action. He asks me if I know Laura, and I say that I have seen her once; he says . . . she just speaks really well to patients. [Also,] the other day [Ben says he] borrowed Zach to do a family conference for him, and he learned so much from him. [I ask him what he learned, and he says] things such as how to word questions are really important.

About a week into his tenure with the palliative care team, Ben noticed that the wording of questions affected how patients and families answered them. He wished to follow experienced palliative care clinicians more closely to learn the intricacies of their question-wording skills.

> [Ben said,] 'For example, I used to ask, "If your heart stops, would you want us to bring you back to life?"—and of course people would say yes. It's as if you're inviting them to say "yes," regardless of what their goals of care are. But when Zach had the code conversation* with them, he asked it, "When your time comes, would you like to die peacefully and naturally?" And this was what made the difference.'

---

* The term "code conversation" refers to conversations about whether or not to resuscitate or intubate patients.

> Abigail agrees with him, says that you usually go [to family meet-
> ings] and you say, 'That was a good conversation.' But then you see
> one [done by palliative care staff] and say, 'Wow, they *really* did it
> amazing.'

When Ben asked patients if they wanted to be brought back to life, he
tended to get affirmative answers; when Zach phrased the question differently, and emphasized that signing a DNR/DNI form would lead to
"natural" and "peaceful" death, patients and families were more willing
to sign it. This was one central lesson that Ben learned as a trainee: how
to use language in a deliberate, premeditated manner in conversations
with patients and families, knowing that he could influence their stated
wishes. Palliative care clinicians worked as conversation analysis
practitioners.[14] They controlled their wording in an effort to elicit the
desired reflections—and, at times, responses—from patients and their
families.

Zach's question phrasing style was common. Other palliative care practitioners that I observed used different words, but the principle of contrasting a "natural" and "peaceful" death with a different and presumably
less favorable dying trajectory was repeated in almost all cases. For example, a Private Hospital palliative care physician asked a patient, "If
your heart were to stop, would you like us to let you progress naturally,
in what I call a 'peaceful, soft landing,' or would you want us to attempt
to resuscitate you and connect you to machines?" These formulae were so
common that researchers tested their effectiveness in a laboratory setting. Using an online simulation, Barnato and Arnold asked 256 adults
to imagine their parent or spouse was admitted to an ICU and put on
life-sustaining treatment for "pneumonia, severe sepsis, and acute lung
injury." Respondents then watched an interactive video, in which an
actor playing an ICU physician answered their questions and provided
information about the patient's condition, prognosis, and planned treatment. At the end of the video, the actor informed the respondents that
their family member had a 10 percent chance of "survival to discharge in
the event of cardiac arrest requiring CPR" and asked them to decide
whether they wanted to forgo CPR. When the actor described the alternative to CPR as "allowing natural death," 49 percent of the respondents

requested resuscitation; when the actor presented the alternative as "Do Not Resuscitate," 61 percent of them requested resuscitation.[15]

It would be wrong to dismiss this deliberate choice of words as a simple manipulation. For one thing, asking "Would you want to be resuscitated?" influences families' and patients' answers no less than offering them choice between "a natural and peaceful death" and "being connected to machines." Any phrasing of any question would tilt the answers in one direction or another. Even clinicians who phrase questions in the most neutral and deferential way take a stance—they make families and patients more likely to start a goat rodeo. We can see, however, that palliative care practitioners' choice of words consistently leaned toward economized dying. When they phrased their questions, they deliberately used words such as "peaceful" and "natural," which increased the probability that patients and families would opt for economization and avoided formulae that prompted requests for more life-prolonging and life-sustaining treatments.

Framing Economizing as an Active Form of Care

Discussing economized dying on the more general level required just as much attention as asking questions. Ultimately, forgoing, discontinuing, or limiting life-prolonging interventions collided with the intuitions of many families, who thought of these interventions as essential to caring. When talking to such families, palliative care clinicians made sure to frame economization as an active form of care. They presented economization not as a negative agenda—the withdrawal of unnecessary care—but as a positive one—the provision of appropriate care, which matched patients' needs.

Take, for example, how Scott approached one of the cases he was called to consult:

> [Scott and I walked] to the step-down unit. . . . [He] picks one of the big folders—the patient's chart—from the shelf [at the nurses station]. He opens the chart and says, "Oh, he's ninety-seven!" He tells me that he just read somewhere that 30 percent of the children born today will make it to a hundred—'Of course, if we don't reach complete nuclear annihilation by then.' 'Would you believe that?' he asks me. 'How old do you think people should be today to have a 30 percent

chance to make it to a hundred?' I hesitate, and he encourages me, 'Guess!' 'Probably very old,' I say. He says 'ninety-six!'

Scott made two implicit statements in this exchange. First, he pointed out that the mortality rate of people in their late 90s is very high; a patient's old age (in this case ninety-seven) already signaled that his life expectancy was very short. The second statement was more subtle: Scott referenced the fact that life expectancy in the United States was rising and in the next decades hospitalizations of severely ill elderly people would become even more common.

> Two numbers [in the chart] especially draw Scott's attention. 'His abdomen is very low,' he says and points at a lab test result, 'and his INR* is really high. With this INR I don't think he'll make it to a hundred, unfortunately.' He starts reading notes [that were written] since [the patient's] admission. They're all handwritten . . . [and] pretty long. At some point [Scott] says, 'Wow! All of this from today?' and adds that based on his numbers he can say it's either hepatorenal syndrome† or ATN.‡ 'I know [the patient] doesn't urinate,' he says, 'but then—how can I know whether it's because he doesn't produce urine, or perhaps he has an obstruction?' He looks at me, silently. 'But right now it doesn't matter, because his INR is so high that I wouldn't be surprised if it'll be a matter of days for him.' Then he flips to the last page of the chart, and there's a note from about an hour ago.
>   The note says that [the patient's primary care physician] talked to the family, and they have reached a decision to discharge [the patient] to hospice at home. Scott skims it, then says, 'So I guess they've made the decision. I don't have much to do here.'

Before seeing patients, palliative care clinicians "gathered information" from their chart. Based on the patient's age, medical history, symptoms (such as the cessation of urination), and two laboratory results that significantly deviated from normality, Scott made his opinion about the

---

* International normalized ratio (INR) is a measure of blood clotting.
† Hepatorenal syndrome involves liver failure, followed by kidney failure.
‡ Acute tubular necrosis (ATN) is a medical condition involving the death of cells in the kidneys, which is one of the most common causes of acute kidney injuries.

patient's prognosis. He was convinced that the patient's life expectancy was very short ("a matter of days"). His declaration that he was not really needed on the case, which he made upon learning that the patient's family and personal physician had decided to transfer the patient to home hospice, showed that he saw his role in this case as garnering the patient and family's consent to hospice.

Scott walked into the patient's room and found him unconscious. He conducted a physical examination and talked briefly to the patient's hired caregiver, who was sitting there. He then walked out and called the patient's primary care physician on the phone. Like several other patients at Private Hospital, this patient was wealthy and had a concierge physician—a doctor who, for annual fees that could reach $20,000, served as the patient's personal physician and committed to being available on-call for anything the patient needed. After the phone conversation, Scott and I walked to a nearby room to write a note in the patient's electronic chart.

> Scott logs into the computer. He says that the patient should have been admitted to hospice much earlier, that this hospital admission was unnecessary, and they should have let him stay at home. 'That's what I don't like [about] his doctor,' he says. 'He could have put him on hospice a long, long time ago. And when I ask him [on the phone] why he didn't, he tells me that it's because the son was not ready for that, [he said,] "You know—orthopedists."'

Trying to build a common language with a palliative care physician, the primary care physician mentioned that the patient's son was an orthopedist and offered implicit criticism of the son's support for more life-prolonging care. The primary care physician placed himself in Scott's camp, implying that, like Scott, he thought the son was being unreasonable.[16] Scott did not confront the physician on the phone, but when talking to me later, he sounded very critical:

> 'It's not the son who is disagreeing with [hospice],' Scott [tells me], 'it's the doctor who didn't know how to frame it for the son. Because when you ask [the son], 'Would you like to withdraw care and send him to hospice'—of course he will say, 'No.' But if you talk with him about how we can come up with a plan that would be the most appropriate for

[your father's] age and condition right now—he'll be much more open to the idea of hospice. As much as I hated all of this humanities talk about rhetoric when I was in college—it really, really matters.'

Scott's view of the son's agency in medical decision making was complex. On the one hand, similarly to the primary care physician, Scott recognized the son as a legitimate decision maker. At no point did he challenge the son's right to participate in medical decisions for his father. On the other hand, Scott knew he could influence the son's decisions by framing what hospice meant, by suggesting that hospice was *not* "withdrawal of care" but rather a form of care that "would be most appropriate to your father's age and condition."[17]

When training younger medical staff, senior palliative care clinicians repeatedly emphasized this need to frame economization as an active form of care. At Academic Hospital, a palliative care fellow who gave a class to medical students and interns told them, "Don't say 'there's nothing else that we can do,' and don't say 'withdrawal of care.' I really don't like these two phrases." Ryan, an attending physician from the same service, added that "withdrawal of care" was a very misleading description of, say, disconnecting a patient from a ventilator (extubating). In contrast to popular imagery, which often portrays extubation as a simple act of "pulling the plug" or turning a switch off, extubating was a complex procedure that required preparation and skill. It included arranging the right morphine doses ahead of time so the patient would not appear in respiratory distress (which might in turn distress family members), administrating the medications properly and on time, and pulling out the tube correctly so that it would not hurt the patient or cause bleeding. Rather than a cessation of care, extubation was a very meticulous and attentive form of care.

In Public Hospital, I observed Linda, a palliative care physician, using a similar framing at the bedside when talking to a patient's Spanish-speaking daughter (Silvia, a medical resident, served as a translator):

> [Linda and Silvia] put their stethoscopes on the patient's chest and listen for about 20 seconds. They touch her arms and then roll down the blanket. They touch and feel her legs, then lift and bend them slowly, each from one side of the bed. [This physical examination]

takes a couple of minutes, then Linda turns to the daughter and says, 'There are many things I think we can do.' Silvia translates, and the daughter's eyes light up with hope: "*Sí?*" she says.

Linda says that 'first, we can give her some more pain med[ication]s, to make sure she's totally comfortable.' Silvia translates, and the daughter nods. 'Second,' Linda says, 'we can see if we can move her to Unit D, so you can have more privacy. Or if this is not possible, we can move the other patient in the room somewhere else, so you can have your own space here.' Silvia translates, and the daughter nods again. 'And then another thing is the oxygen mask,' Linda says. 'Usually, after a while, patients don't feel comfortable with the oxygen mask on their face. So one thing that we can do is to remove the mask and put a fan right next to them, which will move the air near her face. There are studies that show that it makes them more comfortable,' Linda says, and adds that 'still, there are some families that don't like this idea and prefer to keep the mask on the patient's face.' After Silvia translates, Linda asks the daughter what she would want. Silvia translates that the daughter would be totally fine with removing the mask.

Even when at first the daughter seemed to identify "things that we can do" as life-sustaining, or even life-saving, interventions, Linda hung onto her framing. By framing the removal of life-sustaining and life-prolonging interventions as active measures of caregiving—as opposed to withdrawal of care—Linda facilitated the daughter's consent to economization.

Contextualizing

A third interactional technique that palliative care clinicians encouraged was contextualizing—namely, recapping the disease process to the patients or the family. In the beginning of a typical meeting with a family, clinicians summarized the patient's medical condition and the events that led to it. This was an act of narration that involved interpretation: clinicians controlled how they presented the case, underplayed or ignored some details, emphasized others, and specified what decisions were on the table.

In one family conference at Public Hospital, members of the palliative care and medicine team met with the family of a young patient who suffered from hepatorenal syndrome. Like many families of young patients, this family was eager to pursue every possible life-prolonging treatment. At the beginning of the meeting, the chief resident provided the family with background on the patient's condition and the disease's progress:

> The chief resident says that . . . the results of the biopsy are that it seems like [the patient's] liver condition is not due to an autoimmune disease, namely, it's not that the body is attacking her liver for some reason, and that it is probably a liver failure due to alcohol use. [I see the husband nodding silently.] The resident says that we were hoping that her liver would recover a bit and that following that, her kidneys might regain function. But this hasn't happened. Right now she is totally dependent on dialysis and her liver is not functioning, so she will most likely need a liver transplant to survive.
>
> The dialysis she's getting is not something that will help recover her kidneys, the resident says. It's something that replaces her kidneys. Sometimes the kidneys restart after a while, and then the dialysis can be stopped; but in any case, it functions instead of the kidneys rather than improving their function. Linda [a palliative care physician] says that another way to frame it is that dialysis is not a treatment for kidney failure, but a treatment that comes instead of kidney function in cases where the kidneys don't work.

By contextualizing—representing the patient's overall disease process—the resident and the palliative care physician gained more control over the discussion. They not only presented the most recent medical conclusions—that the cause of the illness was alcohol and not an autoimmune disease—but also mentioned the hopes that they once had for liver and kidney recovery, which did not materialize. They emphasized that the patient was in decline and also clarified (twice) that dialysis would not be a long-term solution. Several days later, the patient's blood pressure dropped so low that she could not be dialyzed safely. The family experienced this as an expected progression of the disease, and the patient died shortly thereafter.

Another example of a contextualization that changed family members' initial intuitions involved Mr. Lipset, a white man in his 70s who had congestive heart failure. I first saw him when I accompanied Carol (a palliative care nurse) to a meeting with him, his son, and his wife. We walked into Mr. Lipset's room, and after introducing ourselves, Carol said we could either hold the meeting in the room or find another location.

> The son, looking a bit angry—or perhaps he's just anxious?—says that his take on the whole thing is that his father simply needs rehab. 'We've already been in this situation,' he says. 'A cardiologist told [my father] that he had six months! And that was two years ago! But then he went to rehab and his physical condition really improved. He came back home and he was extremely energetic, in great condition. But then, you know, he didn't do much with himself, and he stayed home all day, in his armchair, watching TV and being lazy—and his condition [deteriorated] again. So if we only get him rehab and improve his condition again—this will change everything.'
> Mr. Lipset is lying in bed, appearing rather thin. He looks at his son and Carol, seems to nod silently as the son says he should go to rehab.
> Carol responds in a very calm tone of voice—quite a sharp contrast to how the son speaks. She says, 'I will answer your question, but I suggest that we move to another room where we can all sit, if this is okay. The social worker will join us there.'

Mr. Lipset's son had a very clear view on what led to his father's condition, and Carol had to respond to it in some way. Leaving Mr. Lipset in his bed, the son, wife, Carol, and I went to the conference room down the hallway. Two residents from the medicine unit joined us; both appeared tired, and one nearly fell asleep as Carol, the son, and the wife talked. Carol introduced herself again and asked about Mr. Lipset's living situation and his life story. She then talked about what the son had said when they were still standing in Mr. Lipset's room, still characterizing it as a "question."

> 'Now I want to answer your question. You are talking about how your dad was two years ago. And two years ago, with rehab, he was able to gain back some of his function. But this is not the case now. Because according to the tests that we did, his heart is very weak. His disease has progressed, and he is not in the same condition he was two years ago. And you can see it by the fact that he doesn't eat well and that he's lost so much weight. Usually you can see a lot by just looking at

people; you can see much more than you would see in a medical test. He is so thin because his heart cannot pump blood to both his kidneys and his brain.'

The son and wife listen quietly, and Carol continues. 'In his condition right now,' she says, 'he is not going to benefit from rehab.'

Carol set the context for the discussion that followed: she confronted Mr. Lipset's family with her diagnosis and presented it as a hard medical fact. This contextualization conditioned the rest of the interaction. From that point on, the conversation was about what they should do given the fact that Mr. Lipset's condition would not improve. Contextualizing was a technique that tamed the son's agency. It did not fully determine his position on Mr. Lipset's care, but it did put certain limits on it.

Practices of question phrasing, framing, and contextualizing mark out the clinicians' implicit approach to what agency means. According to this approach, human agency is circumstantial. It not only depends on patients' and families' personal qualities, but also on the interaction between them and the clinicians. The clinicians knew they could influence patients and families during family conferences, and they deliberately used their influence to affect patients' and families' agency.

Handling "No"s

Seeking the Communicator

I have so far used a clumsy phrase—"patients and families"—to refer to all the people who discussed decisions with the medical staff. There were many cases, however, in which families disagreed among themselves, which made economization—and conversation in general—very difficult. Different family members presented different views about the patients and how they would want to be treated. I witnessed several cases—and heard numerous stories about others—where a palliative care team and a family reached agreement on how to treat a certain patient, only to confront a "new" opinionated daughter, son, or sibling who flew in from the other side of the country and opposed all the decisions they had reached. Even when all family members participated in family meetings from the beginning, they might see things very differently. Frustrations, tension, and anger from time immemorial often surfaced when families faced such difficult decisions, which made conversations very hard to control.

The most basic strategy the palliative care teams adopted in cases when families disagreed among themselves was to identify a single key family member and ask her (or him) to be the family representative. There was no single criterion for who this person should be, but generally the staff preferred she would also be the patient's legal surrogate decision maker, know the patient well, and have authority within the family. They reduced the plethora of potentially contradictory opinions of multiple people to the voice of one person, and they encouraged families to discuss things and settle internal disagreements before meeting with the medical staff. This was an important dimension of taming patients' and families' agency: by designating one representative for each family, the palliative care clinicians made the families' agency more consistent, coherent, and manageable.

As an example, recall Carol's conversation with Mr. Lipset's son. Carol chose to talk to Mr. Lipset's son and wife without Mr. Lipset, although Mr. Lipset was mentally clear enough to participate in a conversation, and he was staying in a private, sufficiently large room. Initially, Carol mentioned they could hold the meeting in his room: "[Carol] says that we can do [the meeting] here or see if there's a family room where we can meet." But after the son said he wanted to send Mr. Lipset to rehabilitation, she suggested that 'we move to another room where we can all sit, if this is okay. The social worker will join us there.'

> 'Would that be okay with you?' [Carol] asks Mr. Lipset, who looks a bit confused from the fast exchange [between Carol and his son]. I personally feel a bit confused too. This is a pretty intense beginning of conversation [the son looking anxious and insisting that his father should go to rehab], which I didn't really expect. Mr. Lipset seems to nod and says, 'It's okay if they meet with you.' Carol says, 'I promise that you'll hear everything that we'll talk about here.' The son nods, and the wife appears to defer to him. We all leave the room.

Most of the conversation during the meeting was between Carol and the son, and the wife was far less involved. At the end of the meeting, after they reached a decision to transfer Mr. Lipset to an inpatient hospice, the son asked Carol about whether and how to communicate the decision to his father.

> [The son] says he's worried about what exactly we're going to tell [Mr. Lipset]. . . . 'I don't want to make him feel . . . that he's going to die soon. So maybe we can tell him that we're moving him to a rehab facility, which is true, because he could get physical therapy there.' Carol hesitates. . . . She says that we can tell him that we're moving him to an inpatient facility where they'll take a good care of him—which is true—and that if he gets better he'll be able to go back home, which is also true. Carol mentions things that they will stop doing [at the hospice]: they're not going to check his blood sugar so frequently—she says [that] since he's at the end of his life, it's not that important to monitor his sugar right now. The son says he's surprised that they have [done that], because he eats so little that he hardly ever needs insulin. Carol mentions a few other medications that they're going to take him off of.
>
> [Back in Mr. Lipset's room], the son is telling Mr. Lipset that they'll try to find him a place where he can do some physical therapy and improve his condition, because he can't go home the way he is now. Nathalie [resident] and Carol walk [in] together. . . . [Carol] shakes Mr. Lipset's hand and tells him that he has a great family. He nods and smiles. Carol says, 'I don't know what you did right with these guys, but apparently you did something right. They really want your best interest,' she says. . . . 'We were talking about how to give you the best care that we can for your condition, and we will now work on finding a place where we can do that.' He nods.

Carol did not choose to talk to the son because he had a more favorable opinion on hospice. At least initially, he seemed adamant to pursue more rehabilitative and curative care to bring his father back to his previous condition. But in this situation, when a "no" appeared to have been uttered, she decided to confront the son with his father's diagnosis in a separate room. Statements such as "he's at the end of his life" were easier to make when the subject of the conversation was not around. Ultimately, it was Mr. Lipset that she bypassed. Carol and the son sought ways to tell him a truth without telling all the truth, and they did not say "hospice" or "dying" in front of him. They enacted a Goffmanian boundary between the backstage—the conference room behind a closed door—and the front-stage—Mr. Lipset's room. The conference room was an area where Carol and the son prepared for their performance in Mr. Lipset's room.[18]

I documented several contrasting cases in which palliative care clinicians insisted on empowering *patients* to speak in order to bypass the agency of their family members.[19] Ms. Ju, a quadriplegic woman in her eighties, was hospitalized at Private Hospital for aspiration pneumonia. After forty-eight hours in the ICU her condition improved, and she was transferred to the step-down unit. The clinical staff was confident about how the rest of her life would look. She was likely to suffer repeated incidents of aspiration pneumonia, which her weakening immune system would be unable to control, and she would be hospitalized more frequently for longer and longer periods.

A day after a meeting with Ms. Ju and her three children, the palliative care team discussed its outcomes.

> Resident: We tried to have [Ms. Ju] participate. She [responded] with her eyes. One blink is yes, two blinks are no, and she also tries to talk.
>
> Attending physician: [interrupts her] The first part of the meeting was futzing with the ventilator, which was clear the son really enjoyed. That was much better for him that we were messing with the vent.
>
> Resident: We couldn't get from the son exactly what he wanted—when we asked him, he said that he didn't prepare a statement for this occasion. [People laugh.] 'I haven't prepared anything, so I have nothing to say'—it was really strange.
>
> Attending physician: The daughter was nicer—I hate to put it in normative terms— . . . but she gave me a little bit of information. . . . I think what's happening is that with old patients who end up being incredibly medically dependent but are not totally impaired [i.e., are able to participate in medical decision making], we tend to notice the really gray line between encouragement and coercion. You know, . . . I gave [the patient] ample opportunity to say, "I'm done here," and she can't quite say it. It's clear . . . she can't say "I've had enough" before the family accepts that.

Several other people in the room agreed with the attending that Ms. Ju probably wanted to transition to comfort care but her children (her son in particular) were pressuring her to keep fighting. (These opinions, however, were not independent of the attending physician's because he left a note in her medical chart, which they read.) The attending physician decided to visit Ms. Ju's room when her children were not around to hear what she genuinely thought. A few hours later, I observed their interaction. The attending physician said that the doctors were "totally fine" with the plan to treat her pneumonia, but that he still thought that 'you didn't get the space to talk about what you wanted yourself.' Yet still, when he asked her, 'Is that true, do you feel this way?' Ms. Ju blinked twice, signaling that she disagreed.

> Outside Ms. Ju's room, I wonder how [the attending physician] would interpret what she just signaled him. As far as I could judge, she completely refuted his suspicion that the son didn't allow her the space to make her own decision. A small circle emerges by the nurses station—the social worker, the case manager, the resident, and the palliative care attending. The attending says that 'there is also a matter of altered agency here. . . . The son influences her a lot, and she doesn't have enough space to say that she's actually had enough. . . . [I] just talked to her when she was alone, but she still doesn't feel comfortable to say it.'

Regardless of what a patient said, it was almost always possible to maintain that others influenced or pressured her or him. While the attempt to talk to the patient alone did not lead to a different conclusion than the one reached in the family meeting, it illustrated a method that palliative care teams used: bypassing one communicator's outright resistance. When a family member said "no," it was always possible to talk to another family member—or to the patient herself. When the patient said "no," it was possible to approach them through family members or other supportive parties.

At the same time, it is not that palliative care clinicians listened to the party that was most open to economized dying. They were, quite simply, likely to engage with those patients and family members who were most open to engagement. Mr. Lipset's son, for example, at first seemed resistant, yet Carol identified him as a potential person with whom she could communicate. By contrast, Ms. Ju's son was "really strange" and hence a disfavored communicator. Still, when palliative care conversations did develop, their outcome usually pushed decisions toward economized dying. Consequently, the people who engaged in these conversations were more likely to be the parties who would lead the transition from curative to comfort care.

Revisiting and Validating

Another technique to deal with resistance was treating it as one phase in a long and still ongoing conversation. Refusals to sign DNR forms, for example, were not taken as final words in a discussion but as positions that could change as time passed, as discussions developed, and as a patient's medical condition persisted or declined. When families did not decide to withhold some life-sustaining treatments on the first meeting, second, third, and fourth meetings could be called, and the topic could be revisited. Take, for example, the case of Mr. Richards, who was hospitalized in minimally conscious condition after suffering a series of strokes. By the time the palliative care team began consulting on his case, he was having seizures. He was fed through a PEG tube, which a surgeon had inserted several weeks earlier; however, in his delirium he kept hitting it and pulling it out. The alternative to removing the tube and stopping artificial nutrition was restraining him to bed, which the medical team was reluctant to do.

At a meeting with the family, the medicine unit's attending physician, Dr. Wright, insisted that they needed to transition Mr. Richards to comfort care. The day after, at a staff meeting of the palliative care team, I saw that many disagreed with his approach.

> Nurse: So we had a family meeting with Dr. Wright yesterday, he was the attending physician [on the floor]. They [the family] really insisted that they wanted [Mr. Richards] to be full code.
> Social worker: You know, I actually appreciated their position there. Wright was there for half an hour, and he came from the place of "okay, this is my agenda, this is what I think we have to do." And he talked for most of the time, and didn't really listen to them. . . . I got the impression that this family was very well educated and very thoughtful, and that they've given it a lot of thought. Wright just didn't listen to them, he was talking all the time, and there was no conversation for about half an hour, until he left. . . . We should keep talking to this family, this conversation is just not over yet.

The family's insistence on keeping Mr. Richards full code despite Dr. Wright's recommendation did not lead the palliative care team to withdraw from the case. Two elements were particularly important. First was the social worker's impression that the family was "very well educated and very thoughtful." Within palliative care practice, thoughtfulness was a highly valued quality—unlike Ms. Ju's son, whom the palliative care clinicians perceived as "strange," the Richards family was appreciated. Second, the palliative care team sensed that the attending physician did not handle the conversation well, did not listen to the family, and did not let the family members express themselves. It seemed like the palliative care team appreciated the family more than it appreciated Dr. Wright. The statement that "the conversation is just not over yet" and the decision to continue meeting with the family were illustrative palliative care moves. Even when a family or a patient insisted on continuing certain life-prolonging interventions, palliative care teams could continue talking to them and revisit their refusals.

When patients consented to economization, however, the palliative care teams did not revisit their decisions but rather validated them. For example, when the daughter of a cancer patient gradually consented to forgo curative and life-prolonging treatments, the palliative care fellow endorsed each of her decisions and emphasized they were "very good."

> The daughter asks about antibiotics; she [the patient] has a UTI, do you think we should not give more antibiotics and fluids to her? Sarah [palliative care fellow] says she doesn't think we should because it wouldn't really help her at this point. The daughter nods. 'Do you think I'm making good decisions?' she asks Sarah. Sarah nods and says quickly, 'I think you're making very good decisions. Very good decisions.'

In another case, a palliative care social worker validated the decision of another woman, who explicitly mentioned that her family was critical of her choice to transition her father to hospice care.

> [The daughter] tears up a bit, but still manages to control herself. She asks Hanna several times if she thinks she's doing the right thing, and Hanna says she does. The daughter says, 'This is not really accepted

where I come from; my cousins were telling me that I'm killing him, and that I need to wait until God helps him, but I understand that going to hospice will be better for him.' Hanna nods in affirmation.

The professional predisposition of palliative care clinicians is to promote economization. From the perspective of palliative care, signing a DNR/DNI form, transitioning to comfort care, and forgoing hospitalizations or other forms of escalation of care are actions that end and seal decision making. By contrast, in many cases palliative care clinicians treat the rejection of economization as an ad hoc position that invites further discussion.

Lubricating and Trialing

Two additional ways to avoid and work around "no"s were *lubricating* and *trialing*. Clinicians "lubricated" in cases where a family was generally open to economize dying but wanted certain procedures done first. Lubricating meant declaring these procedures the last that would be performed before transitioning the patient to comfort care. For example, the family of Ms. Hauser, a patient with a brain tumor whose ability to participate in conversation declined very fast, leaned toward accepting a care plan of hospice and no further escalation of care. Yet during a palliative care consult they said they wanted to do a magnetic resonance imaging (MRI) scan before transitioning her to hospice:

> The daughter . . . asks if it won't make sense to do an MRI, just to know if the tumor has grown and how much. [Palliative care physician] nods, says, 'I wouldn't recommend it, and I'll tell you why. We do MRIs when we think that the result that we'll get can change our decisions on a certain case. And in this case, if the MRI says that the tumor has grown, it's not going to change our plan for her. So I wouldn't *recommend* [emphasizes] an MRI in this case. But I actually just had a conversation about when to do an MRI in such cases. [Sometimes] families need it for reassurance, and this is something that I can understand. Is it important for you?' he asks the daughter.
> The daughter says that she thought that if they just knew whether the tumor has grown by 8 percent or 2 percent, it would give them a

sense of what's going on, how the disease is progressing. [The physician] nods, says that he can understand that, if it's important to her, he's open to the possibility.

MRIs are expensive procedures, and insurance companies do not pay for them unless a doctor confirms that they are necessary. The daughter said she needed the MRI to satisfy some general curiosity the family had about the disease's progression—a reason that an insurance company would be unlikely to accept.

> The daughter asks if the insurance would cover that, . . . tells [the palliative care physician] about [Ms. Hauser's] coverage. . . . [He says,] 'Usually we don't have problems with this company, I think they'll approve it, we'll just have to think how to justify it to them. The other thing is whether it's worth it for the patient, because the MRI is a really intense experience: it's lying down on the table there, and it's noisy. It's not pleasant. And I see that you're feeling better today,' he tells [Ms. Hauser], 'which is great, but is it going to be okay with you?' She doesn't answer, and the son says, 'She'll be fine with that—she's a fighter.' Physician says, 'Okay, I can write this order.' Thinking out loud, he says, 'We can tell them [the insurance company] that if the tumor has grown significantly, we would still want to get an oncology consult, perhaps to resect it, and if not—then we'll proceed with the hospice plan.' He says quietly, 'I can order the MRI, we should just think about how to bill for it.' And then adds instantly, 'I mean, not bill-bill. Just how to present it to the insurance company.'

"Lubricating" often involved massaging orders. Lubrication helped smooth and expedite the decision-making process and was particularly helpful in giving families a "final push" before they endorsed economization. In this case as in many others, it was a way to give the family the peace of mind required to economize.

> Outside, [the physician] tells the resident, 'It's such a pleasure to talk to these people. Every one out of ten patients that I see—I just have to have families like that, otherwise the conservative Republican comes out of me, and you can ask Roi that it can happen.' We laugh, and she [the resident] smiles politely. . . . He tells [the resident]

that he prefers to do this MRI: 'Maybe I'm biased because I've just made a similar decision with another patient, which was a different case [but a similar decision because in both cases he decided to do an MRI although he didn't consider it medically necessary]. But I think it makes sense here. It's a short hospitalization, overall, and if what I need to do to make sure that [the patient] gets discharged on time is to get this MRI—it sounds like a reasonable decision.'

Studying sales interactions, sociologist Asaf Darr analyzed the role gifts play in finalizing transactions. The salespeople that Darr studied offered "closing gifts" when buyers were close to making their final decisions—for example, by adding a software package as a gift to a customer who considered buying a computer. Darr also observed "post-sale gifts," which sellers gave buyers *after* completing transactions. "The best explanation for the post-sale gifting," Darr wrote, "is socio-psychological in nature. The seller wants to express gratitude for an easy and large sale and to reward the buyer for playing her social role as a buyer to perfection."[20]

Lubricants were located somewhere between pre- and post-sale gifts. The palliative care physician agreed to order an MRI scan as Ms. Hauser's family was accepting hospice as a care plan and while there was still a certain chance they would change their minds. The physician's reasoning for lubricating the decision with an MRI dovetailed with Darr's interpretation. First, 'it was a pleasure to work with these people' denoted that they had fulfilled an exemplary role as family members of a patient and reached a decision he thought was responsible, reasonable, and feasible, and all in a timely manner. (As the physician noted, the hospitalization was short.) Second, ordering the MRI was legitimate because it saved money by expediting decision making: it helped streamline medical decisions and ultimately the patient's discharge.

Similarly to lubricants, *trials* facilitated economization. The key difference between them was that lubricants were about placing a limit by allowing *one last procedure*, while trials were about limiting the *time period* physicians would provide such procedures. When setting a trial, clinicians could determine, for example, that they would wait several additional days before transitioning a patient to comfort care. As a palliative care physician put it in an interview,

One of the tricks of a palliative care doc is what's called "a trial of therapy." If you're not gonna win the argument—not that it's a win or loss thing—but if you're not gonna, you know, for lack of better words, get your way, set a limit [on] when we are going to reevaluate what we're doing.

Becky, a palliative care physician in Public Hospital, suggested using a trial in the case of Mr. Su, an elderly Vietnamese American man who was ventilator-dependent in the ICU. In a staff meeting of the palliative care team, she said,

It's hard, because he's intubated, so he can't speak. You can't really communicate directly with him . . . so getting at what he wants is really hard in this situation, even though he's awake. He was really out of it for me, and I don't even know how to say hello in Vietnamese. I should ask my friends. So my hope is to coach the [ICU] team . . . to suggest that they frame this as a time-limited trial. . . . He's really dependent on the ventilator, and what this might mean is that he'll go to a long-term acute care facility, and . . . I don't even know what will cover the long-term acute care [LTAC]. [Maybe it] means that he's gonna go to another state somewhere to be on an LTAC. . . . There are only several facilities that take medical patients for long-term acute care. It's a handful of beds, and way more people waiting for them than there are beds.

Becky hesitated to transfer Mr. Su to an LTAC facility for several reasons. First, she was unsure who would pay for the facility (although generally, Medicaid covered it). Second, she suspected that the patient would have to move far away from his family because there were not enough LTAC beds in the area. And finally, she was generally reluctant to consign Mr. Su to a long ventilator-dependent life without knowing what he wanted. She suggested the trial as a compromise: keeping Mr. Su on the ventilator for an agreed-upon period, which would allow him some time to improve; then, if improvement did not occur, extubating him. Such trials were negotiation tools that palliative care clinicians used with families as well as with other clinicians: by stipulating a date in which everybody will review their past decisions and evaluate whether the curative treatment they offered has

proven itself, they increased the probability that people would ultimately embrace economization.

> [In a palliative care staff meeting:] [The physician] says that she
> made a recommendation to the primary team to increase Ms. Seale's IV
> dose of pain meds, and that it will be helpful to meet with the team
> and define the concept of time-limited trial in TPN.* 'She [Ms.
> Seale] has just started getting a TPN, which is not unreasonable,
> but we should decide now how long we're going to try this course.'

Trials were particularly significant in cases where, in principle, the
treatment provided could continue indefinitely. By setting time limits on
a treatment, palliative care clinicians tried to create agreement among
families and clinicians over what would count as sufficient medical improvement that would merit additional life-prolonging efforts and by
what date this improvement should show. Trials also fostered shared
definitions of what would be an indication that a patient's condition was
indeed irreversible and the time to economize dying had come. The
construction of such trials facilitated a smoother decision to withdraw
life-sustaining measures.

Two Forms of Withdrawal

There are, however, cases where despite the palliative care clinicians' skill
and effort the families (or patients) still refused to economize. One
morning, Private Hospital's palliative care team discussed the death of
such a patient.

Hospice Liaison: Mr. Abel died yesterday.
   . . .
Physician: Without being fully coded?
Nurse: Nancy dealt with [the case], so I suspect that the ICU got called
   [and attempted resuscitation]. [Smiling:] You can't save every starfish,
   and that one was gonna go down with drama, because his wife was creepy.
Physician: He crashed on Sunday [two days earlier]. Hard.

---

* Total parenteral nutrition (TPN) is nutrition provided intravenously.

The nurse's starfish comment—a reference to a popular motivational story[21]—portrayed the team as surrounded by cases of patients dying painful and terrible deaths, unable to save all of them. The nurse accepted that every once in a while, despite her best efforts—and for reasons that were beyond her control (such as a 'creepy wife')—she failed to "save" patients and economize their dying.

In this case, the patient died while the team was still trying to convince his wife to move him to comfort care. But there were other cases where palliative care clinicians chose to withdraw before the patient passed away. They often talked about conceding and knowing when to withdraw from a case as an important skill in and of itself, which sometimes created a possibility to reengage in the future. There were two main ways palliative care teams withdrew from cases. In *complete withdrawals*, the palliative care teams accepted that a certain patient would, as one physician put it, "go down with all guns blazing." They either removed the patient from their list and stopped visiting her, or restricted their contributions in the case to mere technicalities such as treating pain and managing symptoms.

Ms. Davis, who had terminal cancer, enrolled in a phase I clinical trial. (Phase I trials involve testing drugs' side effects and determining their safe dosage; these trials often mean immense suffering and virtually never provide life prolongation.) The palliative care team took her enrollment in the trial as a sign that she was completely dedicated to pursuing the most extreme and aggressive treatments in existence. From their perspective, this was the ultimate and most unequivocal rejection of economization.

> Pharmacist: Ms. Davis is now on a clinical trial, phase I experimental chemo.
> Fellow: [looks at her chart] I see she has nausea, and maybe we can treat her for the nausea and then step back.
> Attending: [laughing] Treat her nausea—and then that's it—she's palliated!

The second form of withdrawal was what I call *engaged withdrawal*. These were cases in which palliative care clinicians still remained involved, even though they did not believe they could contribute to the decision-making process. Engaged withdrawals usually meant that an individual clinician continued seeing and talking to a family or a patient even after the rest of the palliative care team had withdrawn completely. It was very hard to predict when an engaged withdrawal would develop. It seemed to be the outcome of idiosyncratic sympathies—something in the patient (or the family) that a clinician found moving, touching, or intriguing, which made her or him continue seeing them.

> Hanna [palliative care social worker] says that Mr. Chang's family has been really, really difficult. 'They take wonderful care of him, but everything goes very hard with them: in meetings there are sometimes ten different people in the room, some of them children, and all of them have questions to ask. . . . They [prepare] flashcards with questions, and they have some system, they take turns asking questions from the flashcards.' 'Like, what questions?' I ask her. 'They ask about this blister that suddenly appeared on his pinky!' she says. 'What should we do with that? And then when you actually look at it you see that it has already disappeared.' She laughs.
>
> [Later] in the office, with Sarah [a fellow] and Kathy [a resident], I hear more details about the last meeting they had with the family, which Hanna apparently felt uncomfortable sharing in the hallway. Sarah says that during that meeting, she kept [saying], "Let's look at the big picture," [but] they asked her to look at the blister that popped up on [the patient's] penis. Sarah laughs. 'I had to look at the blister and tell them that it's okay.' Hanna says that they even insisted that she [the social worker] look at it too, and she closed her eyes, leaned forward, tried not to burst out laughing, and said, 'I think it's good, I think it looks really good!'
>
> Hanna says that the hepatology team stopped passing there in rounds—they're avoiding the family as much as they can. The family looks through the door, waiting for them to come as they walk down the hallway, and then the team just sneaks by the room, without entering it.

The palliative care team labeled the family as "detail oriented"—and while this case was an extreme example, they referred to many other families and individuals similarly. Such families insisted on discussing specific problems rather than talking about the patient's overall condition or disease trajectory; consequently, it was hard to talk to them about dying. But Hanna stayed in touch with the family even when it was clear she had little ability to influence them:

> 'And the family asks me, "are they skipping us on rounds?" And I say, "Oh no, what makes you think so? Of course they're not passing over you!" Nobody can bear them,' Hanna says, 'but I actually like them.'
> 'How can you handle them?' Sarah asks her. 'They just fascinate me,' Hanna replies, 'their system of who speaks when and asks what questions is just incredible.'

Hanna found the family intriguing and entertaining, which made her continue seeing them. Other clinicians "couldn't bear them." In another case at another hospital, a palliative care nurse continued seeing an ICU patient who battled multiple organ failures and used his dialysis catheter to inject heroin. Like Hanna, she felt personally attached to him, even though she did not believe she would convince him to embrace economization.

Knowing how and when to withdraw was no less important than knowing how to talk to people. In a lecture at the continuing education conference that I attended, a senior palliative care physician emphasized that even when clinicians felt very strongly about economization, they needed to know how to step back.

> 'It's common to become frustrated. A doctor came and told me, "I'm having a family meeting every day, and we're not getting anywhere." So I tell him, "Stop. Take a step back." All cases resolve. Even Mrs. Jones will die eventually. Take a step back, relax, stop having family meetings if they're not going anywhere. Sometimes disengagement will help you.'

Disengagement not only allowed clinicians to relax and recuperate, but also gave the families and patients some time in which they did not have to push back against economization. It eased tensions and gave everyone an opportunity to put down their defenses and think independently. In the long run, this could also serve the purpose of economizing dying.

Conclusion

From a palliative care perspective, treating patients' and families' wishes objectively did not mean abstaining from influencing them. Clinicians recognized their role in constructing patients' and families' agencies and saw influencing them as part of their job. In the process, they avoided using certain vocabulary and formulae, deliberately employed other vocabulary and formulae, controlled the medical information they provided about the patient's condition and treatment, chose which party in the family to talk to, revisited decisions to escalate care, and used lubricants and trials to smooth the decision-making process.

These practices did not mean that clinicians fully controlled decision making. The clinician's acknowledgment that one could not "save every starfish" and the multiple instances where palliative care clinicians withdrew were testimonies to patients' and families' relative autonomy. At the same time, the clinicians heavily influenced this autonomy. The consent achieved in clinician–family–patient interactions was circumstantial. What people thought and wanted partly depended on how the clinicians approached them, how they phrased their questions, what interpretations they shared, and what medical options they presented. Consent was not a voluntary endorsement that autonomous patients and families gave to certain plans of care; rather, it was a recursive negotiation process in which statements that patients made could be gradually transformed into an embrace of economized dying. Family meetings were sites where agencies consolidated, and clinicians had a great impact on this consolidation process.

Some of the different cases that this chapter presented reveal the social inequalities structured into such construction processes. Palliative care practice is mostly verbal—the bulk of palliative care work consists of talking. Conversational skills, friendliness, reason, intuitive understanding, and ability to control and express one's emotions are all socially variable qualities that some people have, but others do not. Expressing oneself in a way that makes sense to clinicians but does not manifest as "strange" or "creepy" in the medical setting does not come easily to everyone, especially when people are dealing with situations as difficult as the death of a close family member. This puts the families and patients who feel comfortable talking, expressing themselves, and showing emotion in an advantaged social position. Not only are they able to articulate themselves better and reach a better and more consolidated sense of who they are and what they want, but they also gain the medical staff's acknowledgment, support, and validation.

Conclusion:
Toward a Sociology of Economization

Consider modern medicine. . . . By his means the medical man preserves the life of the mortally ill man, even if the patient implores us to relieve him of life, even if his relatives, to whom his life is worthless and to whom the costs of maintaining his worthless life grow unbearable, grant his redemption from suffering. . . . Whether life is worthwhile living and when—this question is not asked by medicine. Natural science gives us an answer to the question of what we must do if we wish to master life technically. It leaves quite aside, or assumes for its purposes, whether we should and do wish to master life technically and whether it ultimately makes sense to do so.

—Max Weber, *Science as a Vocation*

THIS BOOK HAS INVESTIGATED the emergence and operations of what I call the "new economy of dying" in the United States. Since the 1960s, multiple social, professional, financial, and political actors have advanced the view that the U.S. health care system is facing a problem of excess, which is particularly pronounced near the end of life: patients approaching the end of their life receive too many life-prolonging interventions, which result in uncontrolled monetary spending and immense suffering. The new economy of dying crystalized around this view. It is "a historically specific regime of valuation," which tackles excess by putting life-prolonging and life-sustaining interventions under systematic scrutiny, drawing on an industry, a professional movement, patient mobilization, a moral orientation, and a policy approach.[1]

The new economy of dying has become so hegemonic and intuitive that its critics risk labeling themselves as irrational and irresponsible. Achieving this hegemony required extensive work: advocating within the medical profession to advance the notion that near the end of life, less treatment makes for better care (Chapter 1); mobilizing the general public to support and participate in the new economy of dying (Chapter 1); lobbying among politicians, state administrations, insurance companies, and hospitals to establish the idea that hospice and palliative care can be financially beneficial (Chapter 2); representing patients' views as aligning with the new economy of dying (Chapter 3); and working at the bedside to bring dying patients and family members to voluntarily consent to less life-prolonging and life-sustaining treatment (Chapters 4 and 5).

Can the case of the new economy of dying in the United States teach lessons about economies and economization processes in general? To conclude, I will take on generalizing the story this book tells by highlighting several dimensions of the term *economization*, which encapsulates much of my argument, and by illustrating its relevance to more extensive theoretical discussions.

The term *economization*, like its awkward derivatives *economizing* and *economized*, is rather obscure, and economic sociologists and philosophers have taken on defining it only recently. Literally, *economization* would mean the emergence, creation, or expansion of an economy. Many scholars have somewhat vaguely associated this process with capitalist market imperialism.[2] From this perspective, an economization of dying would mean that free market logic has encroached on morality and that profit-driven monetary calculations now exclusively dominate the management of dying processes.

This is not the route I have taken in this book. As I described it, the new economy of dying involves moral as well as financial values. Existential reflections on what people find meaningful in life coexist with corporations' profit considerations. Moral doubts on the worth of life in severe illness feed financial doubts on the utility of sustaining these lives. Rather than encroaching upon moral and existential reflections, hospital administrations capitalize on them: they save money by hiring palliative care physicians and encouraging people to think over their values regarding end-of-life care.

This argument underlines two problems in defining economization as the encroachment of markets on morality. First, as several generations of economic sociologists have argued, markets and morality are not mutually exclusive.[3] Creating market institutions—such as money, rules of exchange, commodities, and private property—depends on and at the same time furthers certain moral acts, values, and views.[4] Numerous case studies that economic sociologists have analyzed over the years support this point. Nineteenth-century insurance companies associated their products with family values and made life insurance policies part of death rites.[5] A French economist, who designed a local strawberry market according to the "perfect market" model, depended on the buyers' and sellers' perception that this model would be more just and fair.[6] And the pioneers of the notoriously cutthroat financial derivatives market in Chicago had to act collectively, lend each other money to facilitate trade, and establish a community that worked to legitimize its activities.[7] Even if we define economization as the process of capitalist market expansion, it is clear that furthering and hinging on moral values is a central component of it.

Second, there is a problem with identifying *the economy* with capitalist markets and economization with capitalist market expansion because this leads to ignoring the diverse phenomena that the term *economy* describes.[8] We can think, for example, of socialist and communist economies, non-market economies that comprise traditional institutions of reciprocal exchange or central distribution,[9] moral economies,[10] and domestic, informal, and non-monetary economies.[11] "The anthropologist, the sociologist or the historian," Karl Polanyi wrote, faces "a great variety of institutions other than markets, in which man's livelihood [is] embedded."[12] The term economization should therefore include a variety of possible economization projects and numerous different economies that emerge from them.[13]

There are, however, reasons why the reduction of *economization* processes to capitalist market expansion is so common. After all, it is mainly economists who have the social power to create an abstraction that towers above the plurality of economies and impresses itself upon them.[14] Rather than studying the works of various *economies*, economists have claimed for themselves *the* study of *the* economy. Their discipline's power lies not only in analyzing and creating markets, but also in topicalizing a general concept of *the* economy and defining it as their jurisdictional domain.[15] Reducing the plethora of existing economies into a single market design is a paramount economization project, which economists have promoted. They have delineated a distinctive life-sphere, claimed it is governed by distinctive rules and truths, and monopolized knowledge on its workings.[16]

Even economic sociologists, who have dedicated themselves to challenging this monopoly, ended up reproducing economics' definition of the economy. Most of economic sociology's pioneers aimed to apply "the frames of reference, variables, and explanatory models of sociology to that complex of activities concerned with the production, distribution, exchange, and consumption of scarce goods and services"[17]—a goal that many still embrace.[18] Yet largely they continued analyzing the economy as a domain of exclusively material activities, which involves monetary and commodity exchange in markets. Despite their intentions, they unquestioningly accepted the abstraction that economists created—"the economy"—as a reality and merely added new variables to its study.[19]

Analyzing *economization* sociologically should address this shortcoming and expand the program of economic sociology beyond its traditional limits. For one thing, writing about economization means problematizing "the economy" and treating it as an outcome of social, political, historical, and fiscal forces, not a given reality.[20] Furthermore, treating economists' definition of the economy as an important part of economization means transcending economists' concepts, reflecting on the circumstances where they developed and spread them, and emphasizing the plethora of economies and economization processes that emerged and declined in the process.

In the introduction, I presented two definitions of the verb "to economize," each implying a different economization project. First, Aristotelian economization meant adopting a prudent disposition toward abundance. This was the stance that early hospice and palliative care advocates propagated: in the face of abundant life-prolonging and life-sustaining interventions that modern medicine has made available, they defined skepticism and prudence as virtues. Second, neoclassical economization meant making rational and calculated choices between alternatives under conditions of scarcity. This framework applied to monetary considerations, for example, when advocates argued that the scarce health care resources spent on futile life-prolonging treatments could be directed elsewhere. It also manifested in how people approached non-monetary questions. Consider, for example, Feudtner and Morrison's statement that one cannot "hold a loved one's hand while they are dying at the same moment that a code team yells 'clear' and attempts to defibrillate the patient's heart" (see Chapter 5).[21] From a neoclassical standpoint, because there is scarcity in resources, time, or the number of interventions that one can provide simultaneously, people are obliged to choose. Neoclassicists prescribe that this choice be rational, methodical, and based on individual preferences.[22]

This book suggests a very inclusive concept of *economy*. It treats the new economy of dying as the regime of valuation that emerged from the amalgam of these two economization projects. In the rest of the conclusion, I recap some of the history and present of the economy of dying in a way that elucidates three main features of economization processes as I see them: first, the delineation of limits and states of scarcity; second, the development of governmental mechanisms; and third, the emergence of hierarchies.

Economization and Limits

Consider a common visualization of the demographic transition (Figure 6.1): a graph indicating the size of the world population rises moderately for over 10,000 years, then spikes without warning around the eighteenth century.[23] The dramatic acceleration marks the beginning of modernity—a period of unprecedented economic, political, and scientific growth. Modernist thinkers described this growth as the fulfillment of what has always been a distinctive human potential: the ability to know, control, and go beyond the human species' natural qualities and environmental confines.[24] This has manifested very clearly in the realm of health and medicine. The power to manage disease, control morbidity, and reduce mortality through sanitation, vaccinations, improved nutrition, and new medical interventions meant that humans mastered and transcended many of the limitations of their biology and environment.[25] Population growth was the outcome of these triumphs. Like economic growth, it indicates a historical trajectory of unbounded advance and progress.

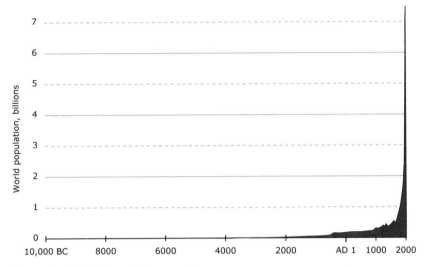

Figure 6.1. World population over time. Source: Wikimedia Commons, Population curve.svg.

The problem of economization, however, has always lurked underneath this trend. As early as the late eighteenth century, Thomas Malthus argued that because population growth outpaced growth in food supply, this spike would collide with a hard ceiling of agricultural productive capacity.[26] By the 1930s, biologist Raymond Pearl modeled patterns of population growth and predicted they would flatten when approaching levels of economic and environmental saturation.[27] Both of them argued that life expectancy and population size were not moving in a unidirectional path of infinite growth but were bounded by limits, which could be modeled.

The delineation (or modeling) of boundaries and limits is central to economization processes. The economization of dying laid out two boundaries. One was financial: economists emphasized that end-of-life spending outpaced economic growth, argued that population aging would amplify the trend, and concluded that economization on end-of-life care was a financial imperative. The other was more existential: it was a concern—which hospice and palliative care advocates, bioethicists, right-to-die groups, and others articulated—that medical triumphs could not surpass the transcendental finitude of meaningful human life. That is, medicine could prolong life only to a certain upper limit, beyond which life would lose all meaning.

These two boundaries aligned. From the advocates' point of view, dying had to be economized because the United States could no longer afford prolonging it *and* because it was immoral to prolong life beyond the upper limit. On paper, this seemed to be a conflict-free economization project: financial economization was not just legitimate but morally necessary because it could help people avoid suffering and allow them to die dignified deaths.[28] As I show in Chapters 3 through 5, however, support for the economization of dying was not universal. Some social groups regarded economization as necessary and even virtuous; others, however, remained unconvinced about the validity and objectivity of the economy's limits and insisted that life could still be meaningfully prolonged and economization was not imperative.

In their frustration, many clinicians attributed such vitalist attitudes to patients' and families' individual whims and irrationalities, or to traits that they thought characterized entire ethnicities, religious groups, and nationalities. These tensions around economization reflected on medicine no less than they reflected on individual patients and families. The fact that clinicians and health organizations experienced resistance to economization as problematic, disturbing, and disruptive revealed how deeply economization had pervaded their professional judgment, moral intuitions, and organizational logic. It showed that much of the health care system and medical profession has come to need and depend on economization, to the point of feeling that opposition was unbearable, immoral, and sometimes impossible to accept. Clinicians and organizations took the limits that the new economy of dying presupposed as objective givens, not as contingent judgments that had their history and sociology—which some people did not share.

Resistance to limits is an indication that the new economy of dying is not completely unquestionable. It also shows, however, how strong this economy is. When a certain social power is weak, people can dismiss or ignore it; resistance happens only when a power is solid to the point of becoming the rule. Patients (and families) resisted because much of the medical profession, health care system, and public discourse accepted, at least to some degree, the limits that economization advocates have propagated. Such generally shared recognition of limits is one cardinal feature of economization.

Economization and Governmental Logics

A second feature of economization is governmental mechanisms, which conduct and direct human behavior vis-à-vis the limits that people recognize. The shape that these mechanisms assume tends to reflect dominant political and social forces.

Consider, for example, Thomas Malthus's argument that population growth would outstrip food supply and inevitably lead to food shortages. The economic governance that Malthus advocated molded into his period's politics, specifically the English gentry's efforts to manage and control the poor through free markets. Malthus considered the threat of hunger as essential to governing poor populations. This threat guaranteed that poor people would regulate themselves, work hard, and have fewer children. Malthusian economization therefore hinged on free-market mechanisms of governance. He deemed "poor relief" laws, which provided minimal income to all, threatening to optimal economic governance.[29]

Similar to Malthus, biologist Raymond Pearl's early twentieth century economization models of population and economic growth mirrored his period's colonial governmental projects.[30] Pearl was interested in the limit that material resources put on population growth. Drawing on the basic insight that when material resources in a certain economy are exhausted, population growth declines, Pearl suggested adjusting population growth to economic growth. For one thing, his work was thoroughly invested in the effort to represent national economies and govern them through social science tools.[31] But more strongly, Pearl inspired ambitious projects to govern population growth in the colonial and postcolonial Global South and adjust the sizes of populations to their potential economic value.[32]

Like these economization projects, projects to economize dying resonated with existing governmental structures. Countries with centralized health care systems orchestrated economization through central planning. The British National Health Service (NHS), for example, adopted a comprehensive metric—quality-adjusted life years (QALY). It administered surveys where people ranked how they valued life in severe illness and disability, calculated the QALY that various treatments added on average, and estimated the costs of these treatments. Based on these calculations, NHS ruled which treatments were cost efficient and merited funding and which did not justify their cost.[33]

The U.S. health care economy, by contrast, has always been highly decentralized. Drawing on the country's traditional individualistic sentiments, first the American Medical Association, then insurance companies and other corporate actors, repeatedly intercepted attempts to centralize and nationalize health care.[34] Part of the reason why health care costs in the United States have been the highest in the world has to do with this historical weakness of central control mechanisms.

The U.S. economization of dying thus had to be individuated. It needed to speak to the business interests of individual corporations, the moral predilections of individual clinicians, the donations of private philanthropists, and the wishes of individual patients. Economization had to affect these actors' views of themselves, their values, and their interests. The chief governance mechanisms of the new economy of dying in the United States have been what sociologist Nikolas Rose called "techniques of self." Economization turned people and corporations inward and conducted them by granting them autonomy. Advocates of the new economy of dying urged people to reflect and think about who they were, what life meant to them, in what circumstances they felt life was meaningless, and when and how they would want to die.

An unprecedented number of medical procedures became matters of patient choice and preference. Even the most technical and automatically applied medical procedures (such as cardiopulmonary resuscitation) transformed into interventions that people could decide on doing or not doing, based on their personal tastes. Documents such as advance directives, the Physician Order for Life-Sustaining Treatment (POLST), living wills, Go Wish cards, and Do Not Resuscitate / Do Not Intubate (DNR / DNI) forms recorded such tastes and preferences formally, and insurance companies began paying physicians to fill them out with patients. This system encouraged "rendering into speech [or writing] who one is." As Nikolas Rose put it, "In the act of speaking, through the obligation to produce words that are true to an inner reality, through the self-examination that precedes and accompanies speech, one becomes a subject for oneself" and to others.[35]

Acts of writing and talking created objects that were physically separate from patients—pieces of paper or electronic files that coded the patients' statements and which clinicians took as representing who the patients were. These forms and documents—like the words spoken in family conferences—came to dominate patients. Patients received treatment based on how these documents and the clinical notes described them.

Corporations' agency was subject to a similar governmental logic. Hospital administrations became preoccupied with the costs they incurred for treating patients at the end of life because they, too, turned inward and reflected on their conduct in the area. The papers that advocacy organizations such as the Center to Advance Palliative Care (CAPC) (see Chapter 2) published did not order hospitals to cut costs on end-of-life care—the advocacy organizations had no authority to do so. Rather, they instructed hospitals on how to monitor and document their end-of-life expenditures in order to make these expenditures more visible and subject to management. As a result, hospitals began questioning themselves. They participated in the new economy of dying out of a conviction that it was serving their interests.

This was the essence of the individuated governmental approach of the new economy of dying. It informed how corporations thought of their financial interests, how patients thought of their lives and existence, and how clinicians perceived their goals as professionals. The outcome was pervasive. A growing number of corporations began thinking of the end of life financially and started counting patients who were nearing death as financial liabilities. Numerous clinicians internalized the palliative care gaze, doubted the benefit of life-prolonging interventions, and applied the economizing logic at the bedside. And a record number of patients (and future patients) contemplated their "end-of-life goals," reflected on their personal values, and ranked and recorded them in formal and legally binding forms. Where economization through central planning had seemed improbable (and has indeed failed several times), an economizing medical specialty—which permeated hospitals, medical schools, insurance companies, and people's common sense—held much promise.

There are, however, reasons to believe that this promise has only been partly fulfilled. Joan Teno and colleagues showed that in 2000–2009, the use of hospice and palliative care rose in tandem with acute care interventions. It is clear that the new economy of dying grew markedly. From 2000 to 2009, the rates of hospice deaths climbed from 21.6 to 42.2 percent of the total deaths in the country, and hospital deaths declined from 32.6 to 24.6 percent. There was also steady growth in the number of hospices and palliative care services during these years (see Chapter 1). However, the mainstream, cure-oriented health economy also grew. Dying patients were more likely to be hospitalized in the last three months before their deaths (62.9 percent in 2000 to 69.3 percent in 2009), more patients received care in intensive care units (ICUs) in the last month of their life (24.3 percent in 2000 to 29.2 percent in 2009), and cancer patients were more likely to receive mechanical ventilation during this last month (5.9 percent in 2000 to 6.7 percent in 2009).[36]

These are indications that the new economy of dying has not replaced the old one, but rather has developed next to it. Intentions and declarations aside, there appears to be no zero-sum game between the two economies. The expansive economy, which prolongs and sustains life, grows concurrently with the new of dying, which purports to cap it. Both economies extract financial value from the process, and both rely on elaborate moral reasoning to legitimize their clinical and financial practices. It is hard to predict how these economies will continue to evolve, but currently it seems that the U.S. health care system is becoming more aggressive not only in prolonging life but also in counteracting its own aggression. It provides a great deal of life-prolonging and life-sustaining care, and then a great deal of comfort care to treat pain, alleviate suffering, and bring people to the place of relinquishing curative treatments.[37]

The dying processes that this contradictory system fosters are heart wrenching. Many patients receive extensive, invasive curative care in a hospital, then move on to have their deaths economized. Clinicians continue treating severely ill patients curatively—by some measures, even more invasively and aggressively than in the past—and when the treatment fails, right before patients die, the clinicians pass them onto hospice. The ratio of hospice patients who spent less than three days in hospice before dying more than doubled over one decade (4.6 percent in 2000 to 9.8 percent in 2009). Transitions between different health care institutions in the last three days of life also rose substantially (10.3 percent in 2000 to 14.2 percent in 2009).[38] For frail and fragile dying patients, these transitions between institutions are extremely unpleasant. It is hard to see how they serve the patients, although it is clear how they benefit the health corporations treating them.

Morality and Hierarchies

In his formative 1917 lecture, "Science as a Vocation," Max Weber asserted that science could not provide answers to the most crucial moral questions that humanity faces. Paraphrasing Tolstoy, he stressed that science "gives no answer to our question, the only question that is important to us: 'what shall we do and how shall we live?'" As Weber subsequently argued, scientific thinking can only help understand the consequences of following certain moral rules.[39]

The relationship between medicine and moral predicaments near the end of life fits so neatly into this framework that Weber used it as an example (see this chapter's epigraph). Medicine, he argued, can answer technical questions—for example, how to prolong the life of a severely ill or badly incapacitated person. It can also clarify how the life of this person would look when prolonged. It cannot, however, rule on whether prolonging this person's life would be right or wrong. Doing so would involve a value judgment, which a rational science cannot make.

The case of the hospice and palliative care specialty complicates this position because its essence has been addressing moral questions through professional means. By pervading people's moral judgment, hospice and palliative care have established "a thought world, expressed in its own thought style, penetrating the minds of its members, defining their experience, and setting the poles of their moral understanding."[40] It has facilitated a pattern of moral reflection, bridged between the general logic of the new economy of dying and people's personal views and experiences, and brought many people to act in accordance with a social project of economization that is greater than their own individual selves. The people who embrace economization do so not out fear or coercion, but, as Émile Durkheim put it, "out of respect to . . . moral authority." "The force of the collectivity," Durkheim wrote,

> is not wholly external [to individuals]; it does not move us entirely from outside. Indeed, because society can exist only in and by means

of individual minds, it must enter into us and become organized within us. That force thus becomes an integral part of our being and, by the same stroke, uplifts it and brings it to maturity.[41]

Far from the mechanical role that Weber attributed to physicians, palliative care clinicians play a most central role as the moral muscles and sinews of economization—the moral authorities that facilitate individuals' internalization of economization. Clearly, the techniques that I have outlined in this book did not always succeed in making people embrace economization. At times, the efforts to economize dying failed. At the same time, on average, palliative care clinicians managed to nudge patients in more economized directions. Had they not been able to do so, hospital administrations would not have hired them.

The new economy of dying that hospice and palliative care promote is particularly intriguing sociologically because it developed in a realm of moral indefiniteness. As the clinicians I studied said on multiple occasions, there are often no clear and categorical rights and wrongs in end-of-life care. People tried to do what they thought was moral in situations that oftentimes did not have clear solutions. To a great extent, the clinicians were damned if they did and damned if they didn't: when prolonging the life of a seriously ill patient, they could be blamed for causing unnecessary suffering or for serving the profit-driven medical-industrial complex. When they allowed a seriously ill patient to pass away, they could be rebuked for managing a death panel, which possibly served their hospital's financial interest. By articulating a reasonably solid moral view and investing people's intuitive sense with it, palliative care clinicians somewhat eased this problem.

The power of palliative care lies in the deeply empathetic way in which it governs patients. This power, however, impacts different people differently. Hospice and palliative care had very particular social origins. The people who promoted the specialty were predominantly white, highly educated, and from middle- and upper-class backgrounds. Palliative care's quasi-psychotherapeutic techniques reflected these people's cultural tastes. Consequently, there were very particular social groups whose intuitions resonated with palliative care and who felt at home when talking to palliative care clinicians. These were the people clinicians enjoyed talking to, whose cultural and social capital matched the expectation to reflect existentially on their values and feelings, who not only could but also *wanted* and *needed* to articulate and voice a certain inner self. These patients were comfortable talking with clinicians in the hospital, and they experienced professional authority as helpful, unintimidating, and not malevolent.

Others were less likely to articulate themselves, have their voices heard, or be validated in the decision-making process. This included people who were unclear about their wishes; who did not trust the medical establishment; who clinicians discredited; who did not have family members or friends who knew them well and who would feel comfortable representing them after the patient lost consciousness; or who lived their life from day to day and, for various reasons, did not like to plan ahead and avoided committing to any future plan. These were the people who were hard to subjectify.

Sociologists tend to document economization projects that discipline unprivileged populations: the poor, the Global South, and the marginalized populations of urban areas.[42] Paradoxically, the economization of dying governed people with valued cultural and social capital far more easily because they were the ones who best communicated with palliative care clinicians. Social privilege made patients more pliable, that is, more likely to be influenced by palliative care, and hence more likely to accede to economizing dying.

Obviously, from a certain moral standpoint being more pliable was advantageous, because the alternative to economized dying was a wild, untamed, and unrestrained dying trajectory—so different from the ideals of "good death" that the hospice and palliative care movement promoted, which have become so dominant in U.S. public discourse. Economized dying was therefore a very tempting trajectory in an otherwise indefinite moral realm. The new economy of dying gave answers to the questions that Weber and Tolstoy raised, providing those who embraced these answers with an opportunity to "live and die with a gentler and lighter spirit."[43]

Methodology

Notes

References

Acknowledgments

Index

Methodology

How the Project Began

I did not plan to write about death. An economic sociologist at heart and by training, my first empirical research was about how states manage their sovereign debts. Then came my first summer in the United States, which I spent reading dozens of arid World Bank reports, reaching nowhere. Come the fall, frustrated and enervated, I embarked on what I thought would be an adventurous excursion away from the world of finance: writing an ethnography on a hospice.

This hospice, however, brought me straight back to economic sociology. On my very first day of fieldwork, I met with its volunteer coordinator to inquire about whether I could volunteer and write about the place. Without me asking anything about money, she sat me down and explained the organization's finances in great detail. She said the hospice was mainly treating Medicare patients, and that Medicare paid a flat daily rate for each of them, regardless of the level and amount of care that they needed. In return, the hospice treated the patients according to the "hospice way of care": it controlled their pain, addressed their other symptoms, and provided them (and their families) with spiritual and social support. The volunteer coordinator said that this model was so successful that private insurance companies began showing interest in it. Insurers often incurred costly bills from seriously ill patients who came to the emergency room (ER) when their condition worsened, so paying hospice a daily rate—and making it responsible for all costs until the patient died—was a way to avoid financial risk. On the hospice's side, things could get quite lucrative, too. Eschewing life-prolonging treatment and long hospitalizations meant reduced expenses, which left a good profit margin when expenses were lower than the Medicare rate.

The situation surprised me. I came to study death, suffering, emotions, and dramatic life-and-death decisions permeated by moral perplexity and doubt. All of those certainly existed in the hospice, and yet there I was, listening to a volunteer coordinator seamlessly weaving them into her employer's financial and business interests. Was economic sociology following me, or were these my own predilections that made me attentive to any mention of pecuniary matters? Whatever it was, my sense that this economy was worthy of research strengthened the further the fieldwork developed and the more I read about the history of U.S. hospices, the ways they combined financial, moral, and professional arguments, and the increasing role they played in managing death and dying in the United States. A year later, the cost of end-of-life care became central to public debates over the Patient Protection and Affordable Care Act of 2010 ("Obamacare") and Sarah Palin accused Obama of instituting "death panels" (see Introduction). It was clear that the topic deserved a deeper and more extensive look.

When I finished drafting my paper on the hospice, I invited its manager for dinner.[1] Although she did not read the paper (I summarized it for her), she managed to identify a major deficiency in my work. My chief interest was the intersection between finance and decisions to forgo life-prolonging treatments. Studying hospices meant looking at patients who no longer received curative care. The decision to stop was already behind them; if I were to pursue the topic seriously, I should go to places where people still had to make this decision.[2]

This was how I started work on this book. The ethnographic parts of this book draw on fieldwork I conducted between October 2011 and October 2012. After the dinner with the hospice manager, I approached several hospital physicians of different specialties, hoping that they would help me decide on which area in medicine I should focus. I quickly noticed that these interviews channeled me in the direction of palliative care. The references to palliative care differed from each other. On one extreme were the physicians who thought of palliative care as a self-contained specialty with clear jurisdictional boundaries. They described palliative care physicians as "death specialists"—the people you would call when one of your patients is dying. One cardiologist, for example, told me that she hardly came across death in her work; when I asked if she never had a patient who died, she responded that when such cases did occur she referred them to palliative care before they passed away. She thought of her own and palliative care's jurisdictions as mutually exclusive—cardiology was about curing, while palliative care was about helping patients die a better death. Other specialists, however, did see death and dying as relevant to their work and treated palliative care clinicians as consultants who could help them when problems related to it arose. An emergency care physician talked to me about nursing home residents with advanced dementia who came to the ER with chronic problems such as recurrent pneumonia. How and how not to treat these patients were questions he grappled with regularly, and he called the palliative care service when he felt addressing them was particularly challenging.

Regardless of how physicians used palliative care, they all recognized that treating the patients they thought were dying was relevant to the specialty. And while it was clear that palliative care clinicians did not have a monopoly over treating dying patients—cardiologists, oncologists, intensive care physicians, and others could choose whether or not to consult palliative care—it was generally accepted that, as the ER physician put it, when it comes to death and dying, palliative care 'is a comprehensive way of looking at care, A-to-Z.' I decided to develop the research in this direction and make it a study of a medical specialty and its more general impact on the U.S. health care economy.

The focus on this specialty reflects a transition in how U.S. hospitals manage death. The first ethnographies of hospital deaths (published during the 1960s and 1970s) did not focus on any individual site within the hospital. People died in a general and nonprofessionally specific space, particularly in medicine units.[3] Ethnographies published in the 1990s tended to cover particular hospital units—intensive care units (ICUs), neonatal wards, and ERs.[4] Even Sharon Kaufman, who aimed to study hospital deaths in general, reported that she ended up spending most of her time in ICUs because this was where most deaths occurred.[5] Medicine's professional sequestration led to spatial separation of deaths, and consequently to sequestration of the ethnographies that documented these deaths.

The development of the palliative care specialty shifted not only the professional management of death in hospitals, but also its spatial distribution. Shadowing palliative care clinicians brought me to many different hospital departments. We visited ICUs and medicine units, we saw oncology, cardiology, neurology, and other patients, and we encountered patients suffering from failures of virtually all organ systems. Exceptions did exist, and some were obvious (orthopedics patients are unlikely to be terminal); others indicated the closure of some medical disciplines to professional outsiders (surgery referrals were relatively rare). Yet overall, studying palliative care meant visiting multiple hospital units, which was indicative of the specialty's character. It did not isolate itself to any particular space, but rather sought to communicate with other specialties and invest them with its logic of care.

Focusing on palliative care and shadowing its practitioners conferred the advantage of directing me to sites where people negotiated life, dying, and death. These were the borderlands between the traditional and cure-oriented economy of dying and the new economy of dying that arose to counteract it. Yet the focus on palliative care meant that I examined the borderlands from the side of the counteraction. When I was following the palliative care logic, I inevitably overlooked some of the work of nonpalliative care clinicians.[6] This book should therefore not be read as a study of all hospital deaths, let alone all deaths; it is an account of the new economy of dying and its relationship to traditional curative medicine.[7]

Data Collection

I wanted to observe palliative care as it worked in different sectors in the U.S. health care economy. I chose a metropolitan area in California that was served by several hospitals that served different populations.[8] Within this area, I interviewed palliative care clinicians from six hospitals. In three of these hospitals—a public hospital, a private hospital, and an academic medical center—I also joined the palliative care teams for a total of eighty workdays.

The three hospitals differed greatly. The public hospital ("Public") was a safety-net institution that served a diverse patient population. Public's patients included homeless and marginally housed people, undocumented and uninsured immigrants, trauma patients of various classes and ethnic backgrounds (like many other public hospitals, Public was the only trauma center in the area), as well as a significant population of lower and lower-middle class people, especially younger people whose precarious employment situation did not afford them health care benefits.[9] Common to this very diverse population was a lack of stable and comprehensive insurance coverage.[10] The hospital's chief budgetary resource was county budgets, which had been under threat for decades.

I joined Public's palliative care service as a volunteer, usually visiting the service once or twice a week. I attended the palliative care team's "rounds" in the morning, where on most days an attending physician, a nurse, a social worker, and two chaplains met and discussed the patients who were listed in the service's "patient census." Then I went to see the patients that the physician thought were communicative enough to benefit from my company. Like most of the clinicians that I met in the hospital, members of the palliative care team were extremely competent professionals; and like other health care providers in the public system, they often expressed frustration about the lack of resources. Public's underinsured and uninsured patients had to wait long periods to be discharged from the hospital to lower levels of care. Beds in the only public nursing home in the area were scarce, and many of these patients did not have a "stable living situation," leading the clinical staff to consider them "unsafe" for discharge. Lack of resources and frustration with the hospital's rigid bureaucracy also made it difficult for the service to retain its nonphysician staff. Over the course of one year, three social workers left the service, and its chaplains were paid very modest salaries by a nonprofit organization and a church.

The academic hospital ("Academic") was a large medical center connected to a medical school, which offered cutting-edge treatments in virtually every medical field. Academic was far better staffed than Public, and could offer more types of treatments to its patients.[11] Academic served as a referral center, treating cases that were "too complicated" to manage in smaller and less specialized hospitals. The hospital prided itself on its professional ranking and prestige, which several people in the palliative care team referred to as a challenge because the fixation on offering the most advanced treatments could make physicians reluctant to talk about end-of-life care. At the same time, Academic had a very large and respected palliative care team. The hospital's doctors and administration seemed to embrace palliative care as one professional frontier among many that the hospital was advancing. Several of the physicians involved in the team were engaged in research on end-of-life care and in advancing palliative care outside the hospital. Like many other physicians at Academic, they worked as leaders in their field, as opposed to clinicians who focus on day-to-day hospital work.

Academic's palliative care service was the largest of the three that I studied. On a typical day, it included an attending physician, two residents, two medical students, a social worker, a chaplain, and two nurses, in addition to chaplaincy and nursing interns who joined the service periodically. It was fairly easy to merge into this large team. I counted as one among many students. As such, I could join the team's rounds in the morning, shadow team members throughout the day, and attend training sessions that were given on days when there was time. I joined the team's work once a week for a period of three months.

The private hospital that I studied ("Private") was owned by a large nonprofit corporation that had acquired it more than a decade before I began fieldwork. Many of Private's physicians referred to its formal non-profit status sarcastically. One physician defined it as "not-for-profit, but definitely for money." Physicians in another unit hung on their office wall a list of the corporation's executive salaries, which were all seven digits. When I referred to Private's not-for-profit status in an interview with a physician, he chuckled and said, "This is such bullshit." The corporation that controlled Private was regularly criticized for diverting resources away from hospitals located in poorer neighborhoods and for its aggressive acquisition policy. Private Hospital itself was considered the corporation's flagship in the area. Virtually all of its patients were insured, and a significant proportion of them had more than one single insurance provider, usually Medicare and a supplementary private insurance. With the gradual privatization of Medicaid and its transition into a managed-care system, which private insurance companies operated, Private began seeing a higher number of patients from lower-class backgrounds.

Employment patterns at Private were different from Public and Academic. Although physicians in the latter two were salaried, many of Private's specialists were affiliated with physician networks, which insurance companies reimbursed directly, usually on a fee-for-service basis. (A growing number of Private's physicians transitioned to salaried contracts, by many accounts, because of the cost and hassle of maintaining a back-office to process and charge multiple bills to multiple insurance companies.)[12] Because these physicians were typically reimbursed on a fee-for-service basis, their financial incentive in end-of-life care was at odds with Private Hospital's. Although Private lost money on seriously ill patients who were hospitalized for long periods (due to the diagnosis related group system, which I described in Chapter 2), many of its specialists profited from such patients because they were sicker and required many interventions—the specialists could visit many patients in a relatively short and profitable time period. My fieldwork at Private lasted four months, in which I joined the palliative care team about once a week. The core of the team included two physicians and a nurse practitioner, and once a week they met with a larger group of clinicians that included social workers, chaplains, Private's hospice liaison, and at times volunteers.

I conducted observations in multiple sites. On some days, I was able to shadow members of palliative care teams and observe them interacting with patients, families, and other clinicians. In Public Hospital, where I also volunteered, I saw and talked to some patients myself. In Academic Hospital, I was able to join teaching sessions, which exposed me to the socialization of young clinicians into the palliative care specialty. In all three hospitals I took part in team meetings ("morning rounds") and in informal conversations among the teams. In addition, I participated in nurse and physician trainings on end-of-life care, observed several "grand rounds" (highly attended lectures to the hospital's staff) on the topic, and conducted observations in classes taught to physician interns. I usually took short notes during the day, then extended them after the day was over. I also had several opportunities to share some of my ideas—in writing or orally—with palliative care people and hear their thoughts about them.

I complemented this fieldwork with in-depth interviews with clinicians whose work pertained to end-of-life care. Most of these interviews lasted fifty to seventy minutes; a few extended beyond three hours. I conducted a total of eighty interviews with physicians, nurses, social workers, chaplains, and some administrative staff. I spoke to people who represented a variety of specialties, including internists, intensive care physicians, oncologists, cardiologists, nephrologists, infectious disease specialists, surgeons, neurologists, and bioethicists. With several exceptions, where I was invited to interviewees' homes or sat with them at cafés, I interviewed people at their workplace. I consolidated my list of interviewees through a targeted snowball sample. Although I did not draw a random sample from a clearly defined population of interviewees, I made sure the sample included people from multiple specialties and professions, as well as people who held various attitudes toward palliative and end-of-life care. That is, I talked to specialists who were relatively open to palliative care as well as to people the palliative care clinicians defined as "naysayers" who hesitated to cooperate with the service.[13] On several occasions I approached specialists the other interviewees had mentioned, whose names had come up in rounds, or whom I met while I was shadowing the palliative care teams. Some interviewees I reached through direct referrals from palliative care clinicians. In these cases as in others, I evaluated what the interviewees told me in light of what other clinicians had reported and what I had observed myself.

I analyzed these interviews as ethnographic documents. They are not to be taken as factual descriptions of events but rather as records of conversations that took place in a specific social setting. Facing me, interviewees were asked to explain their views of end-of-life care, describe cases in which they were involved, and reflect on how these cases were approached. Their responses were "presentations of self," which they performed for a sociologist who inquired about end-of-life care.[14] They could not fully control any and every aspect of their self-presentation, yet much of their reflection was declarative: they made statements about end-of-life care that were anchored in their experiences and illuminated how they thought the topic should be thought and talked about.

They ordered their experience of end-of-life care in a certain narrative structure, and this structure was my main object of analysis. I could clearly see, for example, physicians who declared their openness to palliative care and their support for its approach as a way of signaling that they are up-to-date professionally. When an oncologist at Private Hospital said that he collaborated with the palliative care team closely, and a palliative care physician chuckled dismissively, 'Yeah, he calls us two days before his patients die,' I could draw conclusions not only about the gap between their accounts, but also about how important it was for the oncologist to leave an impression on me that he was acquainted with and profession-ally committed to palliative care. His statements validated palliative care and his own professional value at the same time: he classified palliative care as a valuable medical approach and himself as an informed physician who uses it in practice.[15]

I originally envisioned this project as a comparative ethnography that would illuminate variations in how hospitals manage the dying process. Yet despite the clear differences between the three hospitals, I found that their palliative care teams applied very similar practices. This finding re-flects the power of professions in general and of palliative care profes-sionalization in particular. Regardless of organizational, sociological, and economic contingencies, and despite idiosyncrasies and personality dif-ferences between clinicians, the palliative care professional toolkit had strong constant features.[16] Still, the clinicians applied these similar prac-tices in fundamentally different material contexts and toward people of very different backgrounds. Rather than a comparative ethnography, this study is therefore a multi-sited ethnography that examines how clinicians apply the palliative way of care in different contexts.

Shadowing palliative care clinicians drew me to historical questions, which mainly concerned how they came to think and practice medicine the way they did. Ethnographic methods are very limited in answering such questions, and interviewing people about their personal histo-ries could only give me access to their present reflections on the past. These were meaningful yet insufficient historical documents. Like many ethnographers, I found myself "writing the history of a present without a past."[17] Somewhat suspicious of the analytical solutions that structural anthropology suggested, I decided to combine ethnography and interviewing with historical methods.[18]

The book's historical materials come from several sources. With research assistants, I reviewed all the congressional hearings on the topic, all the articles that were published on the topic in the two leading U.S. medical journals, all the articles published in the *New York Times*, and a selection of noteworthy publications in other newspapers.[19] I also compiled an exhaustive list of books that were published on the topic beginning in the 1950s. Whenever possible, I generated quantitative estimates of the volume of relevant publication, which I used to evaluate the growth of the professional and public discussions on end-of-life care. I followed the activities and publications of the main advocacy organizations for hospice and palliative care, as well as the lively discussions on the two main blogs on palliative care—Geripal and Pallimed. In several places, I drew on public opinion surveys and demographic and organizational data that advocacy organizations, research institutes, and government agencies had published. As I was conducting my fieldwork, I became aware of an excellent archive of bioethics consultations that dated back to the mid-1980s. I read, summarized, and coded about half of the archive and based much of Chapter 3 on it.

Positionality

Studying palliative care has been an unusual experience. With the possible exception of psychiatry, it is hard to think of a medical specialty that is as open to multidisciplinary and nonscholarly perspectives as palliative care. Much of the thinking that inspired the specialty's pioneers originated from outside of medicine, and many of its leaders have written on moral, psychological, cultural, sociological, and policy issues, addressing the general public as they addressed their own profession.

The specialty's openness had a clear advantage for me: compared with other medical specialties, palliative care is very accessible to nonclinicians. Their expertise is mainly conversational and involves talking with severely ill patients, families, and other clinicians about end-of-life care.

Besides being able to follow and understand most of this work, I also felt that I shared a common language with many of the clinicians that I studied. We thought and cared about similar issues: social interactions and how differences in class, race, ethnicity, and age affected them, the relationship between organizational constraints and the personal and emotional dimensions of care, and the policy implications of palliative care work.[20] On the bookshelves of some of the practitioners whom I interviewed were the same books that I kept in my office: Kaufman's *And a Time to Die* (2006), Christakis's *Death Foretold* (1999), Anspach's *Deciding Who Lives* (1993), Timmermans's *Sudden Death and the Myth of CPR* (1999), Starr's *The Social Transformation of American Medicine* (1982), and Bosk's *Forgive and Remember* (1979). I interviewed and shadowed people who published research, columns, and blog posts that were full of sociological insight. They knew and were interested in the sociology of health and medicine.

This was also a challenge. Implicitly or explicitly these people held solid sociological views—far more solid than my own—about the nature of "cultural" attitudes toward death, the sociological characteristics of U.S. medicine, and the ways the U.S. health care system should manage death and dying. Writing about hospice and palliative care clinicians meant interpreting their sociological interpretations sociologically—or, to paraphrase Clifford Geertz, "winking at their wink."[21] Theirs is a very powerful wink. For one thing, the palliative care interpretation is very convincing. Its advocates and practitioners have established palliative care not only as a *beneficial* way to care for the dying, but also as a *moral* one. It is hard to think critically about palliative care practitioners because they are the "good guys," the medical professionals who not only want to humanize their profession and allow people to die a "good death," but are also reflective enough to consider multiple definitions of "good death" and stress the importance of respecting them all.

Many of the clinicians whom I studied hoped my work would help them improve their practice. They wanted my critique to have clear bottom lines that would identify problems and suggest solutions. I, on the other hand, preferred the comfort of the ivory tower and wanted to be an outsider, who would think and write free from the heavy responsibility that the clinicians carried.[22] This book does not propose applicable professional or policy reforms. Unlike most writers on the topic, I consider myself neither an ally of palliative care nor an opponent or a "critical friend."[23] My goal has been neither to praise nor condemn palliative care but to outline how it came to be and how it operates, how certain views of what is good care at the end of life became widely accepted, who has promoted these views, how they intersect with professional, financial, and political interests, and how they inform the ways people think about themselves and the care that they want.

This goal notwithstanding, the book may have political repercussions. It is hard to write on a topic as tense and dense as end-of-life care without having some impact on public discussion—intended or unintended. I am aware of the possibility that certain people would use and abuse my work to make arguments that I would never support. I should therefore clarify: No part of this book is meant to invalidate the palliative care approach, claim it is immoral, or advocate against it. As Paul Rabinow once wrote, making things "visible and vulnerable to analysis" is not the same as denouncing them.[24] Its professional peculiarities notwithstanding, palliative care is part and parcel of U.S. medicine, and it tackles problems that medicine in particular, and science in general, have confronted for over half a century. There is no way to avoid engaging these problems, although much can and should be said about how the United States has done so.

Notes

Introduction

Epigraph: Douglas (1986), 4.

1. Parsons (1951), 466–467.
2. Freidson (1970), 258.
3. Payer (1988), 124–125. See also Bunker (1970), Sontag (1978), Notzon et al. (1987), Institute of Medicine (1997, 47), Rosenthal (2017), and Ehrenreich (2018).
4. Freidson (1970), 257–258. For more recent accounts, see Kaufman's (2015) discussion of internal cardiac defibrillators, hemodialysis, and kidney transplants, and Light's (2010) critique of the pharmaceutical industry.
5. Cancer progresses fairly predictably in its advanced stages, which makes the final decline toward death relatively foreseeable.
6. This figure rose by 13.5 percent between 2000 and 2009 (Teno et al. 2013, 473).
7. American Board of Medical Specialties (2017).
8. Palliative care advocacy organizations have worked on expanding the practice into other institutions of curative care, such as outpatient clinics, nursing homes, and nursing facilities.
9. See Quill and Abernethy (2013).
10. This figure refers to hospitals with 300 beds or more. In 2014, an estimate of 44.6 percent of the total deaths in the country took place in hospice (see National Hospice and Palliative Care Organization 2015, chapter 1).
11. National Hospice and Palliative Care Organization (2017).
12. For other examples see Zelizer (2005, 2011), Bandelj et al. (2017), Fourcade and Healy (2007), Quinn (2008), and Chan (2012).
13. On moral entrepreneurship see Becker (1986), 147–149; Armstrong (1998).
14. See Abbott (2014).
15. See Kierkegaard (1993), 73.
16. For a comprehensive discussion of the sociological significance of death see Bauman (1992).
17. Cicero is cited in Stockton (1971), 166.

18. Some ethicists have taken this goal with much alacrity; see Callahan (1987, 2009), Singer (2009).

19. This approach elaborates on Anspach (1993) and Zussman (1992). Both of these contributions rejected ethicists' normative and prescriptive discussions, which focused on what *should* be done, in favor of empirical examinations of what clinicians do in practice. Anspach and Zussman substituted moralism with a sociology of morality; they examined how people approached moral problems, not whether or not their actions are moral. I share this stance, although I treat ethicists' normative discussions as performative (Callon 1998)—that is, as a prescription that informs and influences people's behavior, if not completely prescribing it.

20. Sarah Palin, "Obama and the Bureaucratization of Health Care," *Wall Street Journal*, September 8, 2009, www.wsj.com/articles/SB10001424052970203440104574400581157986024.

21. John Boehner and Thaddeus McCotter, "Statement by House GOP Leaders Boehner and McCotter on End-of-Life Treatment Counseling in Democrats' Health Care Legislation," Speaker Paul Ryan's Press Office, July 22, 2009, https://web.archive.org/web/20170521133714/http://www.speaker.gov/press-release/statement-house-gop-leaders-boehner-and-mccotter-end-life-treatment-counseling. Perhaps most outrageous was conservative pundit Betsy McCaughey's allegation in a radio interview that the provision "would make it mandatory, absolutely require, that every five years people in Medicare have a required counseling session that will tell them how to end their life sooner." See Earl Blumenauer, "My Near Death Panel Experience," *New York Times*, November 14, 2009, www.nytimes.com/2009/11/15/opinion/15blumenauer.html.

22. Don Gonyea, "Muted Reaction to Obama Health Care Town Hall," *NPR Morning Edition*, August 12, 2009, https://www.npr.org/templates/story/story.php?storyId=111797233.

23. The award was given by PolitiFact.com; see Holan (2009).

24. Institute of Medicine (2014), ix.

25. To the surprise of many end-of-life care advocates, a later attempt to pass a Medicare end-of-life care benefit did ultimately succeed. See Centers for Medicare & Medicaid Services (2016).

26. This is what Michel Foucault (2008) termed "state-phobia": "the idea that the state possesses in itself and through its own dynamism a sort of power expansion, an intrinsic tendency to expand, an endogenous imperialism constantly pushing it to spread its surface and increase in extent, depth, and subtlety to the point that it will come to take over entirely that which is at the same time its other, its outside, its target, its objects, namely: civil society" (187).

27. In particular, Glaser and Strauss (1965), Sudnow (1967), Zussman (1992), Anspach (1993), Timmermans (1999), Christakis (1999), Kaufman (2006), and Shapiro (2012).

28. In 1983, twenty-five-year-old Nancy Cruzan had a car accident that left her with devastating brain damage. Initially optimistic, her parents agreed that doctors could insert a feeding tube and provide her with artificial nutrition. Four years later, however, with no visible improvement in her condition, which "doctors defined as a persistent

vegetative state," the parents asked to have the tube removed. The hospital refused, so the parents launched a legal battle that lasted an additional four years, reached the Supreme Court, and led to a cornerstone ruling on the right to die. Cruzan was removed from artificial nutrition and passed away.

In 1990, twenty-nine-year-old Terri Schiavo collapsed at home due to unknown causes. Like Cruzan, her doctors diagnosed a persistent vegetative state: she could breathe independently but needed artificial nutrition. The prolonged legal battle over her diagnosis, neurological condition, prospects of recovery, and appropriate treatment rallied the conservative Christian right and liberal right-to-die activists, making the matter more politically contentious than ever. Schiavo's husband supported disconnecting her from artificial nutrition while her parents opposed it. After multiple dramatic turns in the plot—and with numerous "right to life" activists holding vigil—Schiavo was disconnected from artificial nutrition and passed away more than fifteen years after her collapse, with her husband sitting at her bedside (Anspach and Halpern 2008).

29. Ariès (1981).
30. "From the physician's standpoint, a case ceases to be medically interesting in the comatose, predeath stage," Sudnow (1967), 91. See also Glaser and Strauss (1968).
31. Kübler-Ross (1969), 36.
32. Kübler-Ross (1969).
33. Compare to the statements of Steinfels (1974); Steinfels and Veatch (1974).
34. These experiences are notably different from what sociologist Alex Broom (2015) describes.
35. See Kaufman (2006).
36. For a popular media example, see Gawande (2014). For an example of health economist arguments, see Peterson (2004), chapter 3. Also see Callahan (1987) for a discussion of limit setting.
37. Roy (2010). On the social construction of social problems see, for example, Jerolmack (2008) and Murphy (2012).
38. See Hart, Sainsbury, and Short (1998), and Timmermans (2005).
39. *Artes moriendi* (Latin: the arts of dying) were treatises published in Europe starting in the fifteenth century that instructed people on how to conduct themselves during the dying process to die well (Ariès 1981, 107–110, 129–130, 303–305). Also see Broom (2015), and Clark (1999), 734.
40. See Polanyi (1957).
41. Polanyi (1968), 98–99.
42. Aristotle (1995), 1258a35.
43. See Xenophon (1994, 11, 9–10); Aristotle (1934, 1177a), cited in Leshem (2013). The household *(oikos)* was a metaphor for larger political frameworks such as the polis (Owens 2015), so the moral virtue of prudency toward abundance (Leshem 2013, 57) also applied to other forms of social organization.
44. Robbins (1945), 16. The definition's origins can be traced back to Menger's foundational book *Principles of Economics* (Menger [1871] 1950). In a later edition, Menger revised this rationalistic definition. It was, however, essentially preserved because

Friedrich Hayek deliberately removed it from the book's English translation (Polanyi 1977, 21–24).

45. Max Weber's definition added a subjective element to this emphasis on scarcity. Like Robbins after him, Weber (1978) saw economic action as one in which "the satisfaction of a need depends, in the actor's judgment, upon relatively *scarce* resources and a *limited* number of possible actions, and if this state of affairs evokes specific reactions. Decisive for such rational action is, of course, the fact that this scarcity is *subjectively* presumed and that action is oriented to it" (339, italics in original). Scarcity is therefore not an objective constraint that people face but a matter of judgment and interpretation.

46. Foucault (2008), chapters 9 and 10.

47. Political philosopher Wendy Brown (2017), for example, defined economization as the dissemination of "the *model of the market* to all domains and activities—even when money is not at issue—[and the configuration of] human beings exhaustively as market actors, always, only, and everywhere as *homo oeconomicus*" (30–31, italics in original; cf. Bourdieu 2008).

48. Mitchell (2002), and Murphy (2017).

49. Espeland and Sauder (2007, 2016).

50. See Fourcade and Healy (2013).

51. See Fourcade (2017).

52. Some have called this dynamic *neoliberal* (Foucault 2008; Brown 2017).

53. See, for example, Ashmore, Mulkay, and Pinch (1989).

54. Murphy (2017), 5–6. Note that Murphy defined economization as a regime of valuation "hinged to the macrological figure of national 'economy'" (6), where economizing something means instrumentalizing it for the purpose of bettering, growing, and optimizing the national economy's performance. As I explain in the conclusion, my own definition is broader. See Appadurai (1986); Boltanski and Thévenot (1999a, b).

55. This transition mirrors the transition liberalism brought to sovereignty, which Foucault (2008) described in his lectures on biopolitics (in particular lecture 2, p. 46). The rise of liberalism meant a shift from a regime where the only limit on sovereign power was external (i.e., a kingdom's borders and the existence of other kingdoms beyond them), to a regime where sovereign power was moderated internally. Sovereign action became legitimate only in as much as it was useful—"the fundamental question of liberalism is: what is the utility value of government and all actions of government in a society where exchange determines the true value of things"—and needed to be minimalistic. For example, while medieval kings used maximal power and violence to control crime, starting the eighteenth century the "mild punishment" principle emerges: the constant question about punishment is whether it is useful. This is the regime of truth that we now see in medicine: the constant internal questioning of an intervention's usefulness. This follows decades in which the only restraint on medical practice was external—diseases that research has not yet conquered. See also Sheldon Wolin's analysis of Machiavelli's politics, which characterizes it as promoting "an economy of violence" (2016, 148–174).

56. For the history of the quality adjusted life-years metric, see MacKillop and Sheard (2018).

57. Cf. Dobbin (1994).

58. Conrad (2005), and Best (2012, forthcoming).

59. See Schneiderman et al. (1990), Jecker and Schneiderman (1992, 1995), and Helft, Siegler, and Lantos (2000).

60. For example, see Brody and Halevy (1995) and Smith (1995).

61. One could argue that the market order stifles economization—a counterintuitive statement given the widespread tendency to identify markets, and capitalist markets in particular, with economies as such (Polanyi 1977, chapter 1). Although markets cultivate economization on the individual level, their twentieth-century advocates have rejected economization as a concerted and planned project organized on a macro national level (cf. Hayek [1944] 2007).

62. Starr (1982), 9–13. See also Freidson (1970), 16.

63. Zola (1972), 487. This is what medical sociologists have called "medicalization" (Zola 1972; also Conrad 2007). Aronowitz (2015) recently showed that medicine is now taking "risk"—the potential that disease would develop—as good enough a reason to intervene (see also Waggoner 2017). On the modernist scientific project to control the human body through medical means, see Callahan (1987), Shilling and Mellor (1996), Turner (1987).

64. On the gap between the public image of cardiopulmonary resuscitation and its actual effectiveness, see Timmermans (1999).

65. Agamben (1998).

66. Zussman (1992), 21.

67. Starr (1982), 392.

68. Rosenberg (1987), 4.

69. We can find similar critiques of medicine as early as the Progressive era (Rosenberg 1987). They did not, however, institutionalize professionally, organizationally, and politically before the 1960s–1980s.

70. Thomas Hoyer, who worked for the Medicare program and was among the people who drafted the hospice Medicare benefit (see Chapter 2), wrote that hospice advocates "viewed the ordinary medical establishment, with its single-minded focus on curative care, with the same skepticism as had Ivan Illich in his 1976 book, *Medical Nemesis*." (Hoyer 1998, 64; cf. Illich 1976). The main people drawn to hospice were from the medicine's professional periphery: nurses, clergy, psychiatrists, and a handful of critical physicians—people whose stakes in the preservation of medicine's professional integrity was lower.

71. Clark (1999).

72. Epstein (1994), 103. Compare to the similar dynamics in the case of autism (Eyal 2013; Eyal et al. 2010).

73. This is comparable to the term "economy," which, as Timothy Mitchell shows, became a concept that denotes a social sphere that economists can analyze and manage (Mitchell 2002, 2005a, 2005b; Fourcade 2006, 2009).

74. Perhaps most famous was the Kübler-Ross model, which created a dichotomy between "denial" and "acceptance," and outlined five stages that terminal patients pass when transitioning from one to the other—denial, anger, bargaining, depression, and acceptance. The model delineated a clear professional goal for hospice care: helping

patients reach acceptance. And while this model attracted much criticism within the hospice movement, it was not exceptional in the ways it determined new goals and criteria for good care: this was something that all hospice advocates did—and had to do—to promote the hospice way of dying. Later on, these concepts and goals spread to the rest of the medical profession. See Borgstrom, Barclay, and Cohn (2013).

75. As I show in Chapter 1, so has the definition of what counts as "the end of life." For a programmatic discussion of the coemergence of disciplines and their objects of analysis, see Latour (1994).

76. This terminology is very specific to the United States. In other countries, such as France, palliative care and hospice care are used interchangeably.

77. The Patient Self-Determination Act, which Congress passed in 1990, required medical providers to inform patients about their right to refuse care and fill out advance directive forms, which appoint surrogate decision-makers and document what life-prolonging treatments patients would and would not want (see note 102 below).

78. Rodwin (2011), 102, 110.

79. Starr (1982), 397.

80. Welch, Schwartz, and Woloshin (2011).

81. See Mahar (2006), Rosenthal (2017).

82. This connected to what Donald Light termed "countervailing powers." The medical profession's dominance and its ability to get "almost everything it wanted" led to buyers' revolt, which targeted the high cost and variable quality of health care as well as its general resulting excesses (Light 1995, 2004). On the historical transition see Star (1982), Schmidt (1999), Scott et al. (2000).

83. By 2016, the Medicaid programs of thirty-nine states had contracted with managed care organizations (MCOs). "In 28 states—including 8 of the 10 states with the most Medicaid beneficiaries . . . —at least 75 percent of all Medicaid beneficiaries were enrolled in MCOs" (Paradise 2017).

84. An illustrative reform is the diagnosis related group (DRG) system discussed in Chapter 2. Consequently, many conditions that had once been treated in the hospital were now treated at home.

85. Rodwin (2011), 142–143.

86. Out of many other examples, see New York Times Editorial Board, "Care at the End of Life," *New York Times*, October 4, 2014, https://www.nytimes.com/2014/10/04 /opinion/care-at-the-end-of-life.html; Ezekiel J. Emanuel, "Better, if Not Cheaper, Care," *New York Times*, January 3, 2013, https://opinionator.blogs.nytimes.com/2013 /01/03/better-if-not-cheaper-care/; Susan Jacoby, "Taking Responsibility for Death," *New York Times*, March 30, 2012, https://www.nytimes.com/2012/03/31/opinion /taking-responsibility-for-death.html.

87. For example, Callahan (1987); Scitovsky and Capron (1986).

88. For example, "Gov. Lamm Asserts Elderly, if Very Ill, Have 'Duty To Die,'" *New York Times*, March 29, 1984, 00016, https://www.nytimes.com/1984/03/29/us/gov-lamm -asserts-elderly-if-very-ill-have-duty-to-die.html. Also see Amanda Bennett's reflection on the cost of her husband's death (Bennett 2012).

89. Kaufman (2006), 131–146.

90. Glaser and Strauss (1968), 148–178.

91. Although hospital deaths are still common, they are in decline (see Kaufman 2006, 89–91). Over one decade (2000–2009), they decreased by nearly a quarter, from 32.6 to 24.6 percent for Medicare fee-for service patients (Teno et al., 2013). The Centers for Disease Control and Prevention data collected on all hospital patients indicates that in 1989–2007, hospital deaths declined from 48.6 to 36 percent of all deaths (National Center for Health Statistics, 2011, 105).

92. I have two main reservations. First, Nick's description of the contemporary "culture of the hospital" is too unequivocal: there are still cases of patients (and families) who resist the heroic measures that physicians prescribe. Second, Nick seemed to accept accounts such as Kübler-Ross's too uncritically. Even in the 1960s, 1970s, and 1980s there were many patients who favored "aggressive" medicine. Recall that Parsons (1951) and Freidson (1970) attributed part of U.S. medicine's bent toward interventionism as stemming from patients' expectations from doctors.

93. On a more basic level, it makes one wonder whether U.S. medicine—and the U.S. health care system in general—can be portrayed as death-denying in the Kübler-Rossian sense. Note that sociologists have long challenged the death denial thesis (Kellehear 1984; Seale 1998; Zimmermann and Rodin 2004; Lavi 2005).

94. Of note, even non-manipulative critics from within the hospice movement, who did not share Palin's politics, warned that hospices might end up imposing the ideas of "good death" on patients. As Timmermans (2005) argued, "relatives and the dying patient still have to 'assent' to the ideology of hospice care aimed at a particular kind of good death" (998).

95. Notice, however, the ethicists who tried to establish clear definition for "futile treatment" during the 1990s. Theirs was an explicit (and ultimately not very successful) attempt to put limits on patient autonomy and determine when physicians can decline requests for life-sustaining and life-prolonging treatments (see Brody and Halevy, 1995; Helft, Siegler, and Lantos 2000).

96. Bellah et al. (2008), xiv. Even more generally, as Nikolas Rose (1998) put it, the ethic of "the free, autonomous self seems to trace out something quite fundamental in the ways in which modern men and women have come to understand, experience, and evaluate themselves, their actions, and their lives" (1).

97. Arney and Bergen (1984); see also Chambliss (1996).

98. Filene (1998), 67–70.

99. For instance, Fox and Swazey (2008).

100. Raz (1986), 204, 369.

101. Friedman (1990).

102. This law requires that health care institutions inform patients about "the right to accept or refuse medical or surgical treatment and the right to formulate advanced directives" [*sic*]. H.R. 4449—Patient Self Determination Act of 1990, 101st Congress (1989–1990). Also see American Hospital Association Board of Trustees, "Management Advisory: A Patient's Bill of Rights," first published in 1973, revised in 1992; www.americanpatient.org/aha-patient-s-bill-of-rights.html.

103. Arney and Bergen (1984), 46.

104. Arney and Bergen (1984). I draw on Lukes's (2005) three-dimensional view of power.

105. See Foucault (1991), Rose (1990), and Rose and Miller (1992).

106. Gramsci (2011), 156.

107. See, for example, Margolin (1997). Similarly, Sharon Kaufman (2006) argued that this notion is built around an "illusion of choice": while medical discourse hails choice rhetorically, in reality patients are heavily constrained by the limited options that medical professionals (such as physicians) and institutions (such as hospitals and insurance companies) give them. If a physician or a hospital does not present a patient with the possibility of having surgery (or conversely, transitioning to hospice care), this possibility remains outside of the patient's realm of choice (47–50). As I show in Chapter 5, I agree with the empirical observation but not with the argument that it reflects an illusion of choice.

108. Heimer and Staffen (1998); Timmermans and Buchbinder (2010).

109. Some define the goal of palliative care as "aligning treatment with a patient's goals," using skills that are "complex and take years of training to learn and apply, such as negotiating a difficult family meeting." Complex conversational skills are necessary because without them, patients' goals will oftentimes diverge and even contradict the economized dying framework (Quill and Abernethy 2013; see also Harris et al., 2016).

110. Althusser ([1971] 2001), 115–120. See also Burawoy (1979), Lahire (2011).

111. This is how Bosk (1979) interpreted the similarities between the surgery services that he studied.

112. See Karsoho et al. (2017).

113. For a discussion of heroic medicine, see Chapple (2010). For euthanasia, see Timmermans's typology of "brokered" deaths (2005) and Lavi (2005).

114. Although I will not focus on heroic deaths in this book, they will constantly appear in the background: these are the deaths that palliative care clinicians would want to make people avoid, out of conviction that they result from bad medicine. There are numerous excellent accounts, from periods before and after the rise of hospice and palliative care, which analyze intensive care and "heroic" deaths very effectively. See, for example, Zussman (1992), Chambliss (1996), Christakis (1999), Timmermans (1999), and Kaufman (2006, 2015).

115. This is the Patient Self-Determination Act of 1990.

116. Douglas (1986).

117. Jerolmack and Murphy (2017).

1. The Palliative Care Gaze

1. On the medical gaze see Foucault (1975).

2. National Hospice and Palliative Care Organization (2017).

3. Clark (2005), 7.

4. Saunders (1999). On the declared promises of medicine in the decades after World War II, see Kaufman (2015).

5. McGehee and Bordley (1976).

6. These patients were admitted after hospital physicians or their family physicians had informed them they had three months or less to live. See Saunders (1965).

7. In *Mirage of Health,* published in 1959, René Dubos dated this approach's origins to the Age of Enlightenment, when the cultural premises underlying modern science emerged. "Condorcet," he writes, "envisaged an era in which man would be free from disease and old age and death would be indefinitely postponed; Benjamin Franklin made similar predictions. To achieve old age had a universal fascination" (18).

8. Quoted in Clark (2005), 7.

9. Weber (2002), 121.

10. Saunders (1969), 57–58.

11. Saunders (1969), 52, italics in original.

12. Saunders (1965), 70.

13. Saunders (1969), 71.

14. This challenging of hierarchies stood in interesting contrast to the fact that Saunders held enormous executive powers at Saint Christopher's. She was not only the ultimate professional authority but also a powerful manager who determined policy almost singlehandedly. See Buck (2005).

15. Medical specialization spiked during those decades. By the early 1970s nearly 80 percent of physicians considered themselves specialists, compared with only 20 percent in 1940 (Twaddle and Hessler 1977, 175, quoted in Conrad and Schneider [1980] 1992, 254).

16. Buck (2005).

17. Saunders (1965).

18. Saunders (1969), 57, 58 (italics mine).

19. Saint Christopher's was located in London; for Saunders, Ireland clearly represented a peripheral, less worldly geographical area.

20. Worcester ([1940] 1961).

21. Worcester ([1940] 1961), 14. Compare, for example, to Gawande (2014); Welch, Schwartz, and Woloshin (2011); and Bloche (2011).

22. Worcester ([1940] 1961), 18.

23. Worcester ([1940] 1961), 44.

24. Baszanger (2012).

25. On Saunder's correspondence, see Clark (1998, 2001), and for her article see Saunders (1960a).

26. Quoted in Jonsen (1998), 14. These conferences coalesced into a community that started the first centers for bioethics in the United States.

27. Poe (1972). This article was also quoted in a congressional hearing: U.S. Senate, "Death with Dignity: An Inquiry into Related Public Issues," Hearing before the Special Committee on Aging, United States Senate, 92nd Congress, 2nd session, August 7, 1972, Part I, p. 17; www.aging.senate.gov/imo/media/doc/publications/881972.pdf.

28. This article was quoted in a congressional hearing: U.S. Senate, "Medical Ethics: The Right to Survival," Hearing before the Subcommittee on Health of the Committee on Labor and Public Welfare, 93rd Congress, 2nd session, On Examination of the Moral and Ethical Problems Faced with the Agonizing Decisions of Life and Death (June 11, 1974).

29. Raymond S. Duff, "On Choosing Death, a Presentation before the Senate Health Subcommittee," in "Medical Ethics," June 11, 1974. Duff was one of the physicians who participated in the hospice pilot program in New Haven mentioned later in this chapter.

30. Filene (1998), 50.

31. Filene (1998), 68. See also Mechanic (1996).

32. In 1975, twenty-one-year-old Karen Ann Quinlan suffered an irreversible brain injury, which left her in a persistent vegetative state. Fearing a homicide charge, hospital officials refused her parents' request to remove Quinlan from the respirator. The New Jersey Superior Court denied a suit that the parents filed, but the state's Supreme Court granted their appeal a few months later. The doctors removed Quinlan from the respirator, she began breathing independently, and she passed away only nine years later. The case attracted much media attention and became a milestone in the history of the Right to Die movement (see Filene 1998, chapter 3).

33. The interface between hospice on the one hand and physician-assisted suicide and euthanasia on the other hand has concerned advocates and practitioners throughout the hospice movement's history. Many of the movement's numerous religious members were unsympathetic to the idea of hastening death. Saunders defined hospice as an approach that neither hastened nor postponed death (Campbell, Hare, and Matthews 1995). Kübler-Ross saw terminal patients' wish to die as an outcome of the failure to treat and support them—if these patients' physical, emotional, and spiritual suffering had been addressed, they would have wanted to live the time they had left in full. In the congressional hearings, she and other advocates navigated around this topic very carefully, if not for their own beliefs then for fear of alienating conservative lawmakers (see Chapter 3). As Ira Byock, the chair of the Academy of Hospice Physicians Ethics Committee put it, "Hospice is a robust alternative to the desperate cries for physician-assisted suicide and euthanasia" (cited in Campbell, Hare, and Matthews 1995). The effort to distinguish hospice from euthanasia and assisted suicide has reverberated through the debates over the "double effect" of opioids. Hospices make regular and wide use of opioids for pain treatment; in some cases these drugs may lead to a patient's death. Ethicists and hospice practitioners have debated whether it is possible to distinguish between the "intended" and "unintended" consequences of opioids. This reflected how important it was for them to differentiate hospice from euthanasia (see, for example, Quill, Dresser, and Brock 1997; Quill, Lo, and Brock 1997; Sulmasy and Pellegrino 1999).

34. Buck (2009).

35. See Bourdieu (1998).

36. On the professional and economic devaluation of feminized care work, see England (2005).

37. See Wald and Leonard (1964), and Wald (1966).

38. This group included Morris Wessel and Raymond Duff (pediatricians), Edward Dobihal (chaplain), Jeanne Quint (a nurse researcher), Claire O'Neil (director of nursing at Yale New Haven Hospital), and Donna Diers (nursing faculty). Max Pepper (physician), Olivia Vlahos (anthropologist), and Kathy Klaus (nurse) joined a few months later.

39. Buck (2005), 119.

40. Buck (2005), 124. This tension is typical to situations where health activists and scientists collaborate; see Epstein (1995), 422.

41. Buck (2005), 138.

42. Buck (2005), 155.

43. Buck (2005), 161.

44. Wald and Dobihal appeared at the Foundation of Thanatology conference, the New York City Presbytery Symposiums, and the Conference on Death and Dying organized in New Jersey (Buck 2005, 166). When the *American Journal of Nursing* printed a programmatic article on hospice care in 1975, Wald and Craven (a nurse at Hospice, Inc.) were its authors.

45. Buck (2005), 167.

46. Buck (2009), 134.

47. Buck (2007), 569.

48. Buck (2009). The centrality of Hospice, Inc., was evident even before then: the first national-level training gathering took place in Connecticut as early as 1975, where fifty-seven groups of aspiring hospice advocates from seventeen states participated (Beresford and Connor 1999).

49. Glaser and Strauss (1965, 1968, 1970); Duff and Hollingshead (1968).

50. Saunders (1999).

51. Kübler-Ross (1969).

52. I borrow the term from Broom (2015).

53. Filene (1998).

54. As Kübler-Ross put it when she testified in Congress, "I would be very leery if the care of the dying patient would become another subspecialty. I would be opposed if we have some modern death houses, which are institutions just for the dying. . . . I would be much more in favor that we train nurses, physicians, and social workers here who love to work with old and dying patients. Then you will not need special institutions for the care of the dying patient, and the majority would be allowed, at least for the final care, to be at home." From "Death with Dignity," I: 17.

55. See Abbott (1988).

56. Buck (2005), 168.

57. "Death with Dignity," I: 23.

58. Baszanger (2012).

59. Holleb (1974), quoted in Baszanger (2012).

60. Krakoff (1979), quoted in Baszanger (2012).

61. Buck (2009).

62. Among these services were "nursing care," "physical or occupational therapy or speech-language pathology," "medical social services," "services of a home health aide who has successfully completed a training program," "medical supplies," "physicians services," "short-term inpatient care," and "counseling . . . with respect to care of the terminally ill individual and adjustment to his death." P.L. 97-248-Sept. 3, 1982: 96 Stat. 359–363.

63. See P.L. 97-248-Sept. 3, 1982: 96 Stat. 359–363. The legislation also included a third period of thirty days that "allowed for errors in prognosis or remissions." Later on, a fourth period of unlimited length was added, making it possible to recertify patients

as hospice eligible even when they stayed for longer than six months in hospice, if their prognosis remained six months or less (Hoyer 1998, 63).

64. See Bourdieu (1990), 122–141.

65. OSI is known today as the Open Society Foundation; I am using the organization's name during the discussed period. The most central among the other funders were the Nathan Cummings Foundation, the Emily Davie and Joseph S. Kornfeld Foundation, the United Hospital Fund, the Fetzer Foundation, the Milbank Memorial Fund, the Commonwealth Fund, and the Fan Fox and Leslie R. Samuels Foundation. See Open Society Institute (2004).

66. Patrizi, Thompson, and Spector (2011).

67. Lynn (1997), 163.

68. RWJF first funded SUPPORT in 1986 and continued through 1994 (Patrizi, Thompson, and Spector 2011, 6). Fifty-five hospitals applied to participate (Schroeder 1999).

69. SUPPORT Principal Investigators (1995), 1594.

70. As one of SUPPORT's principal investigators reflected, "At that time, the expert consensus was that uncertainty over determining patients' prognoses and inadequate understanding of patients' wishes were the key barriers to improving end-of-life care" (Schroeder 1999).

71. SUPPORT Principal Investigators (1995), 1595–1596.

72. In the study, 68 to 69 percent of families and patients said the care they received was "excellent" or "very good" (SUPPORT Principal Investigators 1995).

73. SUPPORT Principal Investigators (1995), 1591.

74. Teno et al. (1994).

75. Phillips et al. (1996).

76. SUPPORT Principal Investigators (1995), 1596.

77. I quote this sentence from the article's abstract. Interestingly, the authors phrased the statement more softly in the article's concluding remarks: "Success will require reexamination of our individual and collective commitment to these goals, more creative effort at shaping the treatment process, and, perhaps, more proactive and forceful attempts at change."

78. As Koren et al. (1989) have shown, negative research results are less likely to be published than positive ones. The fact that these results were published and widely advertised reflects that SUPPORT was unusual. With so many resources invested in data collection and advertising—and many people aware of the project and awaiting its outcomes—the stakes were too high to avoid publication.

79. Patrizi, Thompson, and Spector (2011), 6.

80. Schroeder (1999).

81. Soros (1998).

82. Clark (2013), 13.

83. Open Society Institute (2004), 18.

84. Patrizi, Thompson, and Spector (2011), 11–12.

85. Aulino and Foley (2001).

86. Open Society Institute (2004), 35.

87. Open Society Institute (2004), 55.
88. PDIA fellow Diane Meier similarly argued, "There's no hope of changing care at the bedside without trained medical faculty in the medical schools—not just scientific content, but also the attitudes, the way of being. If doctors don't learn it from experts in palliative medicine, they won't learn it" (Open Society Institute 2004, 19).
89. Open Society Institute (2004), 44.
90. Open Society Institute (2004), 44.
91. Institute of Medicine (1997).
92. Clark (2013), 167–168.
93. These reports from the Institute of Medicine were *Improving Palliative Care for Cancer* (2001), *Describing Death in America: What We Need to Know* (2003), and *When Children Die: Improving Palliative Care and End-of-Life Care for Children and Their Families* (2003).
94. I counted Gerri Frager, who held both registered nurse and doctor of medicine degrees, as a physician.
95. Clark (2013), 14. In addition, only 6 percent of the fellows were African American and 3 percent were Asian, although this hardly signified a change from the hospice movement's early days.
96. Clark (2013), 191–193.
97. Open Society Institute (2004), 36–38.
98. Laporte, Sherman, and Matzo (2001), and Ferrell and Coyle (2001). Another notable figure was Betty Ferrell, who had received a PDIA grant to advance palliative care in nursing homes. This was the HOPE program; see Clark (2013), 94–95.
99. See Clark (2013), 193–194.
100. Altilio and Otis-Green (2011). Also see Clark (2013), 239.
101. Clark (2013), 192.
102. Clark (2013), 17. Burt, a Yale legal and ethics scholar, was one of PDIA's board members.
103. Open Society Institute (2004), 27.
104. Connor (2007–2008).
105. Morrison and Meier (2015). The number has been in constant increase: a 2008 study found that 52.8 percent of the hospitals it surveyed had palliative care services, 72.2 percent of hospitals with over 249 beds had palliative care services, and 84 percent of the medical schools were associated with at least one hospital that had a palliative care service (Goldsmith et al. 2008).
106. Morrison and Meier (2015). Grades were awarded according to the percentage of hospitals with over fifty beds that reported a palliative care service in each: A = over 80 percent of the hospitals reported a palliative care service; B = 61 to 80 percent; C = 41 to 60 percent; D = 21 to 40 percent; F = 20 percent or less.
107. CAPC gave a D grade to Alabama, Alaska, Arkansas, Mississippi, Oklahoma, and Wyoming. West Virginia, Tennessee, Kentucky, Georgia, South Carolina, Kansas, and Texas received Cs. There are, however, intervening variables, which may explain this correlation: rural states, which tend to vote conservative, are also more likely to have compromised access to health care in general and end-of-life care in particular.

108. Open Society Institute (2004), 65.

109. See Fligstein and McAdam (2012).

110. Weisfeld et al. (2000); and Patrizi, Thompson, and Spector (2011).

111. Clark (2013), 71.

112. Golodetz (1997). I thank Cindy Bruzzese, executive director of the Vermont Ethics Network, for providing me a copy of the report.

113. Timmermans (2007), 2; and Timmermans (2005).

114. Open Society Institute (2004), 162.

115. Open Society Institute (2004), 212.

116. Open Society Institute (2013), 60. Kashi and Winokur 2003; Talking Eyes Media 2003. For examples of Deidre Scherer's art, see http://dscherer.com/portfolios /traveling-exhibitions/.

117. See Aulino and Foley (2001).

118. Clark (2013), 36–37.

119. Open Society Institute (2004), 60.

120. Clark (2013), 73–74.

121. Clark (2013), 73–74.

122. In Sartre's terms, hospice expanded "the field of possibilities" toward which an individual such as Soros could act (Sartre 1968, 93).

123. Relmand (1980).

124. Timmermans and Berg (2003), 86.

125. Kaufman (2015), 8–9.

126. Open Society Institute (2004), 29.

127. Bourdieu (1990), 68–70.

128. After the American Board of Medical Specialties recognized Hospice and Palliative Care as a medical subspecialty, physicians who wanted to specialize in the field were required to spend a year as "fellows," which they split between various institutions and teams, and then pass a board examination. Their medical training therefore typically consists of four years in medical school, a year of internship, two years of residency, and a year of fellowship that they spend practicing hospice and palliative care.

129. Adam Reich (2014, 103) has reported the use of this expression by nonpalliative care clinicians as well.

130. See Chambliss (1996).

131. Alex Smith, a palliative care physician and coeditor of the palliative care blog *GeriPal*, reacted to *JAMA*'s 2016 special issue on "death, dying, and end of life:" "We've put in hard work in palliative care to change the frame from 'death, dying and end of life' to 'living well with serious illness.' Wouldn't it be nice to see a theme issue about promoting quality of life for people with serious illness and their caregivers?" From Alex Smith, "Reaction to *JAMA* Theme Issue on Death, Dying, and End of Life," *Geripal,* January 21, 2016, www.geripal.org/2016/01/reaction-to-jama-theme-issue-on-death .html. The Center to Advance Palliative Care has done research on how to best present or "brand" the palliative care subspecialty to people without embracing the label of the death harbingers. See Alex Smith, "What's in a Name? How Do You Explain 'Palliative Care'?" *Geripal,* July 26, 2011, www.geripal.org/2011/07/whats-in

-name-how-do-you-explain.html; and Alex Smith, "How Do You Explain Hospice?" *Geripal,* July 6, 2012, www.geripal.org/2012/07/how-do-you-explain-hospice.html.

132. See Anspach (1988).

133. Featherstone, Hepworth, and Turner (1991).

134. Eva's Jewish identity and my own Hebrew name probably led her to make this reference.

135. Jerolmack and Khan (2014).

136. In 2010–2011, the Center to Advance Palliative Care launched a project entitled Improving Palliative Care (IPAL), which aims to integrate palliative care in a variety of professional settings. As of 2016, the project focused on three such settings: intensive care, emergency medicine, and outpatient care. The project's site is located at www .capc.org/ipal/.

137. In the hospitals that I studied residents usually addressed the attending physicians by their first name. This resident's reference to "Dr. Martin" was particularly interesting because she was a senior resident—and far closer to Scott in status. Also note that I referred to him as "Scott" throughout the interview. It probably reflects the respect and acknowledgment of a still existing status difference.

138. Lizzy Miles, "Pallimed Roundup: Advice to Graduating Fellows in Hospice and Palliative Medicine," *Pallimed,* June 20, 2016, www.pallimed.org/2016/06/pallimed -roundup-advice-to-graduating.html.

139. Institute of Medicine (2014), S-1, S-8.

2. Financial Economization

Epigraph: Callahan (2011b).

1. As I showed in Chapter 1, "the end of life" substituted "death and dying" as hospice and palliative care's main object of management around the early 1990s. For the sake of simplicity, when writing about the movement's entire history, I refer to "the end of life" as its main turf.

2. See Çalişkan and Callon (2009, 2010).

3. Or in Bruno Latour's terminology, "matter of concern" (2004).

4. For discussions of monetizing love and intimacy: Zelizer (2005); children: Zelizer (1985); the environment: Fourcade (2009); and human body parts: Healy (2006), Anteby (2010).

5. I therefore use the verb "financialized," the noun "financialization," and the adjective "financial" very differently from other economic sociologists. For other uses see Krippner (2005) and Van der Zuan (2014).

6. See Livne (2014). This argument is in line with Zelizer and the morals and markets literature, which documented how rather than blocking monetization categorically, moral views structure and inform how monetization take place (e.g., Fourcade, 2011).

7. Kübler-Ross (1969).

8. Kübler-Ross (1969), 30.

9. Kübler-Ross did, however, express such a stance implicitly in a later congressional hearing. See U.S. Senate, "Death with Dignity: An Inquiry into Related Public

Issues," Hearing before the Special Committee on Aging, 92nd Congress, 2nd session, August 7, 1972, Part I, p. 6, https://www.aging.senate.gov/imo/media/doc/publications/871972.pdf. For later, contemporary counterexamples, see Mahar (2006); Welch, Schwartz, and Woloshin (2011).

10. "Death with Dignity," I.

11. "Death with Dignity," I: 3.

12. "Death with Dignity," I: 16–17.

13. Kübler-Ross (1977), quoted in Cohen (1979), 85. The Brompton Cocktail (or "Mixture") contained morphine hydrochloride, cocaine, gin or brandy, aqua chloroformi, and syrup of chlorpromazine (Saunders 1960a, quoted in Clark 1999).

14. I base these statements on reviews of the following lists: A. Kutscher (1969, 1974); M. Kutscher (1975); Poteet (1976); Sell (1977); Miller and Acri (1977); Fulton (1977, 1981); Simpson (1979, 1987); and Fennell (1983). These lists included 24,421 titles in total (some appeared in more than one list). I thank Eunice Yau for her diligent and thorough research assistance. Public discussion of the high cost of funerals exploded following Jessica Mitford's riveting bestselling account on the topic (1963).

15. Feifel (1959, 1977).

16. Kalish (1977).

17. Wald (1988), cited in Buck (2011), 209.

18. See, for example, Vernon (1970). Beyond their moral antipathy toward money matters, remember that these activists lacked financial expertise. Just like Kübler-Ross, they were idealists, not economists. When they did opine on finance they did so as concerned medical professionals who were financial dilettantes, not as reformers who wanted to revolutionize U.S. health care finance.

19. For example, McNulty and Holderby (1983), 166: "community-based, all volunteer programs that do not have to fit into an organizational structure provide, perhaps, the purest form of hospice care."

20. Knowles (1984), 12.

21. Comptroller General (1979), 21.

22. This hospice's salaried staff included only two part-time nurses and one part-time secretary, and it reported $190,000 of professional services donated to it. It is likely that forty other hospices, which were mentioned by the Comptroller General but did not send it financial data, relied on donations and volunteer work as well (Kavanagh 1983).

23. Davidson (1978), 54–55.

24. Cohen (1979); Osterweis and Szmuszkovicz Champagne (1978); Wentzel (1981, 107); Davidson (1978, 51); U.S. House of Representatives, Statement of Dennis Rezendes, Executive Secretary, National Hospice Organization to the Subcommittee on Health, Committee on Ways and Means, June 18–27, 1979, p. 407.

25. Stoddard (1978), 188.

26. Buck (2011).

27. Buck (2007), emphasis mine.

28. Buck (2007).

29. Buck (2007).
30. Beresford (2007). See also U.S. Senate, A Report of the Special Committee on Aging: Developments in Aging: 1978, 1978, Part I, p. 52. https://www.aging.senate.gov/imo /media/doc/reports/rpt179.pdf.
31. Beresford (2007).
32. Beresford (2007).
33. Beresford (2007).
34. Beresford (2007). An early indication of this chasm was Florence Wald's forced retirement from Hospice, Inc., in 1975. See Buck (2005).
35. For example, see Bradshaw (1996).
36. Siebold (1992) pointed out that "by 1988 only 531 out of a possible 1,500 [hospice] programs were approved" by Medicare (143). This indicates that the introduction of the Medicare benefit weeded out a significant number of hospices that did not conform to its standards. Some of these hospices wanted to treat terminal patients whose life expectancy was longer than six months, or patients who needed traditionally curative measures (e.g., radiation, surgeries) for pain control, or patients who required inpatient care. Given Medicare's limited rates and rigid standards, it was extremely hard to let each patient's unique and individual needs drive decision making.
37. Steinhauser, Maddox et al. (2000).
38. This was Charles Garfield from Berkeley, California. See Joan Libman, "Death's Door: Hospice Movement Stresses Family Care for the Terminally Ill," *Wall Street Journal*, March 27, 1978, cited in Paradis and Cummings (1986).
39. A volunteer hospice nurse who participated in the meetings noted that smaller hospices "objected to structure and accountability of any kind." A founder of a Michigan hospice said that meetings of hospice advocates who strategized on how to lobby Congress "were tense and high energy, with fervent debate bordering on anger because people were so passionate. We'd stay 10 hours and then a group of us would march up the hill to the Capitol. Some staffer would come in and say, 'that will never get passed.' So we'd have to go back and start over" (Beresford 2007, 12–13).
40. Buck (2009); Siebold (1992).
41. For example, Garrett (1978); Wentzel (1981), 12; Rosman (1977), 205–208. Also, see Representative Robert N. Giaimo's testimony in Hearings before a Subcommittee of the Committee on Appropriations, U.S. House of Representatives, 95th Congress, 1st session, April 6, 1977, p. 595, https://tinyurl.com/ya23b7h9; and Hoffman (2012). As many hospice protagonists noticed, "the success of hospice proponents in negotiating funding for . . . reimbursement is affected by their ability to demonstrate hospice care systems' cost-saving potential" (Osterweis and Szmuszkoviz Champagne, 1978).
42. Notice, however, that many costs were externalized to families. Hospices during the period operated in many forms—as inpatient and outpatient services, and as independent and hospital-affiliated organizations—but in general, they leaned toward making home hospice their principal model of care, as part of the effort to demedicalize and deinstitutionalize death and shift the primary site of death from hospitals to patients' homes. The financial and personal costs of making people care for their dying relatives

usually disappeared in rhetoric that glorified care at home (see Levitsky, 2014). Some hospice advocates did recognize that many patients needed inpatient care, which the Medicare benefit insufficiently covered (Siebold 1992). Later on, an Institute of Medicine (1997) report acknowledged that the "growing unpaid workforce [of family caregivers] generally is invisible; undertrained; and stressed physically, emotionally, and financially" (158).

43. Comptroller General (1979), 29.
44. Hospice Project Task Force (1980). At the same time, the report recommended an update to the home health agency authorization guidelines to make them more suitable for the number of home visits by registered nurses that were required for terminal cancer patients, and to encourage hospices "to obtain authorization for appropriate services and bill the MediCal program." It also recommended establishing standards for hospice certification.
45. Rezendes, for example, cited a small demonstration project that the NHO conducted with Blue / Cross Blue Shield and the American Hospital Association in Rochester, New York, which showed that care under a home care hospice program "resulted in $152,236 in savings." Statement of Dennis Rezendes, Subcommittee on Health, Committee on Ways and Means, House of Representatives, April 18, 27, 1979, p. 409. Also see Amado, Cronk, and Mileo (1979).
46. As two chief investigators in the National Hospice Study observed, "the legislation was formulated on the basis of limited information. While there were case study reports and anecdotally based vignettes describing hospices . . . no systematic data were available" (Mor and Barnbaum 1983, 81).
47. Quoted in "Washington Briefs," *American Journal of Hospice Care,* November / December 1985, 9.
48. Beresford (2007), 13.
49. Beresford (2007), 14.
50. U.S. House of Representatives, "Medicare in Florida: Looking to the Future," Hearing before the Select Committee on Aging, 98th Congress, 1st Session, December 28, 1983, p. 77.
51. Mor and Barnbaum (1983).
52. Siebold (1992), 145.
53. A 1978 report of the Institute on Health and Healthcare Delivery expressed concern that "given the carrot of possible reimbursement . . . the potential for misuse of the hospice philosophy and concept is obviously high" (32).
54. National Hospice and Palliative Care Organization (2017).
55. Whoriskey and Keating (2014).
56. Wentzel (1981), 105.
57. The shareholder value of Vitas, the largest for-profit hospice in the country, rose over 400 percent in 2013–2018.
58. National Hospice and Palliative Care Organization (2017).
59. Among the founders of this hospice was Donald ("Don") Gaetz, who later became a Republican lawmaker. Gaetz accused the NHO members who criticized the for-profit model of running a "smear campaign" (Paradis and Cummings 1986, 380). There is

evidence that compared with not-for-profit hospices, for-profit hospices offer fewer services (Carlson, Gallo, and Bradley, 2004) and employ professional staff with less training (Cherlin et al., 2010). For-profits are also less likely to provide benefits for their communities in the form of charity care or training programs, and they tend to treat more profitable patients (specifically patients who need longer hospice stays and patients who live in nursing homes). Finally, for-profits have higher levels of patient disenrollment, which may indicate that they are admitting borderline cases that are less costly to treat (Aldridge et al. 2014).

60. Whether hospice is indeed cheaper than conventional care is still unclear, and depends on the type of hospice care provided, hospice patients' length of stay, and how costs are defined. See, for example, Mor and Kidder (1985); Emanuel and Emanuel (1994).

61. As Fligstein would put it, with relatively clear state regulations and a significant number of corporate actors participating in it, the hospice market stabilized and institutionalized (1996, 2001).

62. In 1964 and 1965, the two last years before Medicare's implementation, 58 percent of the people who died at 65 or older had no hospital insurance, and 69.8 percent of them had no surgical insurance. See Timmer (1969).

63. Barnato (2007).

64. Zussman (1992).

65. Riley and Lubitz (2010).

66. Piro and Lutins (1973), 37.

67. Civetta (1973), 267.

68. Civetta (1973), 267–268.

69. Civetta (1973), 268–269. This was also the logic behind the Therapeutic Intervention Scoring System (TISS)—a method that Civetta and his colleagues designed to evaluate the severity of illness and ensure that ICU beds were used to treat only those who need them (Cullen et al. 1974).

70. Cullen et al. (1976), 982.

71. Cullen et al. (1976), 986.

72. Cullen et al. (1976), 986–987.

73. Turnbull et al. (1979), 20.

74. Turnbull et al. (1979), 20.

75. See, for example, Thibault et al. (1980).

76. Christakis (1999).

77. "It is easy enough . . . to designate a patient as terminal or as dying *retrospectively*," wrote health economist Anne Scitovsky, "but an entirely different matter to do so *prospectively*" (1984), 594, emphasis in original.

78. Scitovsky (1984), 605.

79. Scitovsky (1984), 602, 603.

80. Scitovsky (1994).

81. Scitovsky (1984).

82. Institute of Medicine (1997), 159, 184.

83. Shugarman, Decker, and Bercovitz (2009).

84. Barnato (2007), 85.

85. For example, Lubitz and Prihoda (1984); Lubitz and Riley. (1993); Hogan, Lunney, and Lynn (2001); Hoover et al. (2002).
86. Long et al. (1984).
87. McCall (1984).
88. Callahan (1987), 15–18.
89. Callahan (1987), 171, emphasis in original.
90. See Callahan (1998).
91. Lamm's 1984 statement was quoted in Scitovsky (1994).
92. Scitovsky (1988).
93. Aldridge and Kelley (2015).
94. Riley et al. (1987).
95. Scitovsky (1988), 656.
96. Bayer et al. (1983).
97. Bayer et al. (1983).
98. Rodwin (2011), 112.
99. This increase in the uninsured was despite the fact that 84 percent of them were employed or were dependents of people who were employed (Hoffman 2012, 130). The percentage of employees of medium and large businesses who received health care coverage from their employer declined from 96 percent in 1983 to 82 percent in 1993 (Hoffman 2012, 182).
100. Hoffman (2012), chapter 8.
101. Rodwin (2011), 124.
102. Hoffman (2012).
103. Mayes (2007).
104. Hoffman (2012), 175.
105. Hoffman (2012), 175.
106. "CMS to Cut Reimbursement Rates by up to 2% for about 2K Hospitals," *California Healthline Daily Edition*, August 5, 2013; https://californiahealthline.org/morning -breakout/cms-to-cut-reimbursement-rates-by-up-to-2-for-about-2k-hospitals/.
107. Gawande (2011), 347.
108. Fligstein (1990).
109. For a comprehensive review see Bazzoli et al. (2004).
110. See Scott, Ruef, Mendel et al. (2000).
111. Burns and Pault (2002).
112. According to the U.S. Census Bureau, before the implementation of the Affordable Care Act (ACA) 17 percent of the people in the United States were uninsured, and many of the 53 percent who had private insurance had very limited coverage (DeNavas-Walt, Proctor, and Smith 2010). Although the ACA improved the situation, it did not solve it, and attempts to repeal parts of it would throw millions of people back into a state of no insurance coverage.
113. See Hacker (2002).
114. Rosenthal (2014).
115. Rodwin (2011), 122–123. This continues a pattern that dates back to the 1980s (McKinlay and Marceau, 2002).

116. Rodwin (2011), 129–130.
117. Parikh et al. (2013), 2348.
118. Soros was referring to patients in the last year of their life. Soros (1998) cited in Clark (2013), 159.
119. On top of the basic finding that a "small percentage of those who die each year accounts for a considerable percentage of total health care spending," the report mentioned a variety of other monetized measures. When extending the period analyzed to several years before death, "the contrast between survivors and decedents" declined; compared with cancer diagnoses, chronic diagnoses such as diabetes and renal failure led to longer periods of high decedent-to-survivor spending ratios. Medicare spending on "decedents" dropped as their age increased. And its spending on "survivors" increased as their age increased. Institute of Medicine (1997), 156–159.
120. The report called on the Health Care Financing Administration to examine the possibility of adding a palliative care diagnostic code and commanded Medicare's decision to test such a code, which "would be helpful in evaluating the nature of hospital palliative care and its cost compared with alternatives." Institute of Medicine (1997), 184.
121. Smith et al. (2003).
122. Morrison et al. (2008).
123. Institute of Medicine (1997), 177.
124. Clark (2013), 160.
125. Gade et al. (2008).
126. Ciemins et al. (2007).
127. Pantilat et al. (2007).
128. This was the outcome of a legal battle with consumer groups (Rodwin 2011, 128).
129. "The primary purpose of creating a hospital-based palliative care service is to improve the quality of care delivered to patients with serious, life-threatening, or terminal illnesses. The main goal is not to save money. However, it is usually the case that tailoring care to reflect patient and family preferences has the *secondary effect* of reducing hospital costs." Pantilat et al. (2007), 3 (emphasis mine).
130. Pantilat et al. (2007), 4.
131. Pantilat et al. (2007), 5.
132. "Compensation for acute care services is such that hospitals are generally rewarded for controlling costs, either by reducing expenses within a given stay, or in some cases, by avoiding admissions entirely." Pantilat et al. (2007), 6.
133. Pantilat et al. (2007), 7.
134. Pantilat et al. (2007), 9.
135. Pantilat et al. (2007), 14. The physicians would be interested in cooperating with the palliative care service, since, for example, it would save them time "in managing complex discharge arrangements" for their sickest patients.
136. Pantilat et al. (2007).
137. See, for example, Warner and Gualtieri-Reed (2014).
138. Callon (1998).

139. These explanations rely on Robbins's classic definition of economic situations as cases where actors are forced to make choices under conditions of scarcity (Robbins 1945), 4.

3. What the Dying Want

Epigraph: Katz (1984), viii–ix.

1. Similarly, consider the following question, which Kübler-Ross (1969) asked a seventeen-year-old terminally ill patient who participated in her study: "Do you think that we, as physicians, should speak to people who face fatal illness about their future? Can you tell us what you would teach us if your mission was to teach us what we should do for other people?" (209–210).

2. This was a fundamentally different role from the one organized medicine assigned to patients in the nineteenth and early twentieth centuries. The only clause of the American Medical Association's ethical code, which encouraged physicians to take their patients' wishes into account, dismissed those wishes as irrational: "Reasonable indulgence should be granted to the mental imbecility and caprices of the sick" (American Medical Association 1847). The 1903 code only referred to "the caprices of the sick."

3. Fox and Swazey (2008). Daniel Callahan, cofounder of the Hastings Center (the first bioethics center in the United States) wrote that end-of-life care was on the top of the center's list of issues deserving attention (Callahan 2011b).

4. Fox and Swazey (2008), 153.

5. Messikomer, Fox, and Swazey (2001), 491; Fox and Swazey (2008), 154–155; Katz (1984); Orentlicher (1992).

6. Rothman (1991), 6; see also Jonsen (1988).

7. Heimer and Petty (2010).

8. See Evans (2002, 2012), Bosk (2008).

9. Kaufman (2006), 28.

10. Schneider (1998), xii. See also the discussions of Ronald Dworkin (1986, 1993) and Gerald Dworkin (1988).

11. Halpern (2001), 201.

12. This narrative was what anthropologist Sherry Ortner (1973) called an "elaborating symbol": it described a scenario that functions as a vehicle for sorting out complex feelings and ideas, "making them comprehensible to oneself, communicable to others, and translatable into orderly action."

13. U.S. Senate, "Death with Dignity: An Inquiry into Related Public Issues," Hearing before the Special Committee on Aging, 92nd Congress, 2nd session, August 7, 1972, Part III, 100, www.aging.senate.gov/imo/media/doc/publications/891972.pdf.

14. Drawing a conclusion about the witnesses' race was difficult. The hearings' texts did not include mentions of race, and in the United States whiteness is usually the assumed racial category. However, because there were witnesses who came from diverse cities and towns, such as Baltimore in Maryland, and in the absence of video recordings of the hearings, I had difficulty making an argument about racial exclusion.

Using a genealogy website (Ancestry.com) and decennial census records, I verified that many of the witnesses quoted here were indeed white. None of the witnesses was verified as non-white. I have indicated in the notes whenever I failed to find records for witnesses; unless stated otherwise, the witnesses were verified as white.

15. The Hasting Center Report also printed Alfred Morgan's letter to the editor, which could very well be what led to his invitation to the hearing. See Morgan (1971).

16. Morgan (1971).

17. U.S. Senate, "Death with Dignity," I: 7, 9, www.aging.senate.gov/imo/media/doc /publications/871972.pdf.

18. U.S. Senate, "Death with Dignity," III: 109–100. (I could not verify Mrs. and Mr. Heine's racial identities.)

19. Figures are from the U.S. decennial census of 1970. All in all, Silver Spring had only forty-nine African American residents who were older than seventy. U.S. Bureau of the Census, *Census of Population: 1970*, Vol. 1, *Characteristics of the Population*, Part 22: *Maryland* (Washington, D.C.: U.S. Government Printing Office, 1973), www2 .census.gov/prod2/decennial/documents/1970a_md-01.pdf.

20. U.S. Senate, "Death with Dignity," III: 104–105.

21. This number was quoted in the *Washington Star* article. U.S. Congress, "Death with Dignity," III: appendix C.

22. U.S. Senate, "Death with Dignity," III: appendix A.

23. U.S. House of Representatives, "Home Care for the Elderly: The Need for a National Policy," Hearing before the Select Committee on Aging, 95th Congress, 2nd session, February 22, 1978, 12–13, 19.

24. U.S. Senate, "Death with Dignity," I: 10, emphasis mine.

25. U.S. House of Representatives, "Administration's Proposed Payment System for Hospice Care," Hearing before the Select Committee on Aging, 98th Congress, 2nd session, May 25, 1983, 31, emphasis in original. (I could not verify Rosenfield's racial identity, although I did find a 1940 census record that classified her mother as white.)

26. U.S. House of Representatives, "Administration's Proposed Payment System," 44.

27. See Latour (1987).

28. Compare to Fourcade and Livne (2013).

29. Kübler-Ross (1969), 11.

30. U.S. Senate, "Death with Dignity," I: 2–3. The quoted passage is from Kübler-Ross (1969), 22–23.

31. Kübler-Ross (1969), 35.

32. Kübler-Ross (1969), 249, 251.

33. Kübler-Ross (1969), 250.

34. Kübler-Ross (1969), 251.

35. Kübler-Ross (1969), 247.

36. Kübler-Ross (1969), 252, 254.

37. Kübler-Ross (1969), 256.

38. Kübler-Ross (1969), 259.

39. Kübler-Ross (1969), chapter 3.

40. The researchers did not provide any information about the patients' ethnic and racial identities, class, gender, or other sociologically relevant variables.

41. Lo, McLeod, and Saika (1986).

42. Shmerling et al. (1988).

43. Institute of Medicine (1997), 45.

44. See "End of Life Care: Inpatient Days per Decedent during the Last Six Months of Life, by Gender and Level of Care Intensity (Level of Care Intensity: Overall; Gender: Overall; Year: 2015)," *Dartmouth Atlas of Health Care* (Lebanon, NH: Dartmouth Institute for Health Policy and Clinical Practice, 2018), www.dartmouthatlas.org /data/topic/topic.aspx?cat=18. See also Carina Storrs. "Hospice: What Is It and When Is It for You?" *CNN*, July 26, 2015. www.cnn.com/2015/06/29/health/hospice -fast-facts/.

45. Cicourel (1964).

46. Patrick et al. (1997).

47. Danis et al. (1996).

48. For example, Hofmann et al. (1997); Teno and Dosa (2006).

49. For example, see the list in Levinsky (1996), 742.

50. Paris, Crone, and Readon (1990).

51. Paris et al. (1999), 383.

52. S. 1766, 101st Congress, 1st session. October 17, 1989.

53. H.R. 4449, 101st Congress (1989–1990).

54. For reasons of confidentiality, I do not disclose further details about the hospital.

55. See Chambliss (1996).

56. Boltanski and Thévenot (1999b), 359–360.

57. As Kleinman (1994) put it, the clinical record is written with an eye for the professional, bureaucratic, and legal needs of the institution.

58. The difference is not statistically significant at 95 percent (p=.069).

59. I thank Lindsay Fedewa for her research assistance.

60. I had heard other clinicians talking about Russian families as particularly resistant to economized dying in previous interviews. Given my own Ashkenazi Jewish background, which my Hebrew accent and last name often betray, I felt I needed to explicitly invite this physician to talk about this group.

61. I thank Fabian Pfeffer for help and advice.

62. Levinsky (1996).

63. Pam Belluck, "Even as Doctors Say Enough, Families Flight to Prolong Life," *New York Times*, March 27, 2005, www.nytimes.com/2005/03/27/us/even-as-doctors-say -enough-families-fight-to-prolong-life.html.

64. Belluck, "Even as Doctors Say." As early as 1996, physician Norman Levinsky wrote that in his experience "it is far more frequent for patients and their families to demand aggressive treatment against the advice of their physicians than for doctors to press to continue therapy that patients or their families want to discontinue" (742). Levinsky doubted that economized patients cases have ever been common; as I show here, however, they occurred regularly in the hospital that I studied.

65. Pew Research Center (2013).

66. Previous research found similar patterns. Compared with white people, African Americans were found to be less likely to discuss treatment preferences before they died, complete a living will, designate a Durable Power of Attorney for health care, embrace care limitation in certain situations, and withhold treatment before death. See Hopp and Duffy (2000). For a comprehensive review, see Institute of Medicine (2014), 3-26-29.

67. Pew Research Center (2013), 55. Questions on personal end-of-life preferences revealed similar, albeit weaker patterns. The survey presented respondents with the scenario of having "a disease with no hope of improvement." In 2013, 35 percent said they would tell their doctor "to do everything possible" to save their lives, even if they suffered a great deal of physical pain, compared with 28 percent in 1990; 46 percent said they would do so even if it was hard for them to function in day-to-day activities (versus 40 percent in 1990). Finally, 37 percent said they would ask to "do everything" even if they were "totally dependent on a family member or other person" for all of their care (versus 31 percent in 1990) (84–85).

68. Van Ryn and Fu (2003).

69. Van Ryn et al. (2006).

70. Spencer and Grace (2016).

71. Van Ryn and Fu (2003).

72. For instance, Sudnow (1967), Timmermans (1999), Glaser and Strauss (1964), and Roth (1972).

73. Sudnow (1967), 105. Another example was the allocation of hemodialysis treatment in the first decades after its invention, as Fox and Swazey (1974) described it: "A person 'worthy' of having his life preserved by a scarce expensive treatment like chronic dialysis was one judged to have qualities such as decency and responsibility. Any history of social deviance, such as a prison record, any suggestion that a person's married life was not intact and scandal-free, were strong counter indications to selection. The preferred candidate was a person who had demonstrated achievement through hard work and success at his job, who went to church, joined groups, and was actively involved in community affairs" (247).

74. Van Ryn and Burke (2000), cited in Spencer and Grace (2016); van Ryn and Fu (2003).

75. See Spencer and Grace (2016).

76. Kaufman (2015), 4, 25.

77. We still categorized the case as one of a conflicted medical team facing an economizing patient, however.

78. Anspach (2010).

79. See Ubel (2000).

80. Prendergast and Luce (1997), 15.

81. Prendergast, Claessens, and Luce (1998), 1163.

82. Levinsky (1996), 741.

83. See, for example, the Institute of Medicine's 2014 proclamation that "availability of palliative care services has not kept pace with the growing demand" (S-3). Patients' demand was what legitimized expanding palliative care.

84. Day (2015).

4. Making the Dying Subject

Epigraph: Montaigne (2003), 96.

1. Later on, it was revealed that McMath was transferred to New Jersey, where the law forbids physicians from determining brain death if they have "reason to believe . . . that such a declaration would violate the personal religious beliefs of the individual." See "The New Jersey Declaration of Death Act," *Kennedy Institute of Ethics Journal* 1, no. 4 (1991): 289–292; https://doi.org/10.1353/ken.0.0096. On the Jahi McMath case, see Rachel Aviv, "What Does It Mean to Die?" *New Yorker*, May 2, 2018; www .newyorker.com/magazine/2018/02/05/what-does-it-mean-to-die.

2. See Friedman (1990). As Bellah and his coauthors put it, people in the United States *choose* the values in which they believe, pursue them, and achieve self-fulfillment based on their success or failure in this pursuit. "American cultural traditions define personality, achievement, and the purpose of human life in ways that leave the individual suspended in glorious, but terrifying, isolation" (Bellah et al. 2008, 6). In Abend's terms, the individual subject is a principal component of *the moral background:* it is an elementary category, which informs how people think and judge themselves and others (Abend 2015).

3. Shim (2010).

4. See Abramson (2015).

5. These two meanings add to a third one, which the first two chapters discussed: *subject* also means *a topic.* This chapter is about medical practitioners who *make "dying" a subject* by applying professional practices that center on dying people.

6. The modern subject, Foucault argued, coemerged with modern techniques of governance. People became subjects at the same historical moment that they were *subjected* to these techniques. This idea was rooted in Althusser's analysis of self-identification as an act in which one *subjects* to external powers. When embracing an identity—that is, defining themselves as individual subjects—people *subject* themselves to their identity. (For example, identifying as a woman, man, or gender nonconforming, American or anti-American, or capitalist or working-class is an act of self-definition *and* subjection to social and political categories.) See Foucault (2007), and Althusser ([1971] 2001).

7. Rose (1998), 22; Lahire (2011).

8. With some exceptions, hospices usually require that their patients relinquish hospital care if their condition declines. By consequence, a patient who wants to be admitted to a hospital almost always needs to sign off of hospice.

9. "Mortality itself," as Timmermans (2007) observed, "cannot be avoided, but individual *causes of death can be determined,* and then manipulated and postponed" (11). See also Zussman (1992), and Kaufman (2006).

10. Still, litigation poses a public relations risk to hospitals and a financial burden to doctors, who may face higher insurance rates if patients file charges against them. The legal risk does not necessarily involve losing a case in court but rather having to deal with a case.

11. Put differently, the issue here is not the sheer violation of law but discomfort with the possible violation of moral principles, such as the sanctity of human life and

the autonomy of individuals. On this distinction, see Durkheim ([1893] 1984), 53–64.

12. Section 3025 of the Affordable Care Act of 2010 required the Center for Medicare & Medicaid Services to reduce payments to hospitals with "excess readmissions."

13. See Heimer and Staffen (1998), and Anspach (1993). As Glazer (1990) observed, women carry most of this burden of care.

14. Taylor (1985), 257.

15. Consider this as parallel to Albert Hirschman's and Amartya Sen's distinction between preferences and meta-preferences. Preferences show in people's actions and choices, yet very few people are reducible to their actions and choices. Those who are would be what Harry Frankfurt called "wantons"—people who "are entirely, unreflectively, in the grip of their whims and passions." The rest are able to "step back . . . and ask themselves whether they really want these wants and prefer these preferences, and, consequently, [are able] to form metapreferences that may differ from their preferences" (Hirschman 1986, 142).

16. Gabriel Abend (2015) argued that one defining property of moral stances is that they beg justification and explanation. Personal tastes or visceral reactions may be completely subjective: one would not be expected to explain why she dislikes tomatoes. But people expect moral positions—veganism, pacifism, or support of social justice—to be grounded in a general position. Personality, then, belongs to a completely subjective and individualistic realm, which does not beg justification.

17. Rose (1998), 22; Lahire (2011).

18. This is in line with the modern development of what Mauss (1985) described as the person as a "psychological being." "The mentality of our ancestors is obsessed with the question of knowing whether the individual soul is substance, or supposed by a substance: whether it is the nature of man, or whether it is only one of the two natures of man; whether it is one and indivisible, or divisible and separable; whether it is free, the absolute source of all action, or whether it is determined, fettered by other destinies, by predestination" (20).

19. See Rose (1998), 22.

20. Althusser ([1971] 2001).

21. Mishler (1984), 70.

22. For the sake of clarity, I am using the archaic distinction between "disease" and "illness" that Kleinman, Eisenberg, and Good (1978) made, following Talcott Parsons. (See also Timmermans and Haas 2008.) *Disease* refers to purely physiobiological phenomena, whereas *illness* is related to "a state of disturbance in the 'normal' functioning of the total human individual" (Parsons 1951, 431).

23. These interactions took place when I served as a volunteer in the hospital's palliative care service. Part of my responsibility was to report on such interactions to the service's staff, which allowed me to examine their reactions.

24. See the discussion in Chapter 3.

25. The Coda Alliance is run by people from "local hospices, hospitals, faith communities, universities, and elder care organizations." See the Go Wish Game website at www.gowish.org.

26. Steinhauser, Christakis et al. (2000).
27. The pronoun "we" is a bit misleading. In all the cases I observed, the Go Wish activity was carried out by nurses, social workers, or lower ranked doctors and medical students.
28. Following Bruno Latour, I define mediators as things that "transform, translate, distort, and modify the meaning or the elements they are supposed to carry." This is different from intermediaries, which "is what transports meaning or force without transformation: defining its input is enough to define its outputs" (Latour 2005, 39). Go Wish cards do not transport patients' preferences as they are, from patients' brains to physicians' ears, but transform them.
29. Some integrated care systems, such as Kaiser Permanente, can keep electronic documentation of such forms on their records. The hospitals that I studied, however, were not integrated care systems, so advance directive forms were carried by the patients, not by the hospital.
30. Fagerlin and Schneider (2004).
31. Silveira, Kim, and Langa (2010).
32. Shapiro (2012). Of note, not all the patients in this ICU were dying, and not all dying patients passed through the ICU.
33. For a comprehensive critique of advance directives (or, more generally, the living will), see Fagerlin and Schneider (2004).
34. Shapiro (2012), 210–211.
35. Generally, surrogate decision makers' instructions had priority over advance directives. Even in cases of patients who had completed very explicit advance directive forms, the family members could overrule it after the patient lost her or his decision-making capacity. When the clinical staff agreed that the family's concerns might have some validity, advance directives were particularly weakened.
36. There is a great deal of research showing that patients' views and treatment preferences change when their medical condition declines, specifically near the end of life (Fried et al. 2006, 2007).
37. Fagerlin and Schneider (2004), 30.
38. Sudore and Fried (2010); Ubel et al. (2005).
39. Sudore and Fried (2010); Reilly, Teasdale, and McCullough (1994).
40. See National Hospice and Palliative Care Organization (2005) for the "California Advance Directive" document.
41. In palliative care narratives, mentions of "large families" function as Chekhov's gun: they appear in the first act and fire in the second, usually when the multiple family members pressure the medical team in multiple different directions.
42. See Smedira et al. (1990); Schneiderman et al. (1992); Teno et al. (1994); Lo et al. (1985); Goodman, Tarnoff, and Slotman (1998); Danis et al. (1991); and SUPPORT Principal Investigators (1995).
43. Silveira, Kim, and Langa (2010).
44. Sudore and Fried (2010).
45. Foucault (2005).
46. Heimer and Staffen (1998).

47. High (1993).
48. Fagerlin and Schneider (2004).
49. The statement that "butting heads" seldom happened was a way to emphasize that full-blown conflicts, where the palliative care physician confronted the family, were the outliers. Usually the palliative care service managed to reach decisions that families endorsed without conflict.
50. See Latour (1999), chapter 2.
51. Kaufman (2006).
52. The two cases of Mr. Becker and Mr. Emery show how regularly women clinicians encounter sexual insinuation when treating male patients.
53. Kaufman (2006), 17–18, emphasis mine.
54. Bourdieu (1984), 413.
55. Bourdieu (1984), 414.
56. Rose (1998), 2.
57. Bourdieu (1984), 401–411.

5. Goat Taming

1. Anspach 1993, chapters 4–5.
2. Consider, for example, the cases I presented in Chapter 4, where clinicians did not economize without the patients' consent, even when they thought it was medically appropriate and the patients could not resist.
3. Recall the palliative care physician's story from Chapter 1, about the terminal liver disease patient's family who had to decide between an economized or a curative course of treatment. "What do you think the family wanted? They wanted the optimistic doctor."
4. Kaufman (2006), 47–50; Margolin (1997); Anspach (1993).
5. Margolin (1997); Anspach (1993).
6. Feudtner and Morrison (2012), 694.
7. Feudtner and Morrison (2012), 694.
8. Notice how, in line with what I described in Chapter 3, the authors here assume that families and patients are leaning toward economized dying more than clinicians. This assumption is particularly interesting because the article reflects the authors' strong support of economization.
9. Feudtner and Morrison (2012), 695. One palliative care physician radicalized this conclusion even further: "I prefer a 'ban' to a 'moratorium,' as a moratorium is temporary, and I don't see any reason for a second life for this particular phrase." From Alex Smith, "Ban the Phrase 'Do Everything': It's Dangerous Nonsense," *Geripal*, September 7, 2012; www.geripal.org/2012/09/ban-phrase-do-everything-its-dangerous.html.
10. See, for example, the interaction of Mr. Becker and the palliative care team, which I described in Chapter 4: "Dr. Ashley asked him if he was in pain (he said he was not) and 'What are you hoping for?' (he said he was hoping to get better)."
11. This attending physician was young and new to the hospital, so Scott felt comfortable instructing him in this way.

12. Ironically, Scott's direct style of asking questions was itself a way to influence Kara's reflections. He employed a similar conversational tool as the ones he and his colleagues use when talking to patients and families. I thank Renée Anspach for this observation.

13. Anspach (1993).

14. For a review, see Goodwin and Heritage (1990).

15. Barnato and Arnold (2013).

16. Rhetoric aside, the two physicians had different commitments and affiliations. Scott was employed by the hospital, and the concierge physician was paid by the patient. Their professional opinions notwithstanding, at the end of the day Scott had to explain his decisions to the hospital administration (and his hospital colleagues), whereas the concierge reported to the patient's son, who was paying his salary. It is not that surprising that the concierge was more reluctant to challenge the son.

17. Scott was also happy to show me that the patient could have been discharged to hospice from his previous admission to Private Hospital:

> Scott says that we can look back in the chart, and he bets the patient was hospice eligible five months ago. A few clicks and he reaches the screen he was looking for. 'See?' he shows me [the patient's] low abdomen number and high INR—'I could have totally admitted him to hospice when he was admitted last time. But his doctor didn't consult me then, so we couldn't have a plan in place.'
>
> I ask him if the fact that the patient had a concierge physician influenced anything. Scott says that these physicians try to do everything that would satisfy their patients, which oftentimes means that they wouldn't call him 'until shit hits the fan.' . . . He says that the patient being in the hospital might be really bad for him anyway. 'Yes, he's on antibiotics, and maybe it helped his infections somehow. But what do I know? Maybe by bringing him to the hospital and putting him on IV antibiotics I've just caused him *C. diff.* [a *Clostridium difficile* infection], and then he's going to spend the last days of his life with horrible diarrhea?'

18. See Goffman (1959).

19. Virtually all the palliative care practitioners I interviewed told me that patients were more likely to embrace economized dying than their families.

20. Darr (2016); Darr and Pinch (2013).

21. This story is adapted from Loren Eiseley's 1969 essay, "The Star Thrower" (www.eiseley.org/Star_Thrower_Cook.pdf). I am quoting a popular version of the story, as found in John M. Dunn, "The Times Are a Changing," *Quest* 61 (3), https://doi.org/10.1080/00336297.2009.10483615:

> A young man was walking down the beach after a major storm had just come through the area. He was dismayed by the huge number of starfish that the storm had washed up on the beach. He knew the starfish were doomed, but thought that there was nothing he could do because of the immense numbers. As he continued down the beach he saw an

old man throw something into the water. As he got closer, he saw the old man walk a little farther down the beach, bend over, pick up a starfish and throw it back into the water. As the younger man approached, the old man stopped again, bent over, picked up another starfish and was about to throw it into the water. The young man stopped and asked, "Why are you doing that? There are thousands of starfish on the beach. You can't possibly make a difference." The old man looked at the starfish in his hand and threw it to safety in the waves. "It makes a difference to this one," he said.

Conclusion

Epigraph: Weber (1946b), 143–145.

1. I have adapted the concept of "historically specific regime of valuation" from Michelle Murphy (2017), 5–6.
2. For example, see Brown (2017).
3. For an early example, see Durkheim ([1893] 1984).
4. Fourcade and Healy (2007). Consider, for example, business ethicists who contend that for the economy to be stable it needs "moral engineers" (i.e., ethicists) to formulate an ethic that would make businesses behave morally and guarantee economic stability (Abend, 2015).
5. Zelizer (1979).
6. Garcia-Parpet (2007).
7. MacKenzie (2006); MacKenzie and Millo (2003). For examples from other market economies see Almeling (2007, 2011); Anteby (2013); Healy (2006); Bandelj et al. (2017); and Zelizer (1994, 2005, 2011).
8. Gayon and Lemoine (2014).
9. Polanyi ([1944] 2001).
10. Thompson (1966, 1971).
11. Folbre (1991); Zelizer (2004, 2005).
12. Polanyi ([1957] 1992), 30.
13. Çalişkan and Callon (2009).
14. Desrosières (2003).
15. See Callon (1998); MacKenzie, Muniesa, and Siu (2007); and Çalişkan and Callon (2009, 2010).
16. See Foucault (2008).
17. This was the general definition that Neil Smelser and Richard Swedberg proposed in the first edition of the *Handbook of Economic Sociology* (1994, 3).
18. For example, see Granovetter (2017).
19. See Krippner's criticism (2002; Krippner et al. 2004) of Granovetter (1985).
20. Çalişkan and Callon (2009); Brown (2017).
21. Feudtner and Morrison (2012), 694.
22. For example, see Robbins (1945); Callon (1998); and Callon and Muniesa (2005).
23. For example, see Coale (1974).
24. See Marx (1964); Kojève (1969).

25. See Olshansky and Ault (1986).

26. Block and Somers (2014), chapter 3.

27. Murphy (2017). Most recently, economist Thomas Piketty argued that economic and demographic growth rates are likely to fall after reaching a twentieth-century peak. See Piketty (2014), chapter 2.

28. See Livne (2014), for example.

29. Block and Somers (2014), chapter 3.

30. See Murphy (2017).

31. Mitchell (2005a).

32. See Murphy (2017).

33. Ashmore, Mulkay, and Pinch (1989).

34. See, for example, Numbers (1978); Hacker (2002).

35. Rose (1990), 244.

36. Teno et al. (2013). Two issues complicate these findings, however. First, this research focused on Medicare fee-for-service patients. It is very likely that the hospitalization rates of managed care patients did not grow as much because, unlike in the fee-for-service system, the financial incentive of their provider is in reducing utilization. Second, the researchers found different patterns for different diagnoses. The ninety-day hospitalization rate for chronic obstructive pulmonary disease (COPD) patients rose very moderately, from 81.6 to 82.8 percent; in patients with dementia, the rate dropped from 69.9 to 65.5 percent; and in cancer patients it rose from 75 percent to 80.3 percent.

37. Observing this pattern, Helen Stanton Chapple (2010) went so far as to characterize hospice and palliative care as mere "relief valves" to the life-prolonging economy (17). Our views diverge. I see hospice and palliative care as a powerful cultural, financial, and organizational movement that has affected U.S. health care and moral views on end-of-life care. Indeed, the very criticism Chapple and her interviewees make are testimonies to this effect.

38. Teno et al. (2013).

39. Weber ([1919] 1946b).

40. Douglas (1986), 128.

41. Durkheim ([1912] 1995), 209, 211.

42. For example, see Brown (2017); Mitchell (2002); Murphy (2017).

43. Kafka (2008), 83.

Appendix

1. See Livne (2014).

2. Interestingly, Cicely Saunders made a very similar point about fifty years earlier when reflecting on her pioneering work at London's Saint Christopher's Hospice (Saunders 1969).

3. Glaser and Strauss (1965); Sudnow (1967).

4. Zussman (1992); Anspach (1993); and Timmermans (1999), respectively.

5. Kaufman (2006). Kaufman conducted her ethnography in the late 1990s; she mentioned that at the end of her fieldwork one of the hospitals she studied recruited a

palliative care specialist. Historically speaking, this book begins where Kaufman's ended.

6. See Karsoho et al. (2017).

7. See note 114 in the Introduction.

8. A similar methodological approach was adopted in Reich (2014). Reich, however, found stark differences among the three hospitals that he studied whereas I emphasize professional consistency, which survives the socioeconomic and organizational differences that do exist.

9. See Dohan (2002).

10. The exception of trauma patients, who came through the emergency department, should be noted. Many of them were insured, and their insurance companies moved them to other hospitals as soon as their condition stabilized.

11. In fact, in cases where Public Hospital did not have the technologies necessary for treatment, it referred its patients to Academic Hospital.

12. In the state of California, as in several other states, it is illegal for nonacademic hospitals to employ their physicians directly. The formal logic behind this regulation is that it decouples the physicians' medical decisions from the hospitals' financial interests. Yet obviously, because this regulation sends physicians to work independently or in networks, it ultimately mingles medical work with a different set of incentives (Rodwin 2011).

13. See Klinenberg (2012).

14. Goffman (1959).

15. On the use of in-depth interviews in multi-sited ethnographies, see Ho (2009).

16. See Bosk (1979).

17. Lévi-Strauss (1963), 3.

18. Similar strategies have become common in ethnography today. See, for example, Reich (2014); Lara-Millán (2014); Murphy (unpublished ms.).

19. The two leading journals were the *Journal of the American Medical Association* (*JAMA*) and the *New England Journal of Medicine*.

20. I was also interested in gender, but palliative care clinicians did not talk about it much. Many palliative care clinicians were interested in how "culture" affects interaction—using the concept in a manner far too general and essentialistic for me to embrace.

21. Geertz (1973).

22. See Bourdieu (1993) and more specifically, Straus (1957).

23. This is how historian David Clark (2013) defined his position in a book he wrote on palliative care in the United States. The book was commissioned by the Open Society Institute's *Project on Death in America* (see Chapter 1).

24. Rabinow (2007), 98.

References

Abbott, Andrew. 1988. *The System of Professions: An Essay on the Division of Expert Labor.* Chicago: University of Chicago Press.

——. 2014. "The Problem of Excess." *Sociological Theory* 32 (1): 1–26.

Abend, Gabriel. 2015. *The Moral Background: An Inquiry into the History of Business Ethics.* Princeton, N.J.: Princeton University Press.

Abramson, Corey M. 2015. *The End Game: How Inequality Shapes Our Final Years.* Cambridge, Mass.: Harvard University Press.

Agamben, Giorgio. 1998. *Homo Sacer: Sovereign Power and Bare Life.* Stanford, Calif.: Stanford University Press.

Aldridge, Melissa D., Mark Schlesinger, Colleen L. Barry, R. Sean Morrison, Ruth McCorkle, Rosemary Hürzeler, and Elizabeth H. Bradley. 2014. "National Hospice Survey Results: For-Profit Status, Community Engagement, and Service." *JAMA* 174 (4): 500–506.

Aldridge, Melissa D., and Amy S. Kelley. 2015. "The Myth Regarding the High Cost of End-of-Life Care." *American Journal of Public Health* 105 (12): 2411–2415.

Almeling, Rene. 2007. "Selling Genes, Selling Gender: Egg Agencies, Sperm Banks, and the Medical Market in Genetic Material." *American Sociological Review* 72 (3): 319–340.

——. 2011. *Sex Cells: The Medical Market for Eggs and Sperm.* Berkeley: University of California Press.

Althusser, Louis. (1971) 2001. *Lenin and Philosophy and Other Essays.* New York: Monthly Review Press.

Altilio, Terry, and Shirley Otis-Green, eds. 2011. *Oxford Textbook of Palliative Social Work.* New York: Oxford University Press.

Amado, Anthony, Beatrice A. Cronk, and Rich Mileo. 1979. "Cost of Terminal Care: Home Hospice vs. Hospital." *Nursing Outlook* 27 (8): 522–526.

American Board of Medical Specialties. 2017. *ABMS Guide to Medical Specialties.* Maryland Heights, Mo.: Elsevier.

American Medical Association. 1847. *Code of Medical Ethics of the American Medical Association.* Chicago: AMA Press.

Anspach, Renée R. 1988. "Notes on the Sociology of Medical Discourse: The Language of Case Presentation." *Journal of Health and Social Behavior* 29:357–375.

———. 1993. *Deciding Who Lives: Fateful Choices in the Intensive-Care Nursery*. Berkeley: University of California Press.

———. 2010. "The 'Hostile Takeover' of Bioethics by Religious Conservatives and the Counter Offensive." In *Social Movements and the Transformation of American Health Care*, edited by J. C. Banaszak-Hol, S. Levitsky, and M. Zald, 144–166. Oxford: Oxford University Press.

Anspach, Renée R., and Sydney A. Halpern. 2008. "From *Cruzan* to *Schiavo:* How Bioethics Entered the 'Culture Wars.'" In *Bioethical Issues: Sociological Perspectives*, edited by B. Katz Rothman, E. Mitchell Armstrong, and R. Tiger, 33–64. Boston: Elsevier JAI.

Anteby, Michel. 2010. "Markets, Morals and Practices of Trade: Jurisdictional Disputes in the U.S. Commerce in Cadavers." *Administrative Science Quarterly* 55:606–638.

———. 2013. *Manufacturing Morals: The Values of Silence in Business School Education*. Chicago: University of Chicago Press.

Appadurai, Arjun. 1986. "Introduction: Commodities and the Politics of Value." In *The Social Life of Things: Commodities in Cultural Perspective*, edited by Arjun Appadurai, 3–63. Cambridge: Cambridge University Press.

Ariès, Phillipe. 1981. *The Hour of Our Death*. New York: Knopf.

Aristotle. 1995. *Politics*. Oxford: Oxford University Press.

———. 1934. *The Athenian Constitution; The Eudemian Ethics on Virtues and Vices*. Cambridge, Mass.: Harvard University Press.

Armstrong, Elizabeth M. 1998. "Diagnosing Moral Disorder: The Discovery and Evolution of Fetal Alcohol Syndrome." *Social Science and Medicine* 47 (12): 2025–2042.

Arney, William R., and Bernard J. Bergen. 1984. *Medicine and the Management of Living: Taming the Last Great Beast*. Chicago: University of Chicago Press.

Aronowitz, Robert. 2015. *Risky Medicine: Our Quest to Cure Fear and Uncertainty*. Chicago: University of Chicago Press.

Ashmore, Malcolm, Michael J. Mulkay and Trevor J. Pinch. 1989. *Health and Efficiency: A Sociology of Health Economics*. Philadelphia: Open University Press.

Aulino, Felicity, and Kathleen Foley. 2001. "The Project on Death in America." *Journal of the Royal Society of Medicine* 94:492–495.

Bandelj, Nina, Frederick F. Wherry, and Viviana A. Zelizer. 2017. *Money Talks: Explaining How Money Really Works*. Princeton, N.J.: Princeton University Press.

Barnato, Amber E. 2007. "End-of-Life Spending: Can We Rationalise Costs?" *Critical Inquiry* 49 (3): 84–92.

Barnato, Amber E., and Robert M. Arnold. 2013. "The Effect of Emotion and Physician Communication Behaviors on Surrogates' Life-Sustaining Treatment Decisions: A Randomized Simulation Experiment. *Critical Care Medicine* 41 (7): 1686–1691.

Baszanger, Isabelle. 2012. "One More Chemo or One Too Many? Defining the Limits of Treatment and Innovation in Medical Oncology." *Social Science and Medicine* 75:864–872.

Bauman, Zygmunt. 1992. *Mortality, Immortality and Other Life Strategies*. Palo Alto, Calif.: Stanford University Press.

Bayer, Ronald, Daniel Callahan, John Fletcher, Thomas Hodgson, Bruce Jennings, David Monsees, Steven Sieverts, and Robert Veatch. 1983. "The Care of the Terminally Ill: Morality and Economics." *New England Journal of Medicine* 309 (24): 1490–1494.

Bazzoli, Gloria J., Linda Dynan, Lawton R. Burns, and Clarence Yap. 2004. "Two Decades of Organizational Change in Health Care: What Have We Learned?" *Medical Care Research and Review* 61:247–331.

Becker, Howard S. 1986. *Outsiders: Studies in the Sociology of Deviance.* New York: Free Press.

Bellah, Robert N., Richard Madesen, William Sullivan, Ann Swidler, and Steven Tipton. 2008. *Habits of the Heart: Individualism and Commitment in American Life.* Rev. ed. Berkeley: University of California Press.

Bennett, Amanda. 2012. *The Cost of Hope: A Memoir.* New York: Random House.

Beresford, Larry. 2007. "The Legacy of the Medicare Hospice Benefit." *Newsline* 18 (3): 8–16.

Beresford, Larry, and Stephen R. Connor. 1999. "History of the National Hospice Organization." *Hospice Journal* 14 (3–4): 15–31.

Best, Rachel. 2012. "Disease Politics and Medical Research Funding: Three Ways Advocacy Shapes Policy." *American Sociological Review* 77 (5): 780–803.

———. Forthcoming. *Common Enemies: Disease Campaigns in America.* New York, NY: Oxford University Press.

Bloche, M. Gregg. 2011. *The Hippocratic Myth: Why Doctors Are under Pressure to Ration Care, Practice Politics, and Compromise Their Promise to Heal.* New York: Palgrave.

Block, Fred, and Margaret R. Somers. 2014. *The Power of Market Fundamentalism: Karl Polanyi's Critique.* Cambridge, Mass.: Harvard University Press.

Boltanski, Luc, and Laurent Thévenot. 1999a. *On Justification: Economies of Worth.* Princeton, N.J.: Princeton University Press.

———. 1999b. "The Sociology of Critical Capacity." *European Journal of Social Theory* 2 (3): 359–377.

Borgstrom, Erica, Stephen Barclay, and Simon Cohn. 2013. "Constructing Denial as a Disease Object: Accounts by Medical Students Meeting Dying Patients." *Sociology of Health and Illness* 35 (3): 391–404.

Bosk, Charles L. 1979. *Forgive and Remember: Managing Medical Failure.* Chicago: University of Chicago Press.

———. 2008. *What Would You Do? Juggling Bioethics and Ethnography.* Chicago: University of Chicago Press.

Bourdieu, Pierre. 1984. *Distinction: A Social Critique of the Judgment of Taste.* Cambridge, Mass.: Harvard University Press.

———. 1990. *The Logic of Practice.* Stanford, Calif.: Stanford University Press.

———. 1993. *Sociology in Question.* Thousand Oaks, Calif.: Sage.

———. 1998. *Acts of Resistance: Against the Tyranny of the Market.* New York: New Press and Polity Press.

———. [1988] 2008. *Homo Academicus.* Stanford, Calif.: Stanford University Press.

Bradshaw, Ann. 1996. "The Spiritual Dimension of Hospice: The Secularization of an Ideal." *Social Science and Medicine* 43 (3): 409–419.

Brody, Baruch A., and Amir Halevy. 1995. "Is Futility a Futile Concept?" *Journal of Medicine and Philosophy* 20:123–144.

Broom, Alex. 2015. *Dying: A Social Perspective on the End of Life*. Burlington, Vt.: Ashgate.

Brown, Wendy. 2017. *Undoing the Demos: Neoliberalism's Stealth Revolution*. Brooklyn, N.Y.: Zone Books.

Buck, Joy. 2005. "Rights of Passage: Reforming Care of the Dying, 1965–1986." PhD diss., University of Virginia.

———. 2007. "Netting the Hospice Butterfly: Politics, Policy, and Translation of an Ideal." *Home Healthcare Now* 25 (9): 566–571.

———. 2009. "'I Am Willing to Take the Risk': Politics, Policy, and the Translation of the Hospice Ideal." *Journal of Clinical Nursing* 18:2700–2709.

———. 2011. "Nursing the Borderlands of Life: Hospice and the Politics of Health Care Reform." In *History as Evidence: Nursing Interventions through Time,* edited by Patricia D'Antonio and Sandra B. Lewenson, 203–220. New York: Springer.

Bunker, J. P. 1970. "Surgical Manpower: A Comparison of Operations and Surgeons in the United States and in England and Wales." *New England Journal of Medicine* 282:135–144.

Burawoy, Michael. 1979. *Manufacturing Consent: Changes in the Labor Process under Monopoly Capitalism*. Chicago: University of Chicago Press.

Burns, Lawton, and Mark V. Pault. 2002. "Integrated Delivery Networks: A Detour on the Road to Integrated Health Care?" *Health Affairs* 21 (4): 128–143.

Çalişkan, Koray, and Michel Callon. 2009. "Economization, Part 1: Shifting Attention from the Economy Towards Processes of Economization." *Economy and Society* 38 (3): 369–398.

———. 2010. "Economization, Part 2: A Research Programme for the Study of Markets." *Economy of Society* 39 (1): 1–32.

Callahan, Daniel. 1987. *Setting Limits: Medical Goals in an Aging Society*. New York: Simon and Schuster.

———. 1998. *False Hopes: Why America's Quest for Perfect Health Is a Recipe for Failure*. New York: Simon & Schuster.

———. 2009. *Taming the Beloved Beast: How Medical Technology Costs Are Destroying Our Health Care System*. Princeton, N.J.: Princeton University Press.

———. 2011a. "End-of-Life Care: A Philosophical or Management Problem?" *Journal of Law, Medicine and Ethics* 39 (2): 114–120.

———. 2011b. "Rationing: Theory, Politics, and Passions." *Hastings Center Report* 41 (2): 23–7.

Callon, Michel. 1998. "Introduction: The Embeddedness of Economic Markets in Economics." In *The Laws of the Market,* edited by Michel Callon, 1–57. London: Blackwell.

Callon, Michel, and Fabian Muniesa. 2005. "Peripheral Vision: Economic Markets as Calculative Collective Devices." *Organization Studies* 26 (8): 1229–1250.

Campbell, Courtney S., Jan Hare, and Pam Matthews. 1995. "Conflicts of Conscience: Hospice and Assisted Suicide." *Hastings Center Report* 25 (3): 36–43.

Carlson, Melissa D. A., William T. Gallo, and Elizabeth H. Bradley. 2004. "Ownership Status and Patterns of Care in Hospice: Results from the National Home and Hospice Care Survey." *Medical Care* 42 (5): 432–438.

Centers for Medicare & Medicaid Services. 2016. "Advance Care Planning (ACP) as an Optional Element of an Annual Wellness Visit (AWV)." *NLN Matters,* no. MM9271, December 22. https://www.cms.gov/Outreach-and-Education/Medicare-Learning-Network -MLN/MLNMattersArticles/downloads/MM9271.pdf

Chambliss, Daniel F. 1996. *Beyond Caring: Hospitals, Nurses, and the Social Organization of Ethics.* Chicago: University of Chicago Press.

Chan, Cheris Shun-Ching. 2012. *Marketing Death: Culture and the Making of Life Insurance Market in China.* Oxford: Oxford University Press.

Chapple, Helen Stanton. 2010. *No Place for Dying.* London: Routledge.

Cherlin, Emily J., Melissa D. A. Carlson, Jeph Herrin, Dena Schulman-Green, Colleen L. Barry, Ruth McCorkle, Rosemary Johnson-Hurzeler, and Elizabeth H. Bradley. 2010. "Interdisciplinary Staffing Patterns: Do For-Profit and Nonprofit Hospices Differ?" *Journal of Palliative Medicine* 13 (4): 389–394.

Christakis, Nicholas. 1999. *Death Foretold: Prophecy and Prognosis in Medical Care.* Chicago: University of Chicago Press.

Cicourel, Aaron V. 1964. *Method and Measurement in Sociology.* New York: Free Press.

Ciemins, Elizabeth L., Linda Blum, Marsha Nunley, Andrew Lasher, and Jeffrey M. Newman. 2007. "The Economic and Clinical Impact of an Inpatient Palliative Care Consultation Service: A Multifaceted Approach." *Journal of Palliative Medicine* 10 (6): 1347–1355.

Civetta, Joseph M. 1973. "The Inverse Relationship Between Cost and Survival." *Journal of Surgical Research* 14:265–269.

Clark, David. 1998. "Originating a Movement: Cicely Saunders and the Development of Saint Christopher's Hospice, 1957–1967." *Mortality* 3:43–63.

———. 1999. "'Total Pain,' Disciplinary Power and the Body in the Work of Cicely Saunders, 1958–1967." *Social Science and Medicine* 49:727–736.

———. 2001. "A Special Relationship: Cicely Saunders, the United States, and the Early Foundations of the Modern Hospice Movement." *Illness, Crisis, and Loss* 9:15–31.

———, ed. 2005. *Cicely Saunders—Founder of the Hospice Movement: Selected Letters 1959–1999.* Oxford: Oxford University Press.

———. 2013. *Transforming the Culture of Dying: The Work of the Project on Death in America.* Oxford: Oxford University Press.

Coale, Ansley. 1974. "The History of the Human Population." *Scientific American* 231: 15–25.

Cohen, Kenneth P. 1979. *Hospice Prescription for Terminal Care.* Rockville, Md.: Aspen.

Comptroller General. 1979. *Hospice Care, A Growing Concept in the United States: Report to Congress.* Washington, D.C.: U.S. General Accounting Office.

Connor, Stephen R. 1996. *Hospice: Practice, Pitfalls, and Promise.* Bristol, Penn.: Taylor & Francis.

———. 2007–2008. "Hospice and Palliative Care in the United States." *OMEGA* 56 (1): 89–99.

Conrad, Peter. 2005. "The Shifting Engines of Medicalization." *Journal of Health and Social Behavior* 46 (1): 3–14.

———. 2007. *The Medicalization of Society: On the Transformation of Human Conditions into Treatable Disorders.* Baltimore: Johns Hopkins University Press.

Conrad, Peter, and Joseph W. Schneider. (1980) 1992. *Deviance and Medicalization: From Badness to Sickness.* Philadelphia: Temple University Press.

Cullen, David J., Joseph Civetta, Burton Briggs, and Linda Ferrara. 1974. "Therapeutic Intervention Scoring System: A Method for Quantitative Comparison of Patient Care." *Critical Care Medicine* 2 (2): 57–60.

Cullen, David J., Linda C. Ferrara, Burton A. Briggs, Peter F. Walker, and John Gilbert. 1976. "Survival, Hospitalization Charges and Follow-up Results in Critically Ill Patients." *New England Journal of Medicine* 294 (18): 982–987.

Danis, Marion, Elizabeth Murtran, Garrett Joanne, Sally Stearns, Rebecca Slifkin, Laura Hanson, Jude Williams, and Larry Churchill. 1996. "A Prospective Study of the Impact of Patient Preferences on Life-Sustaining Treatment and Hospital Cost." *Critical Care Medicine* 24 (11): 1811–1817.

Danis, Marion, Leslie I. Southerland, Joanne M. Garrett, Janet L. Smith, Frank Hielema, C. Glenn Pickard, David M. Enger, and Donald L. Patrick. 1991. "A Prospective Study of Advance Directives for Life-Sustaining Care." *New England Journal of Medicine.* 324:882–888.

Darr, Asaf. 2016. "Gift Giving in Mass Consumption Markets." *Current Sociology* 65 (1): 92–112.

Darr, Asaf, and Trevor Pinch. 2013. "Performing Sales: Material Scripts and the Social Organization of Obligation." *Organization Studies* 34 (11): 1601–1621.

Davidson, Glen W. 1978. *The Hospice: Development and Administration.* Washington, D.C.: Hemisphere.

Day, Adrienne. 2015. "Ends and Means." *Stanford Social Innovation Review* 13 (2): 66–67.

DeNavas-Walt, Carmen, Bernadette D. Proctor, and Jessica C. Smith. 2010. *Income, Poverty, and Health Insurance Coverage in the United States: 2009.* U.S. Census Bureau, Current Population Reports, P60-238. Washington, D.C.: U.S. Government Printing Office. https://www.census.gov/prod/2010pubs/p60-238.pdf.

Desrosières, Alain. 2003. "Historiciser l'action publique: L'état, le marché et les statistiques," In *Historicités de l'action publique,* edited by P. Laborier and D. Trom, 207–221. Paris: PUF.

Dobbin. Frank. 1994. *Forging Industrial Policy.* Cambridge: Cambridge University Press.

Dohan, Daniel. 2002. "Managing Indigent Care: A Case Study of a Safety-Net Emergency Department. *Health Services Research* 37 (2): 361–376.

Douglas, Mary. 1986. *How Institutions Think.* Syracuse, N.Y.: Syracuse University Press.

Dubos, René. 1959. *Mirage of Health: Utopias, Progress, and Biological Change.* New Brunswick, N.J.: Rutgers University Press.

Duff, Ray, and August Hollingshead. 1968. *Sickness and Society.* New York: Harper & Row.

Durkheim, Émile. (1893) 1984. *The Division of Labor in Society.* New York: Free Press.

———. (1912) 1995. *The Elementary Forms of Religious Life.* New York: Free Press.

Dworkin, Gerald. 1988. *The Theory and Practice of Autonomy.* Cambridge: Cambridge University Press.

Dworkin, Ronald. 1986. "Autonomy and the Demented Self." *Milbank Quarterly* 64 (2): 4–16.

———. 1993. *Life's Dominion: An Argument about Abortion, Euthanasia, and Individual Freedom.* New York: Vintage Books.

Ehrenreich, Barbara. 2018. *Natural Causes: Life, Death and the Illusion of Control*. London: Granta.

Emanuel, Ezekiel J., and Linda Emanuel. 1994. "The Economics of Dying: The Illusion of Cost Saving at the End of Life." *New England Journal of Medicine* 330 (8): 540–544.

England, Paula. 2005. "Emerging Theories of Care Work." *Annual Review of Sociology* 31:381–399.

Epstein, Steven. 1994. *Impure Science: AIDS, Activism, and the Politics of Knowledge*. Berkeley: University of California Press.

———. 1995. "The Construction of Lay Expertise: AIDS Activism and the Forging of Credibility in the Reform of Clinical Trials." *Science, Technology and Human Values* 20:408–437.

Espeland, Wendy Nelson, and Michael Sauder. 2007. "Ranking and Reactivity: How Public Measures Recreate Social Worlds." *American Journal of Sociology* 113 (1): 1–40.

———. 2016. *Engines of Anxiety: Academic Rankings, Reputation, and Accountability*. New York: Russell Sage Foundation.

Evans, John H. 2002. *Playing God? Human Genetic Engineering and the Rationalization of Public Bioethical Debate*. Chicago: University of Chicago Press.

———. 2012. *The History and Future of Bioethics: A Sociological View*. Oxford: Oxford University Press.

Eyal, Gil. 2013. "For a Sociology of Expertise: The Social Origins of the Autism Epidemic." *American Journal of Sociology* 118 (4): 863–907.

Eyal, Gil, Emine Oncular, Neta Oren, and Natasha Rossi. 2010. *The Autism Matrix: The Social Origins of the Autism Epidemic*. Cambridge, United Kingdom: Polity.

Fagerlin, Angela, and Carl E. Schneider. 2004. "Enough: The Failure of the Living Will." *Hastings Center Report* 34 (2): 30–42.

Featherstone, Mike, Mike Hepworth, and Bryan S. Turner, eds. 1991. *The Body: Social Process and Cultural Theory*. Newbury Park, Calif.: Sage.

Feifel, Herman, ed. 1959. *The Meaning of Death*. New York: McGraw-Hill

———, ed. 1977. *New Meanings of Death*. New York: McGraw-Hill.

Fennell, Francis. 1983. *New Horizons on the Hospice Scene: Report for Presentation to the Auckland Medical Research Foundation*. Auckland, New Zealand: Auckland Medical Research Foundation.

Ferrell, B. R., and N. Coyle, eds. 2001. *Textbook of Palliative Nursing*. Oxford: Oxford University Press.

Feudtner, Chris, and Wynne Morrison. 2012. "The Darkening Veil of 'Do Everything'." *Archives of Pediatric and Adolescent Medicine* 166 (8): 694–695.

Filene, Peter. 1998. *In the Arms of Others: A Cultural History of the Right-to-Die Movement in America*. Chicago: Dee.

Fligstein, Neil. 1990. *The Transformation of Corporate Control*. Cambridge, Mass.: Harvard University Press.

———. 1996. "Markets as Politics: A Political-Cultural Approach to Market Institutions." *American Sociological Review* 61 (4): 656–673.

———. 2001. *The Architecture of Markets: An Economic Sociology of Twenty-First Century Capitalist Societies*. Princeton, N.J.: Princeton University Press.

Fligstein, Neil, and Doug McAdam. 2012. *A Theory of Fields.* Oxford: Oxford University Press.

Folbre, Nancy. 1991. "The Unproductive Housewife: Her Evolution in Nineteenth-Century Economic Thought." *Signs* 16 (3): 463–484.

Foucault, Michel. 1975. *The Birth of the Clinic: An Archaeology of Medical Perception.* New York: Vintage Books.

———. 1991. "Governmentality." In *The Foucault Effect: Studies in Governmental Rationality,* edited by G. Burchell, C. Gordo, and P. Miller, 87–104. Hemel Hempstead, United Kingdom: Harvester Wheatsheaf.

———. 2005. *The Hermeneutics of the Subject. Lectures at the Collège de France 1981–1982.* New York: Picador.

———. 2007. *Security, Territory, Population: Lectures at the Collège de France 1977–1978.* New York: MacMillan.

———. 2008. *The Birth of Biopolitics: Lectures at the Collège de France 1978–1979.* New York: Palgrave McMillan.

Fourcade, Marion. 2006. "The Construction of a Global Profession: The Transnationalization of Economics." *American Journal of Sociology* 112 (1): 145–194.

———. 2009. *Economists and Societies: Discipline and Profession in the United States, Britain, and France, 1890s to 1990s.* Princeton, N.J.: Princeton University Press.

———. 2011. "Cents and Sensibility: Economic Valuation and the Nature of 'Nature.'" *American Journal of Sociology* 116 (6): 1721–1777.

———. 2017. "The Fly and the Cookie: On the Moral Condition of 21st Century Capitalism." *Socio-Economic Review* 15 (3): 661–678.

Fourcade, Marion, and Kieran Healy. 2007. "Moral Views of the Market Society." *Annual Review of Sociology* 33:285–311.

———. 2013. "Classification Situations: Life-Chances in the Neoliberal Era." *Accounting Organizations and Society* 38 (8): 559–572.

Fourcade, Marion, and Roi Livne. 2013. "Lost in Translation: Social Structure and the Qualification of Expertise in U.S. Courts." Paper presented at the annual meeting of the Society for Social Studies of Science, San Diego, California.

Fox, Renée C., and Judith Swazey. 1974. *The Courage to Fail: A Social View of Organ Transplants and Dialysis.* Chicago: University of Chicago Press.

———. 2008. *Observing Bioethics.* Oxford: Oxford University Press.

Freidson, Eliot. 1970. *Profession of Medicine: A Study of the Sociology of Applied Knowledge.* New York: Harper & Row.

Fried, Terri R., Amy L. Byers, William T. Gallo, Peter H. Van Ness, Virginia R. Towle, John R. O'Leary, and Joel A. Dubin. 2006. "Prospective Study of Health Status Preferences and Changes in Preferences over Time in Older Adults." *Archives of Internal Medicine* 166:890–895.

Fried, Terri R., John O'Leary, Peter Van Ness, and Liana Fraenkel. 2007. "Inconsistency over Time in the Preferences of Older Persons with Advanced Illness for Life-Sustaining Treatment." *Journal of the American Geriatric Society* 55:1007–1014.

Friedman, Lawrence M. 1990. *The Republic of Choice: Law, Authority, and Culture.* Cambridge, Mass.: Harvard University Press.

Fulton, Robert. 1977. *Death, Grief, and Bereavement: A Bibliography, 1845–1975.* New York: Arno Press.

———. 1981. *Death, Grief, and Bereavement II: A Bibliography.* New York: Arno Press.

Gade, Glenn, Ingrid Venohr, Douglas Conner, Kathleen Mcgrady, Jeffrey Beane, Robert H. Richardson, Marilyn P. Williams, Marcia Liberson, Mark Blum, and Richard Della Penna. 2008. "Impact of an Inpatient Palliative Care Team: A Randomized Controlled Trial." *Journal of Palliative Medicine* 11 (2): 180–190.

Garcia-Parpet, Marie-France. 2007. "The Social Construction of a Perfect Market: The Strawberry Auction at Fontaines-en-Sologne." In *Do Economists Make Markets? On the Performativity of Economics,* edited by Donald MacKenzie, Fabian Muniesa, and Lucia Siu, 20–53. Princeton, N.J.: Princeton University Press.

Garrett, Dorothy M. 1978. "Needs of the Seriously Ill and Their Families: The Haven Concept." *Aging* 289/290:12–15.

Gawande, Atul. 2011. "The Cost Conundrum." In *The Sociology of Health and Illness,* 5th ed., edited by Peter Conrad and Valerie Leiter, 344–354. New York: Worth.

———. 2014. *Being Mortal: Medicine and What Matters in the End.* New York: Metropolitan.

Gayon, Vincent, and Benjamin N. Lemoine. 2014. "Maintenir l'ordre économique." *Politix* 1:7–35.

Geertz, Clifford. 1973. *The Interpretation of Cultures: Selected Essays.* New York: Basic Books.

Glaser, Barney G., and Anselm L. Strauss. 1964. "The Social Loss of Dying Patients." *American Journal of Nursing* 64:119–121.

———. 1965. *Awareness of Dying.* Chicago: Aldine.

———. 1968. *Time for Dying.* Chicago: Aldine.

———. 1970. *Anguish: A Case History of a Dying Trajectory.* Mill Valley, Calif.: Sociology Press.

Glazer, Nona Y. 1990. "The Home as Workshop: Women as Amateur Nurses and Medical Care Providers." *Gender and Society* 4 (4): 479–499.

Goffman, Erving. 1959. *The Presentation of Self in Everyday Life.* New York: Anchor Books.

Goldsmith, Benjamin, Jessica Dietrich, Qingling Du, and R. Sean Morrison. 2008. "Variability in Access to Hospital Palliative Care in the United States." *Journal of Palliative Medicine* 11 (8): 1094–1102.

Golodetz, Arnold, et al. 1997. *Vermont Voices on Care of the Dying: A Report from the Journey's End Project of the Vermont Ethics Network.* Montpelier, Vt.: Vermont Ethics Network.

Goodman, Martin D., Michael Tarnoff, and Gus J. Slotman. 1998. "Effect of Advance Directives on the Management of Elderly Critically Ill Patients." *Critical Care Medicine* 26:701–704.

Goodwin, Charles, and John Heritage. 1990. "Conversation Analysis." *Annual Review of Anthropology* 19:283–307.

Gramsci, Antonio. 2011. *Prison Notebooks.* Vol. 1. New York: Columbia University Press.

Granovetter, Mark. 1985. "Economic Action and Social Structure: The Problem of Embeddedness." *American Journal of Sociology* 91:481–510.

——. 2017. *Society and Economy: Framework and Principles*. Cambridge, Mass.: Harvard University Press.

Hacker, Jacob. 2002. *The Divided Welfare State: The Battle over Public and Private Social Benefits in the United States*. Cambridge: Cambridge University Press.

Hacking, Ian. 1999. *The Social Construction of What?* Cambridge, Mass.: Harvard University Press.

Halpern, Jodi. 2001. *From Detached Concern to Empathy: Humanizing Medical Practice*. New York: Oxford University Press.

Harris, John A., Lindsey A. Herrel, Mark A. Healy, Lauren M. Wancata, and Chithra R. Perumalswami. 2016. "Milestones for the Final Mile: Interspecialty Distinctions in Primary Palliative Care Skills Training." *Journal of Pain and Symptom Management* 52 (3): 345–352.

Hart, Bethne, Peter Sainsbury, and Stephanie Short. 1998. "Whose Dying? A Sociological Critique of the 'Good Death.'" *Mortality* 3 (1): 65–77.

Hayek, Friedrich A. von. (1944) 2007. *The Road to Serfdom*. Chicago: University of Chicago Press.

Healy, Kieran. 2006. *Last Best Gifts: Altruism and the Market for Human Blood and Organs*. Chicago: University of Chicago Press.

Heimer, Carol A., and JuLeigh Petty. 2010. "Bureaucratic Ethics: IRBs and the Legal Regulation of Human Subjects Research." *Annual Review of Law and Social Science* 6:601–626.

Heimer, Carol A., and Lisa R. Staffen. 1998. *For the Sake of the Children: The Social Organization of Responsibility in the Hospital and the Home*. Chicago: University of Chicago Press.

Helft, Paul R., Mark Siegler, and John Lantos. 2000. "The Rise and Fall of the Futility Movement." *New England Journal of Medicine* 343:293–296.

High, Dallas M. 1993. "Why Are Elderly People Not Using Advance Directives?" *Journal of Aging and Health* 5 (4): 497–515.

Hirschman, Albert O. 1986. "Against Parsimony: Three Easy Ways of Complicating Some Categories of Economic Discourse." In *Rival Views of Market Society and Other Recent Essays*, 142–160. New York: Viking.

Ho, Karen. 2009. *Liquidated: An Ethnography of Wall Street*. Durham, N.C.: Duke University Press.

Hoffman, Beatrix. 2012. *Healthcare for Some: Rights and Rationing in the United States since 1930*. Chicago: University of Chicago Press.

Hofmann, Jan C., Neil S. Wenger, Roger B. Davis, Joan Teno, Alfred F. Connors, Norman Desbiens, Joanne Lynn, and Russell S. Phillips. 1997. "Patient Preferences for Communication with Physicians about End-of-Life Decisions." *Annals of Internal Medicine* 127 (1): 1–12.

Hogan, Christopher, June Lunney, and Joanne Lynn. 2001. "Medicare Beneficiaries' Cost of Care in the Last Year of Life." *Health Affairs* 20 (4): 188–195.

Holan, Angie Drobnic. 2009. "PolitiFact's Lie of the Year: 'Death Panels.'" *Politifact*, December 18, 2009. www.politifact.com/truth-o-meter/article/2009/dec/18/politifact-lie-year-death-panels/.

Holleb, Arthur I. 1974. "A Patient's Right to Die . . . The Easy Way Out?" *CA: A Cancer Journal for Clinicians* 24 (4): 256.

Hoover, Donald R, Stephen Crystal, Rizie Kumar, Usha, Sambamoorthi, and Joel C. Cantor. 2002. "Medical Expenditures during the Last Year of Life: Findings from the 1992–1996 Medicare Current Beneficiary Survey." *Health Services Research* 37 (6): 1625–1642.

Hopp, Faith P., and Sonia A. Duffy. 2000. "Racial Variations in End-of-Life Care." *Journal of the American Geriatric Society* 48 (6): 658–663.

Hospice Project Task Force. 1980. *Report to the 1980 California Legislature on the Hospice Project*. Berkeley: California State Department of Health.

Hoyer, Thomas. 1998. "A History of the Medicare Hospice Benefit." *Hospice Journal* 13 (1–2): 61–9.

Illich, Ivan. 1976. *Medical Nemesis: The Expropriation of Health*. New York: Pantheon.

Institute on Health and Healthcare Delivery. 1978. *The Hospice as a Social Health Care Institution*. Los Angeles: Hillhaven Foundation.

Institute of Medicine. 1997. *Approaching Death: Improving Care at the End of Life*. Washington, D.C.: National Academies Press.

———. 2014. *Dying in America: Improving Quality and Honoring Individual Preferences near the End of Life*. Washington, D.C.: National Academies Press.

Jecker, Nancy S., and Lawrence J. Schneiderman. 1995. "When Families Request that 'Everything Possible' be Done." *The Journal of Medicine and Philosophy* 20 (2): 145–163.

———. 1992. "Futility and Rationing." *American Journal of Medicine* 92 (2): 189–196.

Jerolmack, Colin. 2008. "How Pigeons Became Rats: The Cultural-Spatial Logic of Problem Animals." *Social Problems* 55 (1): 72–94.

———. 2013. *The Global Pigeon*. Chicago: University of Chicago Press.

Jerolmack, Colin, and Shamus Khan. 2014. "Talk Is Cheap: Ethnography and the Attitudinal Fallacy." *Sociological Methods and Research* 43 (2): 178–209.

Jerolmack, Colin, and Alexandra K. Murphy. 2017. "The Ethical Dilemmas and Social Scientific Trade-offs of Masking in Ethnography." *Sociological Methods and Research*, March 30, https://doi.org/10.1177/0049124117701483.

Jonsen, Albert R. 1988. *The Abuse of Casuistry: A History of Moral Reasoning*. Berkeley: University of California Press.

———. 1998. *The Birth of Bioethics*. New York: Oxford University Press.

Kafka, Franz. 2008. *Letter to My Father*. Lulu, N.C.: Howard Colyer.

Kalish, Richard K. 1977. "Dying and Preparing for Death: A View of Families." In *New Meanings of Death*, edited by Herman Feifel, 216–232. New York: McGraw-Hill.

Karsoho, Hadi, David K. Wright, Mary Ellen Macdonald, and Jennifer R. Fishman. 2017. "Constructing Physician-Assisted Dying: The Politics of Evidence from Permissive Jurisdictions in Carter v. Canada." *Mortality* 22 (1): 45–59.

Kashi, Ed, and Julie Winokur. 2003. *Aging in America: The Years Ahead*. New York: PowerHouse Books.

Katz, Jay. 1984. *The Silent World of Doctor and Patient*. New York: Free Press.

Kaufman, Sharon. 2006. *And a Time to Die: How American Hospitals Shape the End of Life*. Chicago: University of Chicago Press.

———. 2015. *Ordinary Medicine: Extraordinary Treatments, Longer Lives, and Where to Draw the Lines*. Durham, N.C.: Duke University Press.

Kavanagh, Evan. 1983. "Volunteers in Hospice." In *Hospice Care: Principles and Practice*, edited by Charles A. Corr and Donna M. Corr, 210–212. New York: Springer.

Kellehear, Allan 1984. "Are We a Death-Denying Society? A Sociological Review." *Social Science and Medicine* 18:713–23.

Kierkegaard, Søren. 1993. "At a Graveside." In *Three Discourses on Imagined Occasions*, 71–102. Princeton, N.J.: Princeton University Press.

Kleinman, Arthur. 1994. "Conflicting Explanatory Models in the Care of the Chronically Ill: The Voice of Medicine and the Voice of the Life World." In *Dominant Issues in Medical Sociology*, 3rd ed., edited by H. Schwartz, 95–104. New York: McGraw-Hill.

Kleinman, Arthur, Leon Eisenberg, and Byron Good. 1978. "Culture, Illness and Care: Clinical Lessons from Anthropologic and Cross-Cultural Research." *Annals of Internal Medicine* 88 (2): 251–258.

Klinenberg, Eric. 2012. *Going Solo: The Extraordinary Rise and Surprising Appeal of Living Alone*. New York: Penguin Press.

Knowles, Christopher A. 1984. "The Role of a Director of Finance in a Hospice: Experience of an Iowa Facility." *American Journal of Hospice Care* 1 (4): 12–14.

Kojève, Alexandre. 1969. *Introduction to the Reading of Hegel: Lectures on the Phenomenology of Spirit*. Ithaca, N.Y.: Cornell University Press.

Koren, Gideon, Heather Shear, Karen Graham, and Tom Einarson. 1989. "Bias against the Null Hypothesis: The Reproductive Hazards of Cocaine." *Lancet* 2 (8677): 1440–1442.

Krakoff, Irwin H. 1979. "The Case for Active Treatment in Patients with Advanced Cancer: Not Everyone Needs a Hospice." *CA: A Cancer Journal for Clinicians* 29 (2): 108–111.

Krippner, Greta R. 2002. "The Elusive Market: Embeddedness and the Paradigm of Economic Sociology." *Theory and Society* 30 (6): 775–810.

———. 2005. "The Financialization of the American Economy." *Socio-Economic Review* 3:173–208.

Krippner, Greta, Mark Granovetter, Fred Block, Nicole Biggart, Tom Beamish, Youtien Hsing, Gillian Hart, Giovanni Arrighi, Margie Mendell, John Hall, Michael Burawoy, Steve Vogel, and Sean O'Riain. 2004. "Polanyi Symposium: A Conversation on Embeddedness." *Socio-Economic Review* 2:109–135.

Kübler-Ross, Elisabeth. 1969. *On Death and Dying: What the Dying Have to Teach Doctors, Nurses, Clergy, and Their Own Families*. New York: Scribner.

———. 1977. "Living with Dying," Speech sponsored by Power Within, Loberto Theater, Santa Barbara, California.

Kutscher, Austin H. 1969. *A Bibliography of Books on Death, Bereavement, Loss, and Grief: 1935–1968*. New York: Health Sciences.

———. 1974. *A Bibliography of Books on Death, Bereavement, Loss, and Grief: Supplement* 1, 1968–1972. New York: Health Sciences.

Kutscher, Martin. 1975. *A Comprehensive Bibliography of the Thanatology Literature*. New York: MSS Information.

Lahire, Bernard. 2011. *The Plural Actor*. Cambridge: Polity Press.

LaPorte Matzo, Marianne, and Deborah W. Sherman, eds. 2001. *Palliative Care Nursing: Quality Care to the End of Life*. New York: Springer.

Lara-Millán, Armando. 2014. "Public Emergency Room Overcrowding in the Era of Mass Imprisonment." *American Sociological Review* 79 (5): 866–887.

Latour, Bruno. 1987. *Science in Action: How to Follow Scientists and Engineers through Society*. Cambridge, Mass.: Harvard University Press.

———. 1994. *We Have Never Been Modern*. Cambridge, Mass.: Harvard University Press.

———. 1999. *Pandora's Hope: Essays on the Reality of Science Studies*. Cambridge, Mass.: Harvard University Press.

———. 2004. "Why Has Critique Run Out of Steam? From Matters of Fact to Matters of Concern." *Critical Inquiry* 30 (2): 225–248.

———. 2005. *Reassembling the Social: An Introduction to Actor-Network-Theory*. Oxford: Oxford University Press.

Lavi, Shai. 2005. *The Modern Art of Dying: A History of Euthanasia in the United States*. Princeton, N.J.: Princeton University Press.

Leshem, Dotan. 2013. "Oikonomia Redefined." *Journal of the History of Economic Thought* 35 (1): 43–61.

Levinsky, Norman. 1996. "The Purpose of Advance Medical Planning—Autonomy for Patients or Limitation of Care?" *New England Journal of Medicine* 335 (10): 741–743.

Lévi-Strauss, Claude. 1963. "History and Anthropology." In *Structural Anthropology*, 1–27. New York: Basic Books.

Levitsky, Sandra R. 2014. *Caring for Our Own: Why There Is No Political Demand for New American Social Welfare Rights*. Oxford: Oxford University Press.

Light, Donald W. 1995. "Countervailing Powers." In *The Wiley Blackwell Encyclopedia of Health, Illness, Behavior, and Society*, edited by W. Cockerham, R. Dingwall, and S. R. Quah. Hoboken, N.J.: Wiley-Blackwell.

———. 2004. "Ironies of Success: A New History of the American Health Care System." *Journal of Health and Social Behavior* 45:1–24.

———, ed. 2010. *The Risks of Prescription Drugs*. New York: Columbia University Press.

Livne, Roi. 2014. "Economies of Dying: The Moralization of Economic Scarcity in U.S. Hospice Care." *American Sociological Review* 79 (5): 888–911.

Lo, Bernard, Gary A. McLeod, Glenn Saika. 1986. "Patient Attitudes to Discussing Life-Sustaining Treatment." *Archives of Internal Medicine* 146:1613–1615.

Lo, Bernard, Glenn Saika, William Strull, Elizabeth Thomas, and Jonathan Showstack. 1985. "'Do Not Resuscitate' Decisions: A Prospective Study at Three Teaching Hospitals." *Archives of Internal Medicine* 145:1115–1116.

Long, Stephen H., James O. Gibbs, Jay P. Crozier, David I. Cooper, John F. Newman, and Arne M. Larsen. 1984. "Medical Expenditures of Terminal Cancer Patients during the Last Year of Life." *Inquiry* 21 (4): 315–327.

Lubitz, James D., and Ronald Prihoda. 1984. "The Use and Costs of Medicare Services in the Last 2 Years of Life." *Healthcare Financing Review* 5: 117–131.

Lubitz, James D., and Gerald F. Riley. 1993. "Trends in Medicare Payments in the Last Year of Life." *New England Journal of Medicine*. 328:1092–1096.

Lukes, Steven. 2005. *Power: A Radical View*. Basingstoke, United Kingdom: Palgrave MacMillan.

Lynn, Joanne. 1997. "Unexpected Returns: Insights from SUPPORT." In *To Improve Health and Health Care, 1997*, edited by Stephen L. Isaacs and James R. Knickman, 161–186. San Francisco: Robert Wood Johnson Foundation.

MacKenzie, Donald. 2006. *An Engine, Not a Camera: How Financial Models Shape Markets*. Cambridge, Mass.: MIT Press.

MacKenzie, Donald, and Yuval Millo. 2003. "Constructing a Market, Performing Theory: The Historical Sociology of a Financial Derivatives Exchange." *American Journal of Sociology* 109 (1): 107–145.

MacKenzie, Donald, Fabian Muniesa, and Lucia Siu. 2007. *Do Economists Make Markets? On the Performativity of Economics*. Princeton, N.J.: Princeton University Press.

MacKillop, Eleanor, and Sally Sheard. 2018. "Quantifying Life: Understanding the History of Quality-Adjusted Life-Years (QALY)." *Social Science and Medicine* 211:359–366.

Mahar, Maggie. 2006. *Money-Driven Medicine: The Real Reason Health Care Costs So Much*. New York: HarperCollins.

Margolin, Leslie. 1997. *Under the Cover of Kindness: The Invention of Social Work*. Charlottesville: University Press of Virginia.

Marx, Karl. 1964. *Economic and Philosophic Manuscripts of 1844*. New York: International Publishers.

Mauss, Marcel. 1985. "A Category of the Human Mind: The Notion of Person; The Notion of Self." In *The Category of the Person: Anthropology, Philosophy, History*, edited by Michael Carrithers, Steven Collins, and Steven Lukes, 1–25. Trans. W.D. Hall. Cambridge: Cambridge University Press.

Mayes, Rick. 2007. "The Origins, Development, and Passage of Medicare's Revolutionary Prospective Payment System." *Journal of the History of Medicine and Allied Sciences* 62 (1): 21–55.

McCall, Nelda. 1984. "Utilization and Costs of Medicare Services by Beneficiaries in Their Last Year of Life." *Medical Care* 22 (4): 329–342.

McGehee, Harvey, and James Bordley. 1976. *Two Centuries of American Medicine*. Philadelphia: Saunders.

McKinlay, John B., and Lisa D. Marceau. 2002. "The End of the Golden Age of Doctoring." *International Journal of Health Services* 32 (2): 379–416.

McNulty, Elizabeth G., and Robert A. Holderby. 1983. "Hospice: A Caring Challenge." Springfield, Ill.: C.C. Thomas.

Mechanic, David. 1996. "Changing Medical Organization and the Erosion of Trust." *The Milbank Quarterly* 74 (2): 171–189.

Menger, Carl. (1871) 1950. *Principles of Economics*. Glencoe, Ill.: Free Press.

Messikomer, Carla M., Renée C. Fox, and Judith P. Swazey. 2001. "The Presence and Influence of Religion in American Bioethics." *Perspectives in Biology and Medicine* 44 (4): 485–508.

Miller, Albert J., and Michael J. Acri. 1977. *Death: A Bibliographical Guide*. Metuchen, N.J.: Scarecrow Press.

Mishler, Elliot G. 1984. *The Discourse of Medicine: Dialectics of Medical Interviews.* Norwood, N.J.: Ablex.

Mitchell, Timothy. 2002. *Rule of Experts: Egypt, Techno-Politics, Modernity.* Berkeley: University of California Press.

———. 2005a. "Economists and the Economy in the Twentieth Century." In *The Politics of Method in the Human Sciences: Positivism and Its Epistemological Others,* edited by George Steinmetz, 126–141. Durham, N.C.: Duke University Press.

———. 2005b. "The Work of Economics: How a Discipline Makes Its World." *European Journal of Sociology* 46 (2): 297–320.

Mitford, Jessica. 1963. *The American Way of Death.* New York: Simon & Schuster.

Montaigne, Michel de. 2003. *Michel de Montaigne: The Complete Essays.* London: Penguin.

Mor, Vincent, and Howard Barnbaum. 1983. "Medicare Legislation for Hospice Care: Implications of National Hospice Study Data." *Health Affairs* 2 (2): 80–90.

Mor, Vincent, and David Kidder. 1985. "Cost Savings in Hospice: Final Results of the National Hospice Survey." *Health Service Research* 20 (4): 407–420.

Morgan, Lucy Griscom. 1971. "On Drinking the Hemlock." *Hastings Center Report* 1 (3): 4–5.

Morrison, R. Sean, Joan D. Penrod, J. Brian Cassel, Melissa Caust-Ellenbogen, Ann Litke, Lynn Spragens, and Diane E. Meier. 2008. "Cost Savings Associated with U.S. Hospital Palliative Care Consultation Programs." *Archives of Internal Medicine* 168 (16): 1783–1790.

Morrison, R. Sean, and Diane E. Meier. 2015. *America's Care of Serious Illness.* New York: Center to Advance Palliative Care.

Murphy, Alexandra K. 2012. "'Litterers': How Objects of Physical Disorder Are Used to Construct Subjects of Social Disorder in a Poor Suburb." *Annals of the American Academy of Political and Social Science* 642 (1): 210–227.

Murphy, Alexandra K. Forthcoming. *When the Sidewalks End: Poverty and Race in an American Suburb.* New York, NY: Oxford University Press.

Murphy, Michelle. 2017. *The Economization of Life.* Durham, N.C.: Duke University Press.

National Center for Health Statistics. 2011. *Health, United States, 2010: With Special Feature on Death and Dying.* Hyattsville, Md.: U.S. Government Printing Office.

National Hospice and Palliative Care Organization. 2005. "California Advance Directive: Planning for Important Health Care Decisions." Alexandria, Va.: Caring Info. www.caringinfo.org/files/public/ad/california.pdf.

———. 2015. "The Medicare Hospice Benefit." Alexandria, Va.: NHPCO. www.nhpco.org/sites/default/files/public/communications/Outreach/The_Medicare_Hospice_Benefit.pdf.

———. 2017. "Facts and Figures: Hospice Care in America." Alexandria, Va.: NHPCO. https://web.archive.org/web/20180210024200/https://www.nhpco.org/sites/default/files/public/Statistics_Research/2016_Facts_Figures.pdf

Notzon, Francis C., Paul J. Placek, and Selma M. Taffel. 1987. "Comparisons of National Cesarean-Section Rates." *New England Journal of Medicine* 316: 386–389.

Numbers, Ronald L. 1978. *Almost Persuaded: American Physicians and Compulsory Health Insurance, 1912–1920.* Baltimore: Johns Hopkins University Press.

Olshansky, Stuart J., and A. Brian Ault. 1986. "The Fourth Stage of the Epidemiologic Transition: The Age of Delayed Degenerative Diseases." *Milbank Quarterly* 64 (3): 355–391.

Open Society Institute. 2004. *Transforming the Culture of Dying: The Project on Death in America*. New York: OSI. www.opensocietyfoundations.org/sites/default/files/a _transforming.pdf.

Orentlicher, David. 1992. "The Illusion of Patient Choice in End-of-Life Decisions." *JAMA* 267 (15): 2101–2104.

Ortner, Sherry B. 1973. "On Key Symbols." *American Anthropologist* 75 (5): 1338–1346.

Osterweis, Marian, and Daphne Szmuszkovicz Champagne. 1978. "U.S. Hospice Movement: Issues in Development." *American Journal of Public Health* 69 (5): 492–496.

Owens, Patricia. 2015. *Economy of Force: Counterinsurgency and the Historical Rise of the Social*. Cambridge: Cambridge University Press.

Pantilat, Steven Z., Michael W. Rabow, Kathleen M. Kerr, and Amy J. Markowitz. 2007. *Palliative Care in California: The Business Case for Hospital-Based Programs*. Oakland: California Health Care Foundation.

Paradis, Lenora Finn, and Scott B. Cummings. 1986. "The Evolution of Hospice in America: Toward Organizational Homogeneity." *Journal of Health and Social Behavior* 27 (4): 370–386.

Paradise, Julia. 2017. "Data Note: Medicaid Managed Care Growth and Implications of the Medicaid Expansion." April 24. Menlo Park, Calif.: Kaiser Family Foundation. http:// files.kff.org/attachment/Data-Note-Medicaid-Managed-Care-Growth-and -Implications-of-the-Medicaid-Expansion

Parikh, Ravi B., Rebecca A. Kirch, Thomas J. Smith, and Jennifer S. Temel. 2013. "Early Specialty Palliative Care—Translating Data in Oncology into Practice." *New England Journal of Medicine* 369 (24): 2347–2351.

Paris, John J., Edwin H. Cassem, G. William Dec, and Frank E. Reardon. 1999. "Use of DNR Order over Family Objections: The Case of Gilgunn v MGH. *Journal of Intensive Care Medicine* 14 (1): 41–45.

Paris, John J., Robert K. Crone, and Frank Readon. 1990. "Physicians' Refusal of Requested Treatment: The Case of Baby L." *New England Journal of Medicine.* 322 (14): 1012–1014.

Parsons, Talcott. 1951. *The Social System*. New York: Free Press.

Patrick, Donald L., Robert A. Pearlman, Helene E. Starks, Kevin C. Cain, William G. Cole, and Richard F. Uhlmann. 1997. "Validation of Preferences for Life-Sustaining Treatment: Implications for Advance Care Planning." *Annals of Internal Medicine* 127:509–517.

Patrizi, Patricia, Elizabeth Thompson, and Abby Spector. 2011. "Improving Care at the End of Life: How the Robert Wood Johnson Foundation and Its Grantees Built the Field." RWJF Retrospective Series. Princeton, N.J.: Robert Wood Johnson Foundation. https://www.rwjf.org/content/dam/farm/reports/reports/2011/rwjf69582.

Payer, Lynn. 1988. *Medicine and Culture*. New York: Owl Books.

Peterson, Peter G. 2004. *Running on Empty*. New York: Picador.

Pew Research Center. 2013. "Views on End-of-Life Medical Treatments." November 21, www.pewresearch.org/wp-content/uploads/sites/7/2013/11/end-of-life-survey-report -full-pdf.pdf.

Phillips, Russell S., Neil S. Wenger, Joan Teno, Robert K. Oye, Stuart Youngner, Robert Califf, Peter Layde, Norman Desbiens, Alfred F. Connors Jr., and Joanne Lynn. 1996. "Choices of Seriously Ill Patients about Cardiopulmonary Resuscitation: Correlates and Outcomes." *The American Journal of Medicine* 100 (2): 128–137.

Piketty, Thomas. 2014. *Capital in the Twenty-First Century.* Trans. Arthur Goldhammer. Cambridge, Mass.: Harvard University Press.

Piro, Paula A., and Theodore Lutins. 1973. "Utilization and Reimbursements under Medicare for 1967 and 1968 Decedents." *Social Security Bulletin* 74–11702 (May). https://www.ssa.gov/policy/docs/ssb/v36n5/v36n5p37.pdf.

Poe, William D. 1972. "Marantology, a Needed Specialty." *New England Journal of Medicine* 286:102–103.

Polanyi, Karl. (1944) 2001. *The Great Transformation: The Political and Economic Origins of Our Time.* Boston: Beacon Press.

———. (1957) 1992. "The Economy as an Instituted Process." In *The Sociology of Economic Life,* edited by M. Granovetter and R. Swedberg, 29–51. Boulder, Colo.: Westview Press.

———. 1968. "Aristotle Discovers the Economy." In *Primitive, Archaic, and Modern Economies: Essays of Karl Polanyi,* edited by George Dalton, 78–115. Garden City, N.Y.: Anchor Books.

———. 1977. *The Livelihood of Man.* New York: Academic Press.

Poteet, G. Howard. 1976. *Death and Dying: A Bibliography, 1950–1974.* Troy, N.Y.: Whitston.

Prendergast, Thomas J., Michael T. Claessens, and John M. Luce. 1998. "A National Survey of End-of-Life Care for Critically Ill Patients." *American Journal of Respiratory and Critical Care Medicine* 158 (4): 1163–11637.

Prendergast, Thomas J., and John M. Luce. 1997. "Increasing Incidence of Withholding and Withdrawal of Life Support from the Critically Ill." *American Journal of Respiratory and Critical Care Medicine* 55 (1): 15–20.

Quill, Timothy E., and Amy Abernethy. 2013. "Generalist Plus Specialist Palliative Care—Creating a More Sustainable Model." *New England Journal of Medicine* 368 (13): 1173–1175.

Quill, Timothy E., Rebecca Dresser, and Dan W. Brock. 1997. "The Rule of Double Effect—A Critique of Its Role in End-of-Life Decision Making." *New England Journal of Medicine* 337:1768–1771.

Quill, Timothy E., Bernard Lo, and Dan W. Brock. 1997. "Palliative Options of Last Resort: A Comparison of Voluntarily Stopping Eating and Drinking, Terminal Sedation, Physician-Assisted Suicide, and Voluntary Active Euthanasia." *JAMA* 278 (23): 2099–2104.

Quinn, Sarah. 2008. "The Transformation of Morals in Markets: Death, Benefits, and the Exchange of Life Insurance Policies." *American Journal of Sociology* 114 (3): 738–780.

Rabinow, Paul. 2007. "Anthropological Observation and Self-Formation." In *Subjectivity: Ethnographic Investigations,* edited by João Biehl, Byron Good, and Arthur Kleinman, 98–118. Berkeley: University of California Press.

Raz, Joseph. 1986. *The Morality of Freedom.* Oxford: Clarendon Press.

Reich, Adam. 2014. *Selling Our Souls: The Commodification of Hospital Care in the United States.* Princeton, N.J.: Princeton University Press.

Reilly, Rebecca B., Thomas A. Teasdale, and Laurence B. McCullough. 1994. "Projecting Patients' Preferences from Living Wills: An Invalid Strategy for Management of Dementia with Life-Threatening Illness." *Journal of the American Geriatrics Society* 42:997–1003.

Relmand, Arnold. 1980. "The New Medical-Industrial Complex." *New England Journal of Medicine* 303 (17): 962–970.

Riley, Gerald, and James Lubitz. 2010. "Long-Term Trends in Medicare Payment in the Last Year of Life." *Health Services Research* 45:565–576.

Riley, Gerald, James Lubitz, Ronald Prihoda, and Evelyne Rabey. 1987. "The Use and Costs of Medicare Services by Cause of Death." *Inquiry* 24:233–243.

Robbins, Lionel. 1945. *An Essay on the Nature and Significance of Economic Science.* London: MacMillan.

Rodwin, Marc A. 2011. *Conflicts of Interest and the Future of Medicine: The United States, France and Japan.* Oxford: Oxford University Press.

Rose, Nikolas. 1990. *Governing the Soul: The Shaping of the Private Self.* London: Routledge.

——. 1998. *Inventing Our Selves: Psychology, Power, and Personhood.* Cambridge: Cambridge University Press.

Rose, Nikolas, and Peter Miller. 1992. "Political Power Beyond the State: Problematics of Government." *British Journal of Sociology* 43 (2): 172–205.

Rosenberg, Charles E. 1987. *The Care of Strangers: The Rise of America's Hospital System.* New York: Basic Books.

Rosenthal, Elisabeth. 2014. "Apprehensive, Many Doctors Shift to Jobs with Salaries." *New York Times*, February 13, 2014. www.nytimes.com/2014/02/14/us/salaried-doctors-may -not-lead-to-cheaper-health-care.html.

Rosenthal, Elisabeth. 2017. *An American Sickness: How Healthcare Became Big Business and How You Can Take It Back.* New York: Penguin Press.

Rosman, Parker. 1977. *Hospice: Creating New Models of Care for the Terminally Ill.* New York: Association Press.

Roth, Julius. 1972. "Some Contingencies of the Moral Evaluation and Control of Clientele: The Case of the Hospital Emergency Service." *American Journal of Sociology* 77 (5): 839–856.

Rothman, David J. 1991. *Strangers at the Bedside: A History of How Law and Bioethics Transformed Medical Decision Making.* New York: Basic Books.

Roy, Ananya. 2010. *Poverty Capital: Microfinance and the Making of Development.* New York: Routledge.

Sartre, Jean-Paul. 1968. *Search for a Method.* New York: Random House.

Saunders, Cicely. 1960a. "Drug Treatment in the Terminal Stages of Cancer." *Current Medicine and Drugs* 1 (1): 16–28.

——. 1960b. "The Management of Patients in the Terminal Stage." In *Cancer*, vol. 6, edited by R. Raven, 403–417. London: Butterworth.

——. 1965. "Last Stages of Life." *American Journal of Nursing* 65 (3): 70–75.

——. 1969. "The Moment of Truth: Care of the Dying Person." In *Death and Dying: Current Issues in the Treatment of the Dying Person*, edited by Leonard Pearson, 49–78. Cleveland, Ohio: Case Western Reserve University.

———. 1999. "Origins: International Perspectives, Then and Now." *Hospice Journal* 14 (3/4): 1-7.

Schmidt, Laura Anne. 1999. "The Corporate Transformation of American Health Care: A Study in Institution Building." PhD diss., University of California, Berkeley.

Schneider, Carl E. 1998. *The Practice of Autonomy: Patients, Doctors, and Medical Decisions.* Oxford: Oxford University Press.

Schneiderman, Lawrence J., Nancy S. Jecker, and Albert R. Jonsen. 1990. "Medical Futility: Its Meaning and Ethical Implications." *Annals of Internal Medicine* 112:949-954.

Schneiderman, Lawrence J., Richard Kronick, Robert M. Kaplan, John P. Anderson, and Robert D. Langer. 1992. "Effects of Offering Advance Directives on Medical Treatments and Costs." *Annals of Internal Medicine.* 117 (7): 599-606.

Schnell, Lisa Jane. 2004. "Learning How to Tell." *Literature and Medicine* 23 (2): 265-279.

Schroeder, Steven A. 1999. "The Legacy of SUPPORT." *Annals of Internal Medicine* 131 (10) 780-782.

Scitovsky, Anne A. 1984. "'The High Cost of Dying': What Do the Data Show?" *Milbank Memorial Fund Quarterly/Health and Society* 62 (4): 591-608. Reprinted in *Milbank Quarterly* 83, no. 4 (2005): 825-841.

———. 1988. "Medical Care in the Last Twelve Months of Life: The Relation between Age, Functional Status, and Medical Care Expenditures." *Milbank Quarterly* 66:640-660.

———. 1994. "'The High Cost of Dying' Revisited." *Milbank Quarterly* 72 (4): 561-591.

Scitovsky, Anne A., and Alexander M. Capron. 1986. "Medical Care at the End of Life: The Interaction of Economics and Ethics." *Annual Review of Public Health* 7:59-75.

Scott, W. Richard, Martin Ruef, Peter J. Mendel, and Carol A. Caronna. 2000. *Institutional Change and Healthcare Organizations: From Professional Dominance to Managed Care.* Chicago: Chicago University Press.

Seale, Clive. 1998. *Constructing Death: The Sociology of Dying and Bereavement.* Cambridge: Cambridge University Press.

Sell, Irene L. 1977. *Dying and Death: An Annotated Bibliography.* New York: Tiresias Press.

Shapiro, Alan. 2000. *The Dead Alive and Busy.* Chicago: University of Chicago Press.

Shapiro, Susan. 2012. "Advance Directives: The Elusive Goal of Having the Last Word." *NAELA Journal* 8 (2): 205-232.

Shilling, Chris, and Philip A. Mellor. 1996. "Embodiment, Structuration Theory and Modernity: Mind/Body Dualism and the Repression of Sensuality." *Body and Society* 2 (4): 1-15.

Shim, Janet. 2010. "Cultural Health Capital: A Theoretical Approach to Understanding Health Interactions and the Dynamics of Unequal Treatment." *Journal of Health and Social Behavior* 51 (1): 1-15.

Shmerling, Robert H., Susanna E. Bedell, Armin Lilienfeld, and Thomas Delbanco. 1988. "Discussing Cardiopulmonary Resuscitation." *Journal of General Internal Medicine* 3 (4): 317-321.

Shugarman, Lisa R., Sandra L. Decker and Anita Bercovitz. 2009. "Demographic and Social Characteristics and Spending at the End of Life." *Journal of Pain and Symptom Management* 38 (1): 15-29.

Siebold, Cathy. 1992. *The Hospice Movement: Easing Death's Pains.* New York: Twayne.

Silveira, Maria J., Scott Y. H. Kim, and Kenneth M. Langa. 2010. "Advance Directives and Outcomes of Surrogate Decision Making before Death." *New England Journal of Medicine* 362:1211–1218.

Simpson, Michael A. 1979. *Dying, Death, and Grief.* New York: Plenum.

———. 1987. *Dying, Death, and Grief: A Critical Bibliography.* Pittsburgh: University of Pittsburgh Press.

Singer, Peter. 2009. "Why We Must Ration Health Care." *New York Times,* July 15, 2009. www.nytimes.com/2009/07/19/magazine/19healthcare-t.html.

Smedira, Nicholas G., Bradley H. Evans, Linda S. Grais, Neal H. Cohen, Bernard Lo, Molly Cooke, William P. Schecter, Carol Fink, Eve Epstein-Jaffe, Christine May, and John M. Luce. 1990. "Withholding and Withdrawal of Life Support from the Critically Ill." *New England Journal of Medicine* 322:309–315.

Smelser, Neil J., and Richard Swedberg. 1994. "The Sociological Perspective on the Economy." In *The Handbook of Economic Sociology,* edited by N. J. Smelser and R. Swedberg, 4–26. Princeton, N.J.: Princeton University Press.

Smith, George P. 1995. "Restructuring the Principle of Medical Futility." *Journal of Palliative Care* 11 (3): 9–16.

Smith, Thomas J., Patrick Coyne, Brian Cassel, Lynne Penberthy, Alison Hopson, and Mary Ann Hager. 2003. "A High-Volume Specialist Palliative Care Unit and Team May Reduce In-Hospital End-of-Life Costs." *Journal of Palliative Medicine* 6 (5): 699–795.

Sontag, Susan. 1978. *Illness as Metaphor.* New York: Farrar, Straus & Giroux.

Soros, George. 1998. "Reflections on Death in America." In *Project on Death in America, July 1994–December 1997, Report of Activities,* 4–6. New York: Open Society Institute.

Spencer, Karen Lutfey, and Matthew Grace. 2016. "Social Foundations of Health Care Inequality and Treatment Bias." *Annual Review of Sociology* 42:101–120.

Starr, Paul. 1982. *The Social Transformation of American Medicine.* New York: Basic Books.

Steinfels, Peter. 1974. "Introduction," in *Death Inside Out,* edited by Peter Steinfels and Robert M. Veatch, 1–6. New York: Harper & Row.

Steinfels, Peter, and Robert M. Veatch, eds. 1974. *Death Inside Out: The Hastings Center Report.* New York: Harper & Row.

Steinhauser, Karen E., Nicholas A. Christakis, Elizabeth C. Clipp, Maya McNeilly, Lauren McIntyre, and James A. Tulsky. 2000. "Factors Considered Important at the End of Life by Patients, Family, Physicians, and Other Care Providers. *JAMA* 284:2476–2482.

Steinhauser, Karen E., George L. Maddox, Judi Lund Person, and James A. Tulsky. 2000. "The Evolution of Volunteerism and Professional Staff within Hospice Care in North Carolina. *Hospice Journal* 15 (1): 35–51.

Stockton, David. 1971. *Cicero: A Political Biography.* Oxford: Oxford University Press.

Stoddard, Sandol. 1978. *The Hospice Movement: A Better Way of Caring for the Dying.* Briarcliff Manor, N.Y.: Stein and Day.

Straus, Robert. 1957. "The Nature and Status of Medical Sociology." *American Sociological Review* 22 (2): 200–104.

Sudnow, David. 1967. *Passing On.* Englewood Cliffs, N.J.: Prentice-Hall.

Sudore, Rebecca, and Terri Fried. 2010. "Redefining the 'Planning' in Advance Care Planning: Preparing for End-of-Life Decision Making." *Annals of Internal Medicine* 153:256–262.

Sulmasy, Daniel P., and Edmund D. Pellegrino. 1999. "The Rule of Double Effect: Clearing Up the Double Talk." *Archives of Internal Medicine* 159 (6): 545–550.

SUPPORT Principal Investigators. 1995. "A Controlled Trial to Improve Care for Seriously Ill Hospitalized Patients: The Study to Understand Prognoses and Preferences for Outcomes and Risks of Treatments (SUPPORT)." *JAMA* 274 (20): 1591–1598.

Talking Eyes Media. 2003. *Aging in America: The Years Ahead.* San Francisco, Calif.: Kanopy Streaming.

Taylor, Charles. 1985. "The Person." In *The Category of the Person: Anthropology, Philosophy, History,* edited by Michael Carrithers, Steven Collins, and Steven Lukes, 257–281. Cambridge: Cambridge University Press.

Teno, Joan M., Joanne Lynn, Russell S. Phillips, Donald J. Murphy, Stuart Youngner, Paul Bellamy, Alfred F. Connors Jr., Norman A. Desbiens, William Fulkerson, and William Knaus. 1994. "Do Formal Advance Directives Affect Resuscitation Decisions and the Use of Resources for Seriously Ill Patients?" *Journal of Clinical Ethics* 5 (1): 23–30.

Teno, Joan M., Pedro L. Gozalo, Julie P. W. Bynum, Natalie E. Leland, Susan C. Miller, Nancy E. Morden, Thomas Scupp, David C. Goodman, and Vincent Mor. 2013. "Change in End-of-Life Care for Medicare Beneficiaries: Site of Death, Place of Care, and Health Care Transitions in 2000, 2005, and 2009." *JAMA* 309 (5): 470–477.

Teno, Joan M., and David Dosa. 2006. "'You Can't Always Get What You Want'—or Can You?" *Canadian Medical Association Journal* 174 (5): 643–644.

Thibault, George E., Albert G. Mulley, G. Octo Barneet, Richard L. Golstein, Victoria A. Reder, Ellen, L. Sherman, and Erik R. Skinner. 1980. "Medical Intensive Care: Indications, Interventions, and Outcomes." *New England Journal of Medicine* 302 (17): 938–942.

Thompson, E. P. 1966. *The Making of the English Working Class.* New York: Vintage Books.

———. 1971. "The Moral Economy of the English Crowd." *Past and Present* 50:76–136.

Timmer, Elaine J. 1969. *Health Insurance Coverage of Adults, Who Died in 1964 or 1965, United States: Statistics on Hospital and Surgical Insurance Coverage for Persons Who Died during 1964 and 1965, by Age, Sex, Color, Geographic Region, Family Income, Living Arrangements, Family Size, and Marital Status.* Public Health Service Publication, No. 1000, Series 10. National Center for Health Statistics. Washington, D.C.: U.S. Government Printing Office.

Timmermans, Stefan. 1999. *Sudden Death and the Myth of CPR.* Philadelphia: Temple University Press.

———. 2005. "Death Brokering: Constructing Culturally Appropriate Deaths." *Sociology of Health and Illness* 27 (7): 993–1013.

———. 2007. *Postmortem: How Medical Examiners Explain Suspicious Deaths.* Chicago: University of Chicago Press.

Timmermans, Stefan, and Marc Berg. 2003. *The Gold Standard: The Challenge of Evidence-Based Medicine and Standardization in Health Care.* Philadelphia: Temple University Press.

Timmermans, Stefan, and Mara Buchbinder. 2010. "Patients-in-Waiting: Living between Sickness and Health in the Genomics Era." *Journal of Health and Social Behavior* 51 (4): 408–423.

Timmermans, Stefan, and Steven Haas. 2008. "Toward a Sociology of Disease." *Sociology of Health and Illness* 30 (5): 659–676.

Turnbull, Alan D., Graziano Carlon, Robinson Baron, William Sichel, Charles Young, and William Howland. 1979. "The Inverse Relationship between Cost and Survival in the Critically Ill Cancer Patient." *Critical Care Medicine* 7 (1): 20–23.

Turner, Bryan S. 1987. "The Rationalization of the Body: Reflections on Modernity and Discipline." In *Max Weber, Rationality, and Modernity,* edited by S. Whimster and S. Lash, 222–241. London: Allen and Unwin.

Twaddle, Andrew C., and Richard Hessler. 1977. *A Sociology of Health*. St. Louis, Mo.: C.V. Mosby.

Ubel, Peter A. 2000. *Pricing Life: Why It's Time for Health Care Rationing*. Cambridge, Mass.: MIT Press.

Ubel Peter A., George Lowenstein, Norbert Schwarz, and Dylan Smith. 2005. "Misimagining the Unimaginable: The Disability Paradox and Health Care Decision Making." *Health Psychology* 24 (4, Suppl.): S56–S62.

Van der Zuan, Natasha. 2014. "Making Sense of Financialization." *Socio-Economic Review* 12:99–129.

Van Ryn, Michelle, Diana Burgess, Jennifer Malat, and Joan Griffin. 2006. "Physicians Perceptions of Patients' Social and Behavioral Characteristics and Race Disparities in Treatment Recommendations for Men with Coronary Artery Disease." *American Journal of Public Health* 96:351–357.

Van Ryn, Michelle, and Jane Burke. 2000. "The Effect of Patient Race and Socio-Economic Status on Physicians Perceptions of Patients." *Social Science and Medicine* 50:813–828.

Van Ryn, Michelle, and Steven S. Fu. 2003. "Paved with Good Intentions: Do Public Health and Human Service Providers Contribute to Racial-Ethnic Disparities in Health?" *American Journal of Public Health* 93 (2): 248–255.

Vernon, Glenn M. 1970. *The Sociology of Death*. New York: Ronald.

Waggoner, Miranda R. 2017. *The Zero Trimester: Pre-Pregnancy Care and the Politics of Reproductive Risk*. Berkeley: University of California Press.

Wald, Florence S. 1966. "Emerging Nursing Practice." *American Journal of Public Health and the Nation's Health* 56 (8): 1252–1260.

———. 1988. "In Search of the Spiritual Component of Hospice Care." In *In Quest of the Spiritual Component of Care for the Terminally Ill: Proceedings of a Colloquium,* edited by F. Wald, 25–33. New Haven, Conn.: Yale University School of Nursing.

Wald, Florence S., and Joan Craven. 1975. "Hospice Care for Dying Patients." *American Journal of Nursing* 75 (10): 1816–1822.

Wald, Florence S., and Robert C. Leonard. 1964. "Towards Development of Nursing Practice Theory." *Nursing Research* 13 (4): 309–313.

Warner, Emily, and Tom Gualtieri-Reed. 2014. "Improving Care for People with Serious Illness Through Innovative Payer-Provider Partnership." New York: Center to Advance Palliative Care (CAPC). https://media.capc.org/filer_public/0f/2f/0f2f8662-15cf-4680-baa8-215dd97fbde6/payer-providertoolkit-2015.pdf.

Weber, Max. (1919) 1946a. "Politics as a Vocation." In *From Max Weber: Essays in Sociology*, edited by Hans H. Gerth and C. Wright Mills, 77–128. New York: Oxford University Press.

———. (1919) 1946b. "Science as a Vocation." In *From Max Weber: Essays in Sociology*, edited by Hans H. Gerth and C. Wright Mills, 129–156. New York: Oxford University Press.

———. 1978. *Economy and Society*. Berkeley: University of California Press.

———. 2002. *The Protestant Ethic and Spirit of Capitalism*. London: Penguin.

Weisfeld, Victoria, Doriane Miller, Rosemary Gibson, and Steven A. Schroeder. 2000. "Essay: Improving Care at the End of Life: What Does It Take?" *Health Affairs Grant Watch* 19 (6): 278–283. https://www.healthaffairs.org/doi/pdf/10.1377/hlthaff.19.6.277.

Welch, Gilbert H., Lisa M. Schwartz, and Steven Woloshin. 2011. *Overdiagnosed: Making People Sick in the Pursuit of Health*. Boston, Mass.: Beacon Press.

Wentzel, Kenneth B. 1981. *To Those Who Need It Most Hospice Means Hope*. Boston: Charles River Books.

Whoriskey, Peter, and Dan Keating. "Dying and Profits: The Evolution of Hospice." *Washington Post*, December 26, 2014, www.washingtonpost.com/business/economy/2014/12/26/a7d90438-692f-11e4-b053-65cea7903f2e_story.html.

Wolin, Sheldon S. 2016. *Politics and Vision: Continuity and Innovation in Western Political Thought*. Princeton, N.J.: Princeton University Press.

Worcester, Alfred. (1940) 1961. *The Care of the Aged, the Dying, and the Dead*. Springfield, Ill.: Charles Thomas.

Xenophon. 1994. *Oeconomicus: A Social and Historical Commentary*. Oxford: Clarendon Press.

Zelizer, Viviana A. 1979. *Morals and Markets: The Development of Life Insurance in the United States*. Brunswick, N.J.: Transaction.

———. 1985. *Pricing the Priceless Child: The Changing Social Value of Children*. New York: Basic Books.

———. 1994. *The Social Meaning of Money*. New York: Basic Books.

———. 2004. "Circuits of Commerce." In *Self, Social Structure, and Beliefs: Explorations in Sociology*, edited by Jeffrey C. Alexander, Gary T. Marx, and Christine L. Williams, 122–144. Berkeley: University of California Press.

———. 2005. *The Purchase of Intimacy*. Princeton, N.J.: Princeton University Press.

———. 2011. *Economic Lives: How Culture Shapes the Economy*. Princeton, N.J.: Princeton University Press.

Zimmermann, Camilla, and Gary Rodin. 2004. "The Denial of Death Thesis: Sociological Critique and Implications for Palliative Care." *Palliative Medicine* 18:121–128.

Zola, Irving K. 1972. "Medicine as an Institution of Social Control." *Sociological Review* 20 (4): 487–504.

Zussman, Robert. 1992. *Intensive Care: Medical Ethics and the Medical Profession*. Chicago: University of Chicago Press.

Acknowledgments

Thanking the people who supported, contributed to, and allowed this book to become reality is an intimidating task: they are many, and words cannot do justice to the debt I owe them. First and foremost are the numerous patients and families who allowed me to sit at bedsides and listen to discussions they had with clinicians about their conditions, treatments, and chances of survival. Some of them I met only briefly, but they still welcomed me to observe very painful, agonizing, and vulnerable moments in their lives. Most if not all the patients involved have since died. Dozens of clinicians sat with me for interviews, and many of them allowed me to shadow them in their day-to-day work. This book would not have been written without their openness and good will, which I admire very deeply.

I began working on the project when I was a sociology graduate student at the University of California, Berkeley. Marion Fourcade was a brilliant teacher, a selfless mentor, and a most dedicated dissertation chair; she was always available and supportive, and her razor-sharp instincts kept me challenged and stimulated. Neil Fligstein's boundless faith and encouragement have accompanied me from the day I landed in Berkeley to this very moment, and his ability to draw the essence from each argument has been eye-opening. Aaron Cicourel read field notes, interview transcripts, and scattered ideas; his rigorous methodological critiques made me concede my weaknesses multiple times. Luckily, he has been doing the same for the rest of the sociological discipline for fifty-some years.

At Harvard University Press, editor Janice Audet shepherded the book from early versions to publication, and her perceptive reading improved it greatly.

Mike Aronson was the first editor to review the project, and his astute comments made a long-lasting impact. Four anonymous reviewers provided detailed and apposite comments on each of the book's chapters, and I am deeply grateful for their thoroughness. Vickie West did a remarkably meticulous job as copyeditor, Sherry Gerstein was an accommodating production editor, and Margo Lakin was a resourceful proofreader. I am also grateful to Esther Blanco-Benmaman, Emeralde Jensen-Roberts, and Stephanie Vyce for their assistance in producing images and navigating the mysterious world of copyrights.

I am fortunate to have dedicated colleagues and friends who read the entire manuscript and provided invaluable feedback: Renée Anspach, Ashley Bates, Rachel Best, Müge Göçek, Katie Hauschildt, Joel Howell, Greta Krippner, Tom Pessah, and Mira Vale. Others read individual chapters at various stages and levels of development, and the insights they provided were crucial in fleshing out different parts of the argument: Gabi Abend, Vicki Bonnell, Michael Burawoy, Veena Dubal, Fidan Elçioğlu, Lisa Feldstein, Luis Flores, Alex Garcia, Jodi Halpern, Heather Haveman, Mimi Kim, Daniel Klutz, Deborah Freedman Lustig, David Minkus, Alex Murphy, Frank Neuhauser, Chithra Perumalswami, Alex Roehrkasse, Kelly Russell, Iddo Tavory, Christine Trost, Cihan Tuğal, Frederic Vandenberghe, Ray de Vries, Elizabeth Welch, and Yuval Yonay. As a student, I had the privilege of having numerous conversations with Dylan Riley and Ann Swidler, and their insights made it into the book in various forms.

At the University of Michigan—the warmest greenhouse a young sociologist could wish for—Renée Anspach, Elizabeth Armstrong, Sarah Burgard, Müge Göçek, Rob Jansen, Greta Krippner, Sandy Levitsky, Karin Martin, Peggy McCracken, Jason Owen-Smith, and Al Young provided me with much advice and guidance. Zaineb Al-Kalby, Jen Eshelman, Nancy Herlocher, Tammy Kennedy, and Rebecca Russell were resourceful administrative and technical problem solvers. Conversations with Barbara Anderson and George Steinmetz made me rethink many empirical and theoretical observations. Fabian Pfeffer helped me with chi-square tests and made sure that I exercised. As graduate research assistants, Mira Vale provided excellent insights in the final stages of work and Dana Kornberg provided invaluable help with indexing and proofreading. Two undergraduate research assistants—Lindsay Fedewa and Eunice Yau—helped with historical data analysis. Amanda Armstrong, Erin Cech, Rob Jansen, Margo Mahan, Alex Murphy, and Heidi Sherick kept me in good spirits, with and without good spirits.

Research for this book was funded by grants and fellowships from the Charlotte W. Newcombe Foundation, Berkeley's Center for Research on Social Change, and the sociology department at the University of California, Berkeley.

My faraway family—Nurit Livne-Shilo and Moshe Livne, Tali and Eitan Gal, and Ran Livne and Yael Pedatzur-Livne—was an enormous source of strength. So was the friendship of Debbie Bernstein, Veena Dubal, Luke Fletcher, Trevor Gardner, Mimi Kim, Vered Kraus, Ben Gebre Medhin, Tom Pessah, Anasuya Sengupta, Becky Tarlau, Fithawee Tzeggai, Ashwin Jacob Mathews, Shemi Shabat, and Yuval Yonay.

Last but not least are one Ashley Bates and one Dalia Bates-Livne, who endured me and the book through long, turbulent, and tremulous years. They did so with much love and patience, always reminding me to play with enthusiasm, not only when it concerns work. Let this bundle of paper and ink be dedicated to you, my Peter Panish innermost box wide open.

Index